STEMI: An Issue of Cardiology Clinics

STEMI: An Issue of Cardiology Clinics

Edited by Layla Byrne

hayle
medical

New York

Hayle Medical,
750 Third Avenue, 9th Floor,
New York, NY 10017, USA

Visit us on the World Wide Web at:
www.haylemedical.com

ISBN: 978-1-63241-925-5

Cataloging-in-Publication Data

STEMI : an issue of cardiology clinics / edited by Layla Byrne.
    p. cm.
Includes bibliographical references and index.
ISBN 978-1-63241-925-5
1. Myocardial infarction. 2. Myocardial infarction--Treatment. 3. Coronary heart disease.
4. Cardiology. I. Byrne, Layla.
RC685.I6 S84 2020
616.123 7--dc23

Table of Contents

Permissions

List of Contributors

Index

Preface

It is often said that books are a boon to mankind. They document every progress and pass on the knowledge from one generation to the other. They play a crucial role in our lives. Thus I was both excited and nervous while editing this book. I was pleased by the thought of being able to make a mark but I was also nervous to do it right because the future of students depends upon it. Hence, I took a few months to research further into the discipline, revise my knowledge and also explore some more aspects. Post this process, I begun with the editing of this book.

STEMI or ST-Elevation Myocardial Infarction is a form of myocardial infarction in which a major artery of the heart is blocked. It is a serious and life-threatening medical emergency which is usually associated with atherosclerosis. Acute STEMI may lead to arrhythmias like ventricular fibrillation, and result in sudden cardiac arrest. At this stage, defibrillation and cardiopulmonary resuscitation are required to restore a normal heart rhythm. Nausea, vomiting, chest discomfort, anxiety, diaphoresis and palpitations are signs of a STEMI. An ECG may support a STEMI diagnosis if ST elevation is observed. It is usually treated with thrombolytics or with the aid of a percutaneous coronary intervention. This procedure is known as angioplasty or stenting. This book elucidates the concepts and innovative models around the diagnosis and treatment of STEMI. The topics included on STEMI are of utmost significance and bound to provide incredible insights to readers. In this book, using case studies and examples, constant effort has been made to make the understanding of the difficult concepts as easy and informative as possible, for the readers.

I thank my publisher with all my heart for considering me worthy of this unparalleled opportunity and for showing unwavering faith in my skills. I would also like to thank the editorial team who worked closely with me at every step and contributed immensely towards the successful completion of this book. Last but not the least, I wish to thank my friends and colleagues for their support.

Editor

Lower serum triglyceride level is a risk factor for in-hospital and late major adverse events in patients with ST-segment elevation myocardial infarction treated with primary percutaneous coronary intervention

Yu-Tsung Cheng[1†], Tsun-Jui Liu[1,2†], Hui-Chin Lai[1,2†], Wen-Lieng Lee[1,2], Hung-Yun Ho[1], Chieh-Shou Su[1,2], Chia-Ning Liu[3] and Kuo-Yang Wang[1,2,4*]

Abstract

Background: Whether serum triglyceride level correlates with clinical outcomes of patients with ST segment elevation myocardial infarction (STEMI) treated by primary percutaneous coronary intervention (pPCI) remains unclear.

Methods: From June 2008 to February 2012, all patients with STEMI who were treated with pPCI in this tertiary referral hospital and then had fasting lipid profiles measured within 24 hours were included and dichotomized into lower- (≦150 mg/dl) and higher-triglyceridemic (>150 mg/dl) groups. Baseline characteristics, in-hospital outcomes, and late major adverse cardiovascular events (MACE) were compared in-between. Independent predictors for in-hospital death and late adverse events were identified by multivariate logistic and Cox regression analyses.

Results: A total of 247 patients were enrolled, including 163 lower-triglyceridemic and 84 higher-triglyceridemic subjects. The angiographic characteristics, pPCI results and in-hospital outcomes were similar between the two groups. However, multivariate logistic analysis identified triglyceride level as a negative predictor for in-hospital death (OR 0.963, 95% CI 0.931-0.995, p = 0.023). At follow-up for a mean period of 1.23 to 1.40 years, compared with the high-triglyceridemic group, low-triglyceridemic patients had fewer cumulative incidences of target vessel revascularization (TVR) (21.7% vs. 9.5%, p = 0.011) and overall MACE (26.1% vs. 11.9%, p = 0.0137). Cox regression analysis confirmed serum triglyceride as a negative predictor for TVR and overall MACE.

Conclusions: Serum triglyceride level inversely correlates with in-hospital death and late outcomes in patients with STEMI treated with pPCI. Thus, when managing such patients, a high serum triglyceride level can be regarded as a benign factor but not a target for aggressive therapy.

Keywords: Triglyceride, Myocardial infarction, Coronary, Revascularization, Restenosis, Outcome

* Correspondence: chiefkywang@gmail.com
†Equal contributors
[1]Cardiovascular Center and Department of Anesthesiology, Taichung Veterans General Hospital, Taichung, Taiwan
[2]Departments of Medicine and Surgery, Yang-Ming University School of Medicine, Taipei, Taiwan
Full list of author information is available at the end of the article

Background

Atherosclerotic cardiovascular disease remains the leading cause of disability and death in the Western world [1]. When coronary arteries are involved, ST-segment elevation myocardial infarction (STEMI) manifests an extreme presentation that carries ominous short- and long-term prognosis in terms of fatal arrhythmia, acute pumping failure, myocardial rupture and chronic left ventricular dysfunction [2]. Timely primary percutaneous coronary revascularization (pPCI) is well established as the most effective therapy for restoring vessel patency, salvaging jeopardized myocardium and preserving cardiac performance [2,3]. However, a substantial proportion of patients are still at risk of early electrical/mechanical complications and late major adverse cardiac events (MACE) from myocardial stunning, unfavorable left ventricular remodeling, culprit lesion restenosis and de novo coronary stenosis [4], raising identification of high-risk patient subsets as an essential issue in the goal to improve the overall outcome of such a disease.

The chief prognostic determiners for patients with STEMI are the sizes of the infarcted and residual viable myocardium. When the culprit vessel is successfully opened by pPCI and the ischemic territory is thereby limited, a number of other factors may play a predictive role in determining the prognosis of these patients. Among such factors low-density lipoprotein (LDL) is closely related with early and late cardiovascular events [5] in patients with acute coronary syndrome; hence the use of aggressive statin therapy for these patients is justified to benefit cardiovascular outcome [6]. In contrast, whether serum triglyceride (TG) correlates with the outcome of STEMI and how it should be managed remains unclear. Some investigations showed that hypertriglyceridemia independently predicted development of coronary artery disease (CAD) [7,8] and myocardial infarction [9] as hypercholesterolemia did [10], whereas others reported low TG levels were associated with poorer prognosis in some cardiac and non-cardiac disease states [11-13]. Given the controversial yet potentially crucial impact of hypertriglyceridemia on the outcome of patients with STEMI treated by pPCI, this study was designed to elucidate the differences in short- and long-term cardiovascular outcomes between patients with high- and low-serum TG levels. The results of this study could clarify the role of serum TG in determining the prognosis of patients suffering from STEMI, and may help guide proper management of such patients to improve their overall outcome.

Methods

Patients

From June 2008 to February 2012, of the 301 patients admitted to this tertiary referral center with a diagnosis of STEMI for primary PCI (pPCI), 247 had a lipid profile checked within 24 hours of admission so were enrolled and categorized into either the lower ($\leq$150 mg/dl, N = 163, or 66%) or the higher (>150 mg/dl, N = 84, or 34%) triglyceride group according to the baseline level of serum triglycerides. Baseline characteristics, angiographic findings, and clinical outcomes were obtained from electronic or written medical records as well as the cardiac catheterization laboratory database and were compared between groups. The study protocol was approved by the human research committee of Taichung Veterans General Hospital (approval No. CE12289), and requirement of informed consent was waived by the institutional review board.

Coronary angiography and percutaneous coronary intervention

The diagnosis of STEMI was made based on conventionally standardized criteria [2]. Coronary angiography was performed from either a radial or femoral approach at the discretion of the interventional cardiologists. Grade of blood flow was determined by TIMI classification system [14]. Angiographic stenosis was defined as a luminal diameter reduction of $\geq$50% by quantitative coronary angiography, and critical stenosis was defined as $\geq$70% narrowing of the coronary artery luminal diameter. Complete coronary occlusion was defined as absence of antegrade flow of contrast media beyond a specific vascular segment. The infarct-related lesion was determined by the relevant ECG leads showing ST-segment elevation (or ST-segment depression along with a tall R wave in lead V1 for posterior infarction) and by the typical vascular morphological features of thrombus-laden or hazy filling defects along with compromise of distal flow. Once angiographic occlusion or critical stenosis of any of the coronary arteries was demonstrated, PCI with or without stenting was performed for the infarct-related artery but not for any other bystander vessel unless hemodynamic instability persisted despite opening of the culprit lesion. The success of pPCI was defined as achievement of the TIMI flow of the infarct related artery to grade II or III. Patients were then taken to our intensive coronary care unit for post-procedural care. Pharmacological treatment, including dual-antiplatelet medication, was in accordance with current guidelines [2]. In-hospital complications, including cardiogenic shock requiring intra-aortic balloon pumping support, new-onset atrial fibrillation, ventricular arrhythmia, and death served as in-hospital outcomes.

Follow-up

Discharged patients were followed up by medical records of clinic visits or telephone contacts for MACE, including data regarding non-fatal myocardial infarction, target vessel revascularization (TVR), need of coronary artery bypass grafting, cardiac death and all-cause mortality. Use of lipid-lowering agents (chiefly statins and fibrates) and non–lipid-lowering drugs (aspirin, clopidogrel, cilostazol, β-blockers, angiotensin-converting enzyme inhibitors, angiotensin receptor antagonists, aldactone receptor blockers) was compared between groups.

Statistical analysis

Continuous variables were expressed as mean ± standard deviation (SD). Normally distributed continuous data were compared between groups by unpaired student's T-test, while non-parametric continuous data were compared by Mann–Whitney U test. Categorical variables were compared by χ^2 analysis with Fisher's exact correction. Univariate followed by multivariate logistic regression analyses were used to identify independent correlates of in-hospital mortality in all patients. Rationale variables selected for regression analysis included the following: demographic characteristics, co-morbid illnesses, echocardiographic indicators, and angiographic features. Variables were tested in a backward conditioned multivariate logistic regression model if their univariate P values were <0.20. Statistical significance was defined as a multivariate P <0.05. The odds ratios and their 95% confidence intervals (CIs) from the multivariate logistic regression analysis were used as estimates of relative risk. Kaplan-Meier survival curves for components of MACE and overall MACE rate were constructed and compared between groups with the Log-Rank test. Multivariate Cox proportional hazard analysis was used to determine the independent predictors of TVR and overall MACE after adjustment for baseline and angiographic variables with unequal distribution. A p-value <0.05 was considered significant for all analyses. Statistical analysis was done using SPSS 11.5 or SAS 9.3.

Results

Patient characteristics

The demographic data of both groups of patients are listed in Table 1. Patients in the lower-TG group were older (67 vs. 56 years, p < 0.01) and had lower body mass index, worse estimated glomerular filtration rate, higher high-density lipoprotein (HDL) as well as lower total cholesterol levels than those in the higher-TG group.

ECG, coronary angiographic findings, pPCI results and in-hospital outcomes

The territory of myocardial infarction determined by ECG was mostly located in the anterior wall in both groups (Table 2). The severity of overall coronary artery disease, the culprit lesion vessel, the ECG-to-balloon time and the therapeutic modalities of pPCI in terms of balloon angioplasty, thrombectomy, and endovascular stenting were similar between the two groups (p = NS in all). Success

Table 1 Baseline characteristics of patients in the lower-TG (≤150 mg/dl) and higher-TG (>150 mg/dl) groups

	Lower-TG group	Higher-TG group	P
N	163	84	
Age, yrs	67.1 ± 13.2	56.1 ± 11.3	<0.001
Female (%)	22 (13.6)	19 (22.6)	0.100
Hypertension (%)	97 (59.5)	61 (72.6)	0.058
DM (%)	46 (28.2)	34 (40.5)	0.071
Smoking (%)	99 (60.7)	56 (66.7)	0.439
BMI, kg/m^2	24.1 ± 3.5	26.3 ± 3.2	<0.001
Previous CAD (%)	22 (13.5)	5 (6.0)	0.113
Previous stroke (%)	15 (9.2)	5 (6.0)	0.522
Carotid stenosis (%)	4 (2.5)	0 (0)	0.303
PAD (%)	3 (1.8)	2 (2.4)	1.000
eGFR, ml/min	46.7 ± 18.5	57.6 ± 20.5	<0.001
Previous hypolipid drugs			
Statin	21 (12.9)	12 (14.3)	0.913
Fibrate	1 (0.6)	3 (3.6)	0.115
Admission lipid profile			
HDL, mg/dl	45.4 ± 10.8	37.4 ± 8	<0.001
LDL, mg/dl	100.9 ± 31.6	106.6 ± 41.4	0.231
TC/HDL	3.65 ± 0.87	5.02 ± 1.36	<0.001
LDL/HDL	2.32 ± 0.81	2.93 ± 1.28	<0.001
TG, mg/dl (range)	83.6 ± 34.3 (13–149)	258.6 ± 136.8 (152–805)	<0.001
Cardiogenic shock (%)	29 (17.8)	7 (8.3)	0.071

BMI, body mass index; CAD, coronary artery disease; DM, diabetes mellitus; eGFR, estimated glomerular filtration rate; HDL, high-density lipoprotein; LDL, low-density protein; PAD, peripheral arterial disease; TC, total cholesterol; TG, triglyceride.

of PCI (post-procedural TIMI-blood flow to ≥grade 2) was accomplished in most of the patients in both groups (p = NS). Though post-procedural left ventricular ejection fraction estimated with either ventriculography or echocardiography was more depressed in the low-TG group (44.8% vs. 46.9%, p = 0.031), myocardial infarct size estimated by peak creatinine kinase (CK) levels was comparable between the two groups. Occurrence of new cardiogenic shock, respiratory failure, atrial fibrillation and ventricular arrhythmia, as well as requirement of emergency coronary bypass surgery was also statistically equivalent in the two groups (p = NS in all). Though in-hospital mortality happened in 6 patients in the lower TG (5 from ventricular arrhythmia and 1 from refractory pumping failure) but 0 in the higher TG group, the difference was not statistically significant (p = 0.098). Further univariate followed by multivariate regression analysis identified peak CK and CAD number >1 as positive, whereas serum TG level as negative predictors of in-hospital death for all of these patients (Table 3).

Table 2 ECG location of STEMI, findings of coronary angiograms and results of primary percutaneous coronary interventions in all patients

	Lower-TG group	High-TG group	P
N	163	84	
ECG infarct area			
Anterior (%)	87 (53.4)	51 (60.7)	0.334
Inferior (%)	72 (44.2)	33 (39.3)	0.548
True posterior (%)	2 (1.2)	2 (2.4)	0.607
High lateral (%)	8 (4.9)	4 (4.8)	1.000
Severity of CAD			
Number of diseased vessels	1.8 ± 0.8	1.8 ± 0.8	0.906
SVD (%)	76 (46.6)	37 (44.0)	0.802
DVD (%)	50 (30.7)	30 (35.7)	0.501
TVD (%)	37 (22.7)	17 (20.2)	0.779
LM involvement (%)	7 (4.3)	1 (1.2)	0.271
Treated (culprit) vessel			
LM (%)	2 (1.2)	1 (1.2)	1.000
LAD (%)	86 (52.8)	51 (60.7)	0.291
LCx (%)	18 (11)	6 (7.1)	0.451
RCA (%)	57 (35)	28 (33.3)	0.908
Ramus medianus (%)	1 (0.6)	0 (0)	1.000
Door to balloon time, min	90.5 ± 42.1	87.7 ± 29	0.587
Interventions			
Balloon angioplasty (%)	161 (98.8)	81 (96.4)	0.341
Thrombectomy			
Aspiration (%)	103 (63.2)	55 (65.5)	0.83
Rheolytic (%)	3 (1.8)	2 (2.4)	1.000
Stenting			
Nil (%)	15 (9.2)	10 (11.9)	0.657
DES (%)	37 (22.7)	21 (25.0)	0.806
BMS (%)	108 (66.3)	52 (61.9)	0.591
DES + BMS (%)	3 (1.8)	1 (1.2)	1.000
Final TIMI flow			
Grade 3 (%)	153 (93.9)	82 (97.6)	0.231
Grade 2 (%)	10 (6.1)	2 (2.4)	0.231
Grade 1/0 (%)	0 (0)	0 (0)	0
In-hospital outcome			
LVEF, %	43.8 ± 10.9	46.9 ± 9.5	0.031
Cardiac markers			
Peak CK, mg/dl	2683.3 ± 2451.8	2735.1 ± 2676.8	0.897
Complications			
New cardiogenic shock (%)	21 (12.9)	6 (7.1)	0.248
Respiratory failure (%)	30 (18.4)	8 (9.5)	0.100
Ventricular arrhythmia (%)	25 (15.3)	8 (9.5)	0.282

Table 2 ECG location of STEMI, findings of coronary angiograms and results of primary percutaneous coronary interventions in all patients (Continued)

New atrial fibrillation (%)	16 (9.8)	3 (3.6)	0.142
Emergency CABG (%)	0 (0)	2 (2.4)	0.115
In hospital Death* (%)	6 (3.7)	0 (0)	0.098

*All were related with refractory heart failure, with 5 of them experiencing ventricular arrhythmia before death. BMS, bare-metal stent; CABG, coronary artery bypass grafting surgery; CAD, coronary artery disease; CK, creatinine kinase; DES, drug-eluting stent; DVD, double vessel disease; LAD, left anterior descending artery; LCx, left circumflex artery; LM, left main coronary artery; RCA, right coronary artery; SVD, single vessel disease; TIMI, thrombolysis in myocardial infarction; TVD, triple vessel disease.

Long-term outcomes

The medications prescribed at discharge were similar in the two groups of patients surviving the STEMI episodes, except that fibrates were given more often in higher-TG patients with the intention to lower serum

Table 3 Independent predictors of in-hospital mortality in patients with STEMI undergoing pPCI

Variable	Hazard ratio	95% C.I.	P*	P†
Variables in the model				
CAD number	4.620	1.006-21.223	0.038	0.049
1 (reference)	1			
>1	4.620	1.006-21.223	0.038	0.049
Peak CK	1.001	1.000-1.001	0.001	0.003
TG	0.963	0.931-0.995	0.049	0.023
Variables not in the model				
Age			0.19	
Male			0.794	
Hypertension			0.339	
DM			0.419	
Cholesterol			0.047	NS
ECG to balloon time			0.753	
LM involvement			0.102	NS
Cardiogenic shock			0.004	NS
Anterior infarction			0.770	
Culprit LAD			0.286	
Culprit LCx			0.844	
Culprit RCA			0.424	
Culprit LM			0.015	NS
TIMI grade			<0.001	NS
Thrombectomy				
Aspiration			0.339	
Rheolytic			0.040	NS

*From univariate regression analysis, †from multivariate regression analysis. CAD, coronary artery disease; CK, creatinine kinase; DM, diabetes mellitus; LAD, left anterior descending artery; LCx, left circumflex artery; LM, left main coronary artery; RCA, right coronary artery; TIMI, thrombolysis in myocardial infarction; TG, triglyceride.

Lower serum triglyceride level is a risk factor for in-hospital and late major adverse events in patients...

5

TG level (Table 4). Kaplan-Meier survival test showed that during a mean follow-up period of 1.23 years for lower-TG and 1.4 years for higher-TG patients (p = 0.126), lower-TG patients had significantly more incidences of TVR (21.7% vs. 9.5%, Log-Rank p = 0.0111) and in turn overall MACE (26.1% vs. 11.9%, Log-Rank p = 0.0137) compared to higher-TG patients, yet the rates of de novo lesions, non-fatal MI, cardiac deaths and all-cause mortality were comparable between groups (Table 4). Multivariate Cox proportional hazard model confirmed that, besides the number of diseased coronary arteries as a positive predictor, serum TG level inversely correlated with TVR (hazard ratio 0.993, 95% CI 0.988-0.998, p = 0.007) and overall MACE (hazard ratio 0.994, 95% CI 0.990-0.999, p = 0.016) in all of our study patients (Table 5).

Discussion

Patients with coronary artery disease presenting as STEMI might develop early fatal/non-fatal complications and late MACE in terms of target lesion revascularization, non-fatal myocardial infarction and cardiac death despite being successfully treated by pPCI. This study, which investigated the possible relations between serum TG and in-hospital as well as late outcomes of such patients, indicated that serum TG level correlates negatively with in-hospital mortality: TG level above 150 mg/

Table 4 Take-home medications and late clinical outcomes

	Lower-TG group	Higher-TG group	P
N	157	84	
Take-home medications			
Aspirin (%)	153 (97.5)	84 (100.0)	0.301
Clopidogrel (%)	154 (98.1)	83 (98.8)	1.000
*RAAS inhibitor (%)	145 (92.4)	77 (91.7)	1.000
Beta Blocker (%)	77 (47.2)	47 (56.0)	0.375
Statin (%)	91 (58)	54 (64.3)	0.414
Fibrate (%)	2 (1.3)	11 (13.1)	<0.001
Follow-up years (mean)	1.23 (0.22-3.78)	1.40 (0.44-3.73)	0.126
MACE			
Non-fatal MI (%)	17 (10.8)	3 (3.6)	0.0731[†]
TVR (%)	34 (21.7)	8 (9.5)	0.0111[†]
De novo lesion (%)	9 (5.7)	4 (4.8)	0.404[†]
Cardiac Death (%)	7 (4.5)	0 (0)	0.1688[†]
All-Cause Mortality (%)	13 (8.3)	1 (1.2)	0.1392[†]
Overall (%)	41 (26.1)	10 (11.9)	0.0137[†]

*Including angiotensin-converting-enzyme inhibitors and angiotensin-II receptor blockers. [†]derived from Log-Rank test. MACE, major adverse cardiovascular events; MI, myocardial infarction; RAAS, rennin-angiotensin-aldosterone system; TVR, target vessel revascularization.

Table 5 Independent predictors of TVR and overall MACE by multivariate Cox regression analysis in all patients

Variable	Hazard ratio	95% C.I.	P
TVR			
TG*	0.993	0.988-0.998	0.007
CAD number*			
1 (reference)	1		
>1	2.717	1.655-4.458	<0.001
Overall MACE			
TG*	0.994	0.990-0.999	0.016
CAD number*			
1 (reference)	1		
>1	2.706	1.730-4.234	<0.001

*Adjusted for age, gender, smoking, diabetes mellitus, left ventricular ejection fraction, peak creatinine kinase level, balloon angioplasty only, bare-metal stent, drug-eluting stent, low-density lipoprotein level, all medications and high-density lipoprotein level. CAD, coronary artery disease; MACE, major adverse cardiovascular event; TG, triglyceride; TVR, target vessel revascularization.

dl predicts fewer incidences of late TVR and in turn overall MACE. These findings illustrate the paradoxically inverse relation between serum TG level and clinical outcome of patients with STEMI treated with pPCI, and may justify exclusion of specific TG-lowering therapy from the standard therapeutic regimen in management of such patients in the long term.

Role of TG in in-hospital outcome of STEMI

The role of serum TG in the pathogenesis of CAD is not as clear as that of serum LDL. A number of clinical studies reported a positive association between TG level and severity of CAD [7,15-17], whereas others demonstrated conflicting results [18-20]. Investigations involving histological research found that triglycerides played a constitutive role in atherosclerotic plaques yet were rarely identified in active coronary artery lesions as a culprit component [21]. These findings suggest that triglycerides might be merely an innocent bystander rather than a direct atherogenic mediator [22-24], and this concept may offer some explanation for our findings that patients with higher TG levels are not at risk of poorer in-hospital outcome after STEMI. In fact, our results demonstrate that there exists a paradoxical trend toward more in-hospital deaths in patients with lower TG levels, though the between-group difference did not reach statistical significance possibly due to limited patient number and confounding by coexistent variables. The role that serum TG plays as an independent negative predictor for in-hospital deaths, finally shown by multivariate regression analysis in this study, has similarly been reported in patients with acute stroke [11-13] and acute coronary syndrome [25], but is not easy to understand compared to the roles played by CK level and CAD number as positive predictors, since these two variables represent surrogates of infarct size and ischemic myocardial territory thus are rationally related with in-hospital mortality. One possible explanation for the inverse relation between TG level and in-hospital mortality comes from the findings that incidences of new atrial arrhythmia, ventricular arrhythmia, respiratory failure and new cardiogenic shock all tended to be higher in the lower TG group, along with the exclusive occurrence of lethal ventricular arrhythmia and refractory heart failure in 6 (3.7%) of lower TG patients but not in any of higher TG group. These results implicate the potential role of serum TG in stabilizing the infarcted, stunned or reperfused myocardium after an acute STEMI episode. Another possibility may be based on the concept that serum TG level is an indicator of nutritional status. Lower TG levels denote poorer nutritional condition which could halt myocardial and whole body recovery from STEMI, in turn subjecting patients to in-hospital deaths. This hypothesis gains support from some epidemiologic studies describing low body mass index and serum cholesterol level as markers of poor health status in older subjects [26-28], and from clinical investigations reporting worse outcome in patients with advanced heart failure or various cardiovascular diseases and low serum cholesterol [29,30] or TG concentrations [11-13]. Further studies are needed to determine the exact pathophysiological relations between serum TG level and in-hospital outcome in patients with STEMI who receive pPCI treatment.

Role of TG in late outcome of STEMI
Previous studies have demonstrated that even after primary PCI a considerable proportion of patients with STEMI still succumb to subsequent MACE due to left ventricular remodeling and coronary restenosis [31]. The distinct pathogenesis of restenosis caused by smooth muscle cell proliferation rather than lipid-related neo-atherosclerosis [32] explains the poor preventive efficacy of lipid-lowering medications, particularly statins, on inhibition of neointimal formation in this entity of lesions [33-35]. Nonetheless, whether higher TG-rich lipoprotein is [36,37] or is not [34] related with the restenotic phenomenon remains debatable. The current study demonstrated that risk of de novo atherosclerosis was similar between groups with higher or lower TG levels but overall MACE rates, contributed mostly from incidence of TVR, were significantly lower in high-TG patients. These results suggest a potential action of serum TG against neointimal proliferation at the STEMI-related lesion sites ever treated by angioplasty or stenting. This phenomenon has ever been reported in an in vitro study describing the distinct effects of various TG particles on either stimulation or suppression of the proliferative activity of vascular smooth

muscle cells [38]. Our findings further indicate that though hypertriglyceridemia is regarded as an independent risk factor for atherosclerosis [39] when coexistent with low HDL- and elevated LDL-cholesterol and needs to be treated after the LDL goal is reached [25], application of such a therapeutic strategy to patients with STEMI post-pPCI is not warranted. On the contrary, the paradoxically inverse relation between hypertriglyceridemia and better late outcome in patients with STEMI treated with pPCI may justify exclusion of specific TG-lowering therapy from the standard therapy in long-term management of such patients. Whether there exists a "J-curve relationship" between serum TG level and the outcome of patients with STEMI treated with pPCI awaits further clarification.

Conclusion
On-admission serum TG levels inversely correlate with in-hospital deaths of patients with STEMI treated with pPCI, and those with TG levels below 150 mg/dl have a worse long-term outcome in terms of TVR and overall MACE than those with higher levels. Thus, serum TG can be regarded as a mediator that protects such patients from short and late cardiovascular events rather than a hazard factor, and hence does not warrant aggressive pharmacological treatment to lower it to the so-called normal level.

Abbreviations
CAD: Coronary artery disease; CK: Creatinine kinase; HDL: High-density lipoprotein; LDL: Low-density lipoprotein; MACE: Major adverse cardiovascular event; pPCI: Primary percutaneous coronary intervention; STEMI: ST-segment elevation myocardial infarction; TIMI: Thrombolysis in myocardial infarction; TG: Triglyceride; TVR: Target vessel revascularization.

Competing interests
The authors declare that they have no competing interests.

Authors' contributions
CYT, LTJ, LHC, SCS, LCN and WKY participated in the design of the study, the collection of patients' clinical data, statistical analysis, and manuscript drafting. CYT, LTJ, HHY, SCS and LWL carried out primary percutaneous coronary intervention, whereas LHC and LCN conducted follow-up of patients and acquisition and interpretation of clinical data. All authors have read and approved the final manuscript.

Acknowledgements
The authors thank Mr. Kuang-Hsi Chang and Ms. Yu-Hsin Wan for their assistance in statistical analysis.
Cardiovascular Center, Taichung Veterans General Hospital, Taichung, Taiwan.

Author details
[1]Cardiovascular Center and Department of Anesthesiology, Taichung Veterans General Hospital, Taichung, Taiwan. [2]Departments of Medicine and Surgery, Yang-Ming University School of Medicine, Taipei, Taiwan. [3]Taipei First Girls High School, Taipei, Taiwan. [4]Chung-Shan Medical University School of Medicine, Taichung, Taiwan.

Lower serum triglyceride level is a risk factor for in-hospital and late major adverse events in patients...

7

References

1. Roger VL, Go AS, Lloyd-Jones DM, Benjamin EJ, Berry JD, Borden WB, Bravata DM, Dai S, Ford ES, Fox CS, Fullerton HJ, Gillespie C, Hailpern SM, Heit JA, Howard VJ, Kissela BM, Kittner SJ, Lackland DT, Lichtman JH, Lisabeth LD, Makuc DM, Marcus GM, Marelli A, Matchar DB, Moy CS, Mozaffarian D, Mussolino ME, Nichol G, Paynter NP, Soliman EZ, et al: Heart disease and stroke statistics–2012 update: a report from the American Heart Association. *Circulation* 2012, 125(1):e2–e220.

2. O'Gara PT, Kushner FG, Ascheim DD, Casey DE Jr, Chung MK, de Lemos JA, Ettinger SM, Fang JC, Fesmire FM, Franklin BA, Granger CB, Krumholz HM, Linderbaum JA, Morrow DA, Newby LK, Ornato JP, Ou N, Radford MJ, Tamis-Holland JE, Tommaso CL, Tracy CM, Woo YJ, Zhao DX, Anderson JL, Jacobs AK, Halperin JL, Albert NM, Brindis RG, Creager MA, DeMets D, et al: 2013 ACCF/AHA guideline for the management of ST-elevation myocardial infarction: a report of the American College of Cardiology Foundation/American Heart Association Task Force on Practice Guidelines. *J Am Coll Cardiol* 2013, 61(4):e78–e140.

3. Figueras J, Alcalde O, Barrabes JA, Serra V, Alguersuari J, Cortadellas J, Lidon RM: Changes in hospital mortality rates in 425 patients with acute ST-elevation myocardial infarction and cardiac rupture over a 30-year period. *Circulation* 2008, 118(25):2783–2789.

4. Perers E, Caidahl K, Herlitz J, Karlson BW, Karlsson T, Hartford M: Treatment and short-term outcome in women and men with acute coronary syndromes. *Int J Cardiol* 2005, 103(2):120–127.

5. Ray KK, Cannon CP, McCabe CH, Cairns R, Tonkin AM, Sacks FM, Jackson G, Braunwald E: Early and late benefits of high-dose atorvastatin in patients with acute coronary syndromes: results from the PROVE IT-TIMI 22 trial. *J Am Coll Cardiol* 2005, 46(8):1405–1410.

6. Patti G, Pasceri V, Colonna G, Miglionico M, Fischetti D, Sardella G, Montinaro A, Di Sciascio G: Atorvastatin pretreatment improves outcomes in patients with acute coronary syndromes undergoing early percutaneous coronary intervention: results of the ARMYDA-ACS randomized trial. *J Am Coll Cardiol* 2007, 49(12):1272–1278.

7. Hokanson JE, Austin MA: Plasma triglyceride level is a risk factor for cardiovascular disease independent of high-density lipoprotein cholesterol level: a meta-analysis of population-based prospective studies. *J Cardiovasc Risk* 1996, 3(2):213–219.

8. Kannel WB, Vasan RS: Triglycerides as vascular risk factors: new epidemiologic insights. *Curr Opin Cardiol* 2009, 24(4):345–350.

9. Eberly LE, Stamler J, Neaton JD: Relation of triglyceride levels, fasting and nonfasting, to fatal and nonfatal coronary heart disease. *Arch Intern Med* 2003, 163(9):1077–1083.

10. Carlson LA, Bottiger LE, Ahfeldt PE: Risk factors for myocardial infarction in the Stockholm prospective study. A 14-year follow-up focussing on the role of plasma triglycerides and cholesterol. *Acta Med Scand* 1979, 206(5):351–360.

11. Weir CJ, Sattar N, Walters MR, Lees KR: Low triglyceride, not low cholesterol concentration, independently predicts poor outcome following acute stroke. *Cerebrovasc Dis* 2003, 16(1):76–82.

12. Pikija S, Trkulja V, Juvan L, Ivanec M, Duksi D: Higher On-admission Serum Triglycerides Predict Less Severe Disability and Lower All-cause Mortality after Acute Ischemic Stroke. *J Stroke Cerebrovasc Dis* 2013, 22(7):e15–e24.

13. Li W, Liu M, Wu B, Liu H, Wang LC, Tan S: Serum lipid levels and 3-month prognosis in Chinese patients with acute stroke. *Adv Ther* 2008, 25(4):329–341.

14. Morrow DA, Antman EM, Charlesworth A, Cairns R, Murphy SA, de Lemos JA, Giugliano RP, McCabe CH, Braunwald E: TIMI risk score for ST-elevation myocardial infarction: A convenient, bedside, clinical score for risk assessment at presentation: An intravenous nPA for treatment of infarcting myocardium early II trial substudy. *Circulation* 2000, 102(17):2031–2037.

15. Assmann G, Schulte H, von Eckardstein A: Hypertriglyceridemia and elevated lipoprotein(a) are risk factors for major coronary events in middle-aged men. *Am J Cardiol* 1996, 77(14):1179–1184.

16. Haim M, Benderly M, Brunner D, Behar S, Graff E, Reicher-Reiss H, Goldbourt U: Elevated serum triglyceride levels and long-term mortality in patients with coronary heart disease: the Bezafibrate Infarction Prevention (BIP) Registry. *Circulation* 1999, 100(5):475–482.

17. Sarwar N, Danesh J, Eiriksdottir G, Sigurdsson G, Wareham N, Bingham S, Boekholdt SM, Khaw KT, Gudnason V: Triglycerides and the risk of coronary heart disease: 10,158 incident cases among 262,525 participants in 29 Western prospective studies. *Circulation* 2007, 115(4):450–458.

18. Wilson PW, Anderson KM, Castelli WP: Twelve-year incidence of coronary heart disease in middle-aged adults during the era of hypertensive therapy: the Framingham offspring study. *Am J Med* 1991, 90(1):11–16.

19. Pocock SJ, Shaper AG, Phillips AN: Concentrations of high density lipoprotein cholesterol, triglycerides, and total cholesterol in ischaemic heart disease. *BMJ* 1989, 298(6679):998–1002.

20. Grundy SM, Vega GL: Two different views of the relationship of hypertriglyceridemia to coronary heart disease. Implications for treatment. *Arch Intern Med* 1992, 152(1):28–34.

21. Gandotra P, Miller M: The role of triglycerides in cardiovascular risk. *Curr Cardiol Rep* 2008, 10(6):505–511.

22. Steinberg D: Building the Basic Science Foundation. In *The Cholesterol Wars: The Cholesterol Skeptics vs the Preponderance of Evidence.* Edited by Steinberg D. New York: Elsevier Ltd; 2007:78.

23. Scott MG, Diane B, Luther TC, Richard SC, Margo AD, James H, Donald BH, Roger I, Russell VL, Patrick MB, James MM, Richard CP, Neil JS, Linda VH: Third Report of the National Cholesterol Education Program (NCEP) Expert Panel on Detection, Evaluation, and Treatment of High Blood Cholesterol in Adults (Adult Treatment Panel III) final report. *Circulation* 2002, 106(25):3143–3421.

24. Talayero BG, Sacks FM: The role of triglycerides in atherosclerosis. *Curr Cardiol Rep* 2011, 13(6):544–552.

25. Khawaja OA, Hatahet H, Cavalcante J, Khanal S, Al-Mallah MH: Low admission triglyceride and mortality in acute coronary syndrome patients. *Cardiol J* 2011, 18(3):297–303.

26. Windler E, Ewers-Grabow U, Thiery J, Walli A, Seidel D, Greten H: The prognostic value of hypocholesterolemia in hospitalized patients. *Clin Investig* 1994, 72(12):939–943.

27. Volpato S, Zuliani G, Guralnik JM, Palmieri E, Fellin R: The inverse association between age and cholesterol level among older patients: the role of poor health status. *Gerontology* 2001, 47(1):36–45.

28. Noel MA, Smith TK, Ettinger WH: Characteristics and outcomes of hospitalized older patients who develop hypocholesterolemia. *J Am Geriatr Soc* 1991, 39(5):455–461.

29. Richartz BM, Radovancevic B, Frazier OH, Vaughn WK, Taegtmeyer H: Low serum cholesterol levels predict high perioperative mortality in patients supported by a left-ventricular assist system. *Cardiology* 1998, 89(3):184–188.

30. Horwich TB, Hamilton MA, Maclellan WR, Fonarow GC: Low serum total cholesterol is associated with marked increase in mortality in advanced heart failure. *J Card Fail* 2002, 8(4):216–224.

31. Keeley EC, Boura JA, Grines CL: Primary angioplasty versus intravenous thrombolytic therapy for acute myocardial infarction: a quantitative review of 23 randomised trials. *Lancet* 2003, 361(9351):13–20.

32. Inoue T, Uchida T, Yaguchi I, Sakai Y, Takayanagi K, Morooka S: Stent-induced expression and activation of the leukocyte integrin Mac-1 is associated with neointimal thickening and restenosis. *Circulation* 2003, 107(13):1757–1763.

33. Veinot JP, Edwards WD, Camrud AR, Jorgenson MA, Holmes DR Jr, Schwartz RS: The effects of lovastatin on neointimal hyperplasia following injury in a porcine coronary artery model. *Can J Cardiol* 1996, 12(1):65–70.

34. Petronio AS, Amoroso G, Limbruno U, Papini B, De Carlo M, Micheli A, Ciabatti N, Mariani M: Simvastatin does not inhibit intimal hyperplasia and restenosis but promotes plaque regression in normocholesterolemic patients undergoing coronary stenting: a randomized study with intravascular ultrasound. *Am Heart J* 2005, 149(3):520–526.

35. Lerakis S, El-Chami MF, Patel AD, Veledar E, Alexopoulos E, Zacharoulis A, Triantafyllou A: Effect of lipid levels and lipid-lowering therapy on restenosis after coronary artery stenting. *Am J Med Sci* 2006, 331(5):270–273.

36. Oi K1, Shimokawa H, Hirakawa Y, Tashiro H, Nakaike R, Kozai T, Ohzono K, Yamamoto K, Koyanagi S, Okamatsu S, Tajimi T, Kikuchi Y, Takeshita A: Postprandial increase in plasma concentrations of remnant-like particles: an independent risk factor for restenosis after percutaneous coronary intervention. *J Cardiovasc Pharmacol* 2004, 44(1):66–73.

37. Kato T, Inoue T, Inagaki H, Hashimoto S, Hikichi Y, Tanaka A, Isobe M, Node K: Remnant-like lipoprotein particle level and insulin resistance are associated with in-stent restenosis in patients with stable angina. *Coron Artery Dis* 2007, 18(4):319–322.

38. Bermudez B, Lopez S, Pacheco YM, Villar J, Muriana FJ, Hoheisel JD, Bauer A, Abia R: Influence of postprandial triglyceride-rich lipoproteins on lipid-mediated gene expression in smooth muscle cells of the human coronary artery. *Cardiovasc Res* 2008, 79(2):294–303.

Culprit-only versus staged complete revascularization for patients with ST-segment elevation myocardial infarction and Multivessel disease

Tongtong Yu, Yuanyuan Dong, Jiahe Zhu, Chunyang Tian, Zhijun Sun and Zhaoqing Sun*

Abstract

Background: Multivessel disease (MVD) is common in patients with ST-segment elevation myocardial infarction (STEMI), but optimal treatment management remains undetermined.

Methods: In this retrospective cohort study, 602 consecutive STEMI patients with MVD were enrolled between January 1, 2010 and October 1, 2014. Three hundred and eighty-two patients underwent culprit-only revascularization and 220 underwent staged complete revascularization. Primary end points were a composite of cardiac mortality or nonfatal reinfarction.

Results: The mean duration of follow-up was 35 months (12–71 months). Following multivariate analysis, staged complete revascularization was associated with a lower rate of the composite of cardiac mortality or nonfatal reinfarction [HR: 0.430, 95 % CI: 0.197–0.940, $P = 0.034$] and unplanned repeat revascularization [HR: 0.343, 95 % CI: 0.166–0.708, $P = 0.004$] compared with culprit-only revascularization.

Conclusions: Compared with culprit-only revascularization, staged complete revascularization significantly reduced the rate of the composite of cardiac mortality or nonfatal reinfarction, and the need for unplanned repeat revascularization.

Keywords: Multivessel disease, Revascularization, ST-segment elevation myocardial infarction

Background

Primary percutaneous coronary intervention (P-PCI) of the culprit artery is widely used in patients with ST-segment elevation myocardial infarction (STEMI). Approximately 50 % of STEMI patients have multivessel disease (MVD) [1, 2]. Non-culprit lesions are not just "bystanders", as a pathophysiological inflammation process in acute myocardial infarction could cause plaque instability [3, 4]. Previous research has also shown that STEMI patients with MVD have higher mortality rates and a greater incidence of non-fatal reinfarction than those without MVD [1, 2]. However, the optimal management of STEMI patients with MVD remains undetermined [5–7]. Although a number of randomized controlled trials (RCTs) [8–11], including the PRAMI [9], CVLPRIT [10] and DANAMI-3—PRIMULTI [11] trials, have indicated the clear benefits of complete PCI, other RCTs [12–14], including the PRAGUE-13 trial [12], found no difference between complete and culprit-only revascularization in STEMI patients with MVD. Furthermore, observational studies [15–21] and meta-analyses [22–24] also demonstrated conflicting results.

The present study aimed to determine the benefits and safety of staged complete revascularization in STEMI patients with MVD undergoing P-PCI.

* Correspondence: sunzhaoqing@vip.163.com
Department of Cardiology, Shengjing Hospital of China Medical University, Shenyang, Liaoning, People's Republic of China

Methods

Study design and setting

This was a retrospective cohort study, and included consecutive STEMI patients who were hospitalized and underwent PCI at Shengjing Hospital of China Medical University (Shenyang, China) between January 1, 2010 and October 31, 2014. Six hundred and two consecutive cases were selected in this large-scale hospital in Northeast China. Firstly, the investigators identified all consecutive PCI patients from PACS (Picture Archiving and Communication Systems) of the interventional imaging data and assigned each case a unique study ID. The investigators then abstracted comprehensive clinical data and procedural data using electronic medical records. Abstracted elements included patient demographic characteristics, past cardiac and noncardiac history, patient clinical characteristics on hospital admission, laboratory measurements, procedure-related complications and use of cardiac medications during the index hospitalization and at discharge. Killip classification was introduced [5]. All venous blood samples were obtained on admission and tested using autoanalyzers in the core laboratory of Shengjing Hospital and standard techniques. Left ventricular ejection fraction (LVEF) was determined by echocardiography during hospitalization. Procedural data from surgical records in PCI cases were completed by operators. Angiographic variables were estimated visually or by a quantitative computer analysis system. Thrombolysis In Myocardial Infarction (TIMI) flow grade was determined as defined previously [25]. Clinical follow-up was assessed in October 2015 by hospital visits or phone interviews with the patient's general practitioner/cardiologist, the patient or his/her family. All events were obtained from the patients' medical records. If these data were unavailable, statuses were ascertained by a telephone call to the patient's referring hospital physician. All events were adjudicated and classified by two cardiologists.

Participants and procedures

We identified 1056 STEMI patients treated with P-PCI. Patients who were eligible for P-PCI met the following criteria: (1) chest pain present less than 12 h from onset of pain to time of catheterization, (2) significant ST-segment elevation (at least 0.1 mV in two or more standard leads or at least 0.2 mV in two or more contiguous precordial leads) or a new left bundle branch block. After confirmation of STEMI, P-PCI was immediately undertaken according to current guideline recommendations and operators' routine practice. Operators decided on the use of aspiration thrombectomy, heparin, or glycoprotein IIb/IIIa inhibitor. The culprit artery was determined using ECG, echocardiography and angiographic findings by each operator. For inclusion in the present study, patients had

to have MVD, which was defined as the presence of angiographic diameter stenosis of 50 % or greater in at least one non-culprit major epicardial coronary artery or its major branches (with diameter ≥2 mm). Exclusion criteria included (1) single vessel disease, (2) cardiogenic shock, (3) any type of stent thrombosis, (4) previous coronary artery bypass grafting (CABG), (5) unsuitable for treatment with P-PCI, (6) chronic total occlusion as the only significant non-culprit lesion, (7) non-culprit lesion in coronary artery branches 2 mm or smaller in diameter. The study population was subdivided into (1) the culprit-only revascularization group (CR group), in which only the culprit lesion received PCI during the index catheterization or hospitalization; (2) the staged complete revascularization group (SR group), in which, after culprit lesion PCI, a planned additional non-culprit lesion PCI was performed during the index hospitalization, or within 1 month after discharge, regardless of symptoms or evidence of ischemia. Periprocedural and postprocedural anti-platelet treatments and other cardiovascular medications were administered in accordance with current guidelines [5, 7].

Clinical end points

The primary end point was a composite of cardiac mortality or nonfatal reinfarction. Secondary end points were all-cause mortality, cardiac mortality, nonfatal reinfarction and unplanned repeat revascularization, including any unplanned repeat PCI or surgical bypass of target or non-target vessels. The safety end points were periprocedure-related complications, including BARC 3 or 5 bleeding, contrast-induced nephropathy, stroke, and acute or subacute stent thrombosis during the index hospitalization. Stroke was defined as an acute event of non-hemorrhagic cerebrovascular origin causing focal or global neurologic dysfunction lasting >24 h, which was confirmed by both clinical and radiographic criteria. Contrast-induced nephropathy was defined as an increase in serum creatinine concentration ≥0.5 mg/dl (44.2 mmol/l) or ≥25 % above baseline 72 h after exposure to the contrast medium. All other end points were defined by standardized definitions [26, 27]. This study complies with the Declaration of Helsinki, and Shengjing Hospital of China Medical University Research Ethics Committee approved the research protocol. Written informed consent was formally obtained from all participants.

Statistical analysis

Quantitative variables with normal distribution were represented as mean ± standard deviation (SD) and compared with the independent samples t-test. Quantitative variables without normal distribution were represented as median [interquartile range, IQR] and compared with the Mann-Whitney U-test. Normal distribution was assessed by the one-sample Kolmogorov-Smirnov Test. Categorical variables were represented as counts and proportions (%) and compared using the chi-square test. Event-free survival was estimated in the two groups from Kaplan–Meier curves and compared using the Log-Rank Test. Cox proportional-hazards regression modeling was used to analyze the effects of variables on event-free survival. Variables in Table 1 with $P \le 0.1$ at the univariate analysis were "entered" into the model (Table 3). These variables included age, gender, current smoker, and previous MI. Results were reported as hazard ratios (HRs) with associated 95 % confidence intervals (CIs). All tests were two-sided, and the statistical significance was defined as $P < 0.05$. All statistical analyses were performed using SPSS version 19 (SPSS Inc., Chicago, Illinois, USA).

Results
Participants
Between January 1, 2010 and October 1, 2014, a total of 1,056 patients were treated with P-PCI for STEMI in our center. Figure 1 represents the flowchart for patient selection. The final study cohort consisted of 602 patients, of whom 382 (63.5 %) received culprit-only revascularization and 220 (36.5 %) received staged complete revascularization. For the SR group, the timing of nonculprit lesion PCI was during the index hospitalization

using a staged procedure ($n = 208$) and after index hospitalization but within 1 month ($n = 12$).

Basic characteristics
Clinical characteristics in the two groups were generally similar and are shown in Table 1. Periprocedural details and discharge medication are shown in Table 2. Patients in the SR group had more stents and longer total stent length. Discharge medication was similar between the two groups (Table 2).

Clinical Outcome
All patients were followed for a mean duration of 35 months (12–71 months). The length of follow-up in the CR group was 34 months (12–69 months), and was 36 months (12–71 months) in the SR group. During the follow-up period, 31 events of cardiac mortality/nonfatal myocardial reinfarction events, 17 events of cardiac mortality, 14 events of nonfatal myocardial reinfarction, 19 events of all-cause mortality, and 42 events of unplanned repeat revascularization were observed in the CR group; 8 events of cardiac mortality/nonfatal myocardial reinfarction, 4 events of cardiac mortality, 4 events of nonfatal myocardial reinfarction, 5 events of all-cause mortality, and 9 events of unplanned repeat revascularization were observed in the SR group. The composite of cardiac mortality or nonfatal reinfarction was significantly lower in the SR group compared with the CR group [HR: 0.427, 95 % CI: 0.196–0.929, $P = 0.032$], and unplanned repeat revascularization showed a similar trend [HR: 0.349, 95 % CI: 0.170–0.717, $P = 0.004$] (Fig. 2; Table 3). After adjusting for covariates (Model 1), the SR group was still associated with a lower rate of the composite of cardiac mortality or nonfatal reinfarction [HR: 0.430, 95 % CI: 0.197–0.940, $P = 0.034$] and unplanned repeat revascularization [HR: 0.343, 95 % CI: 0.166–0.708, $P = 0.004$] compared with the CR group (Table 3). There were no statistically significant differences in the other endpoints between the two groups (Table 3). Periprocedure-related complications were not significantly different (Table 4).

Discussion
The present study determined the effects of different treatment strategies on STEMI patients with MVD in a real-world clinical setting. The main findings were as follows: (1) staged complete revascularization significantly reduced not only the rate of the composite of cardiac mortality or nonfatal reinfarction, but also the need for unplanned repeat revascularization; (2) no significant differences in all-cause mortality, cardiac mortality or nonfatal reinfarction were observed between the treatment strategies; (3)

Table 1 Demographics and baseline clinical characteristics, means ± SD, or N (%)

	CR, $n = 382$	SR, $n = 220$	P
Age, yrs	64.6 ± 12.0	62.7 ± 11.5	0.052
Male	257 (67.3)	164(74.5)	0.061
Medical history			
Diabetes	101 (26.4)	70 (31.8)	0.159
Hypertension	194 (50.8)	120 (54.5)	0.374
Hypercholesterolemia	100 (26.2)	56 (25.5)	0.845
Current smoker	194 (50.8)	128 (58.2)	0.080
Previous PCI	14 (3.7)	10 (4.5)	0.595
Previous MI	13 (3.4)	14 (6.4)	0.091
Killip class II/III on admission	27 (7.1)	13 (5.9)	0.582
Systolic blood pressure on admission, mmHg	128.2 ± 22.0	129.9 ± 24.0	0.392
Heart rate on admission, bpm	77.3 ± 16.8	77.8 ± 14.5	0.703
LVEF, %	54.0 ± 9.1	53.6 ± 9.1	0.662
Symptom to balloon time, h	6 (4,9)	6 (3,9)	0.851
Anterior MI	165 (43.2)	103 (46.8)	0.389
Three-vessel disease	160 (41.9)	106 (48.2)	0.134
Intra-aortic Balloon Pump	31 (8.1)	17 (7.7)	0.866

MI myocardial infarction, *bpm* beats per minute, *h* hour

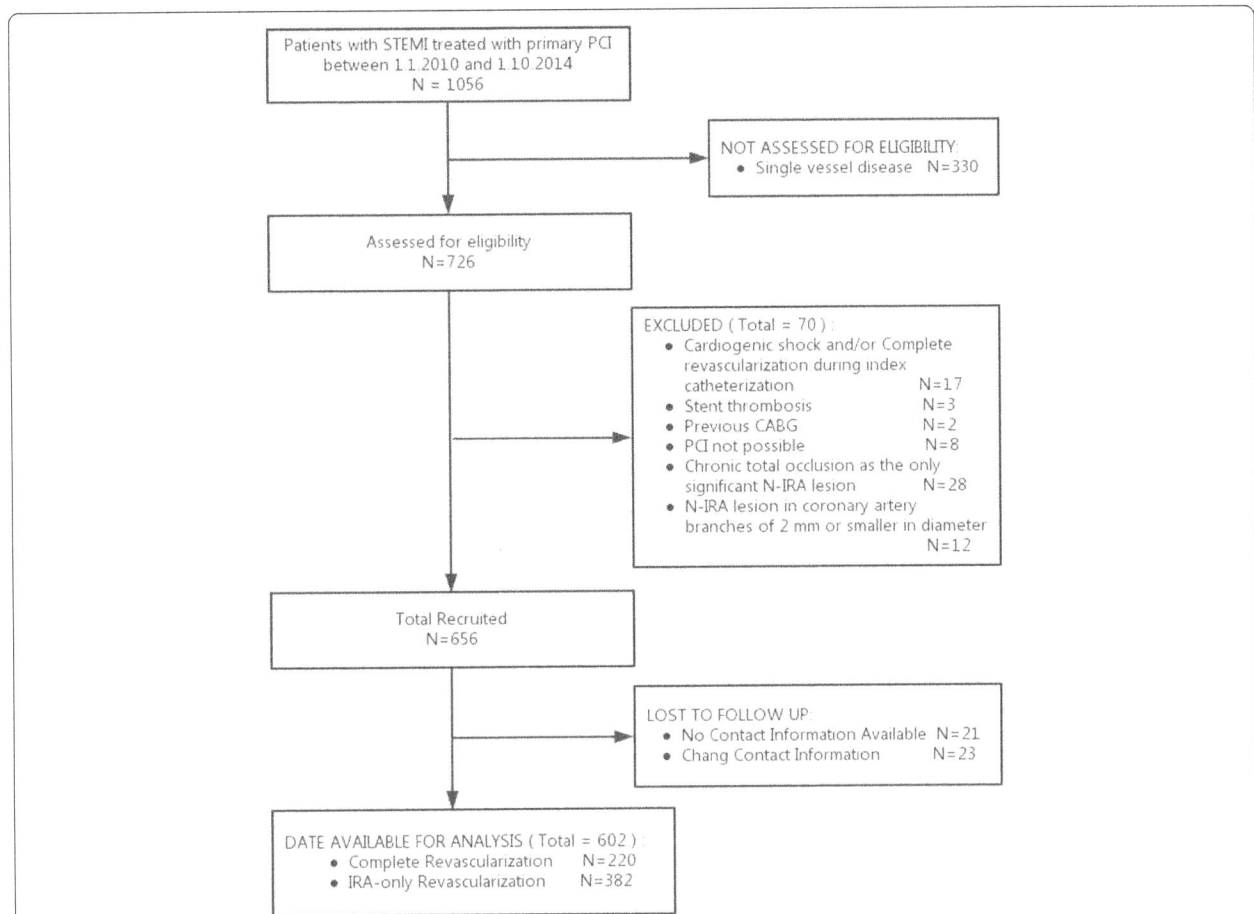

Fig. 1 Flow diagram of participant selection. 330 with single vessel disease, 70 with other exclusion criteria, and 44 without follow-up were excluded. The final study cohort consisted of 602 patients, of whom 382 received culprit-only revascularization and 220 received staged complete revascularization. STEMI, ST-segment elevation myocardial infarction; PCI, percutaneous coronary intervention; CABG, coronary artery bypass grafting; N-IRA, non-Infarct-Related Artery

staged complete revascularization did not significantly increase periprocedure-related complications.

Toyota et al. analyzed 1311 STEMI patients with MVD undergoing P-PCI from the CREDO-Kyoto AMI Registry in Japan (681 in the staged PCI group versus 630 in the culprit-only PCI group), and reported that staged PCI was associated with a lower 5-year composite of cardiac mortality and myocardial infarction compared with culprit-only PCI [HR: 0.67, 95 % CI: 0.44–0.99, P = 0.045] [19]. Our findings also showed a lower composite of cardiac mortality and nonfatal reinfarction in the SR group. A similar conclusion was found in the CvLPRIT and DANAMI-3—PRIMULTI trials [10, 11]. However, no studies have found significant differences in cardiac mortality [8–12, 19] between the treatment groups. Furthermore, most studies [8–12, 17, 19, 20] found no significant differences in nonfatal reinfarction, except for the PRAMI trial [9] and a recent meta-analysis [23]. Our study also failed to find significant differences in cardiac

mortality and nonfatal reinfarction between the two groups. It was demonstrated that staged complete revascularization significantly reduced the need for unplanned repeat revascularization; however, the Japanese study [19] and CvLPRIT trial [10] found no significant differences, and the proportion of patients with three-vessel disease may have played an important role. There was a higher proportion of three-vessel disease in the CR group in our study than in the other two previous studies. In other words, the higher the proportion of three-vessel disease, the higher the proportion of ischemia-driven unplanned repeat revascularizations. Meta-analyses have also confirmed that multivessel PCI will reduce the need for repeat revascularization [22–24]. Different to other studies [17–19], our study found no significant differences in all-cause mortality. It is possible that the follow-up duration in our study was too short to detect significant differences in all-cause mortality: 3-year follow-up in our study,

Table 2 Periprocedural details and discharge medication, median (IQR), or N (%)

	CR, $n = 382$	SR, $n = 220$	P
Percutaneous coronary intervention			
TIMI flow grade 0/1 on arrival	288 (75.4)	165 (75.0)	0.914
TIMI flow grade 3 post-PCI	375 (98.2)	218 (99.1)	0.369
Number of stents	1 (1,2)	3 (2,4)	<0.001
Stent type			0.211
No stenting	9 (2.4)	1 (0.5)	
Bare metal	2 (0.5)	1 (0.5)	
Drug-eluting	371 (97.1)	218 (99.1)	
Total stent length for all lesions treated, mm	36 (24,57)	79 (54,109)	<0.001
Lesion site in culprit vessel			0.700
Left anterior descending artery	169 (44.2)	95 (43.2)	
Left circumflex artery	48 (12.6)	33 (15.0)	
Right coronary artery	165 (43.2)	92 (41.8)	
Thrombus aspiration catheter used	55 (14.4)	27 (12.3)	0.464
Use of glycoprotein IIb/IIIa inhibitor	142 (37.2)	127 (42.3)	0.217
Medical treatment at discharge			
Aspirin	376 (98.4)	217 (98.6)	0.840
Clopidogrel	373 (97.6)	213 (96.8)	0.544
Ticagrelor	5 (1.3)	5 (2.3)	0.373
Statin	358 (93.7)	203 (92.3)	0.498
Beta-blockers	224 (58.6)	115 (52.1)	0.121
Angiotensin-converting enzyme inhibitors/Angiotensin receptor blockers	224 (58.6)	133 (60.5)	0.662
Calcium-channel blocker	24 (6.3)	9 (4.1)	0.255
Nitrate	39 (10.2)	16 (7.3)	0.228
Nicorandil	20 (5.2)	6 (2.7)	0.145

compared with 5-year and 7-year follow-up in the other two studies [18, 19]. In addition, the sample size in our study was relatively small, 602 individuals compared with 8822 and 1311 in the other two studies [18, 19]. Accordingly, adequately powered randomized studies should be performed to obtain meaningful conclusions, such as in the COMPLETE trial (Clinical-Trials.gov NCT01740479).

The safety concerns regarding complete revascularization include the risk of procedural complications, longer procedural time, contrast nephropathy, and stent thrombosis which may increase in a prothrombotic and pro-inflammatory state in the presence of STEMI. Despite this, our study showed no increase in major bleeding, contrast-induced nephropathy, stroke, acute or subacute stent thrombosis. This was consistent with previous studies [8, 10–12, 19].

There are still several problems related to the treatment of STEMI. First, is staged complete revascularization better than "one-time" complete revascularization? While analysis from the HORIZONS-AMI trial preferred staged complete revascularization [15], other studies found "one-time" complete revascularization safe and effective [20, 21]. Second, what is the appropriate timing of staged revascularization? Different studies had different time cut-off points; however, no study could confirm a favored time cut-off point. Third, should fractional flow reserve (FFR) or a non-invasive physiological stress test be used to determine indications for staged revascularization in addition to angiography? FFR measurements of non-culprit lesions could be performed immediately [28] or several days or weeks [7] after treatment of the culprit vessel. To date, studies with FFR as the reference [11, 13, 14] did not have clearer conclusions than those without FFR as the reference [8–10]. The COMPARE ACUTE trial (Clinical-Trials.gov NCT01399736), an ongoing prospective randomized study comparing a FFR-guided multivessel PCI undertaken during primary PCI of the culprit vessel only, may help us to define the role of FFR in STEMI patients with MVD. Fourth, do the benefits extend to non-culprit stenoses of less than 70 % or 50 %? The level of non-culprit stenosis at which the risks of PCI surpass the benefits is still uncertain. In addition to FFR, intra-coronary imaging such as an intravascular ultrasound study (IVUS) and optical coherence tomography (OCT) could be useful tools for non-culprit lesion revascularization. IVUS and OCT could help us describe *in vivo* the pathological morphology of plaque associated with an impaired myocardial blush and slow flow leading to a worse prognosis [29]. As for the use of IVUS and OCT, a per-patient tailored therapy may be achieved.

Limitations

This study had several limitations. First, the study was retrospective and observational, thus potential confounders and selection bias could not be completely adjusted. Second, this was a single center study. Third, the significance of non-culprit lesions was assessed only on angiography, and ischemia tests such as FFR were absent. Fourth, the long symptom to balloon time in this study may have had an impact on the study results, as analysis of the HORIZONS-AMI trial results suggested that a delay in mechanical reperfusion therapy during STEMI is associated with greater injury to the microcirculation [30], and another study showed that a symptom-onset-to-balloon time >4 h was an independent predictor of one-year mortality [31]. Finally, the incidence of the primary composite end-point was quite low during the follow-up period. The low number of events may be a limitation in the overall interpretation of the study results.

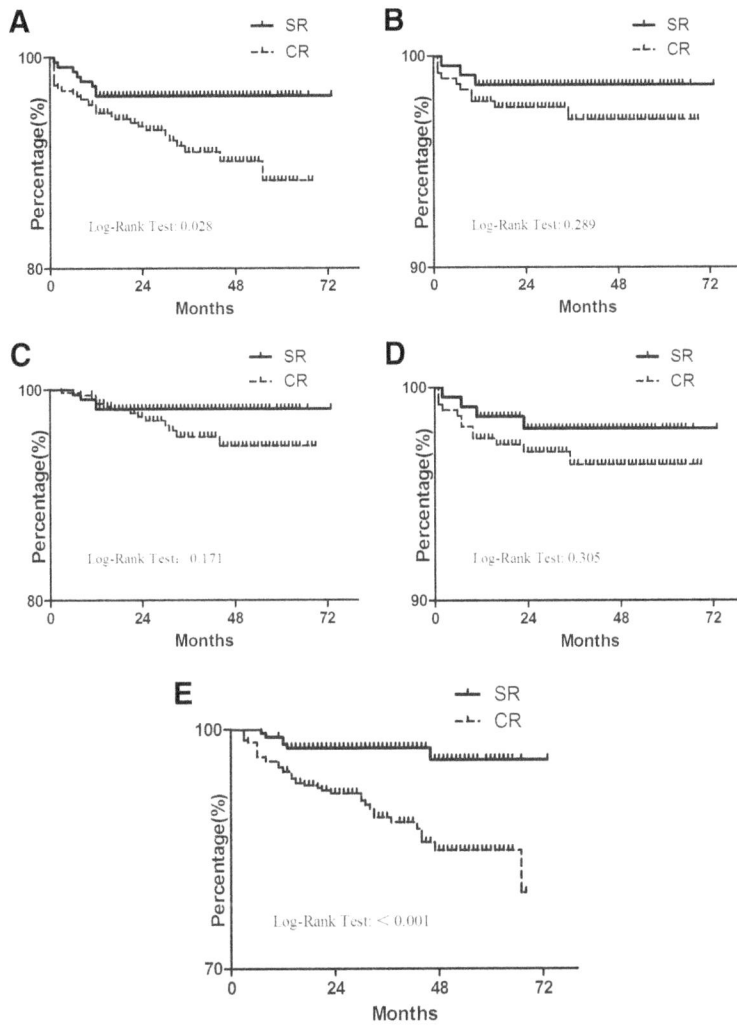

Fig. 2 Kaplan-Meier survival curves free from (**a**) cardiac mortality/nonfatal reinfarction, (**b**) cardiac mortality, (**c**) nonfatal reinfarction, (**d**) all-cause mortality, (**e**) unplanned repeat revascularization according to the different groups. SR, staged complete revascularization group; CR, culprit-only revascularization group

Table 3 Univariate and multivariate analysis of the effects of different treatment strategies at follow-Up, N (%)

	No. patients with event		Univariate analysis		Multivariate analysis*	
	CR	SR	HR (95 % CI)	P	HR (95 % CI)	P
Primary end points						
Cardiac mortality/Nonfatal reinfarction	31 (8.1)	8 (3.6)	0.427 (0.196–0.929)	0.032	0.430 (0.197–0.940)	0.034
Secondary end points						
Cardiac mortality	17 (4.5)	4 (1.8)	0.400 (0.135–1.190)	0.100	0.440 (0.147–1.319)	0.143
Nonfatal reinfarction	14 (3.7)	4 (1.8)	0.467 (0.153–1.418)	0.179	0.442 (0.143–1.365)	0.156
All-cause mortality	19 (5.0)	5 (2.3)	0.442 (0.165–1.185)	0.105	0.489 (0.181–1.321)	0.158
Unplanned repeat revascularization	42 (11.0)	9 (4.1)	0.349 (0.170–0.717)	0.004	0.343 (0.166–0.708)	0.004

*Adjusted for age, diabetes, hypertension, Killip class II/III on admission, systolic blood pressure on admission, heart rate on admission, symptom to balloon time, and anterior MI

Table 4 Periprocedure-related complications, N (%)

	CR (n = 382)	SR (n = 220)	P
BARC 3 or 5 bleeding	2 (0.5)	4 (1.8)	0.124
Contrast-induced nephropathy	13 (3.4)	5 (2.3)	0.433
Stroke	3 (0.8)	0	0.188
Acute or subacute stent thrombosis	1 (0.3)	0	0.448

Conclusions

In STEMI patients with MVD, staged complete revascularization for angiographically significant non-culprit lesions was associated with a significantly lower composite of cardiac mortality or nonfatal reinfarction and unplanned repeat revascularization.

Abbreviations
bpm: Beats per minute; CI: Confidence interval; CR: Culprit-only revascularization group; h: Hour; HR: Hazard ratio; LVEF: Left ventricular ejection fraction; MI: Myocardial infarction; MVD: Multivessel disease; PACS: Picture Archiving and Communication Systems; P-PCI: Primary percutaneous coronary intervention; RCT: Randomized controlled trial; SR: Staged complete revascularization group; STEMI: ST-segment elevation myocardial infarction; TIMI: Thrombolysis In Myocardial Infarction

Acknowledgements
No one who contributed towards the article who does not meet the criteria for authorship.

Funding
This research project was supported by grants from the Social Development Research Program of Liaoning Province (2011225020).

Authors' contributions
ZS conceived and designed the experiments. TY, YD, JZ and CT performed the experiments. TY analyzed the data and wrote the paper. ZS revised the paper. All authors have reviewed and agreed on the contents of this paper.

Competing interests
The authors declare that they have no competing interests.

References
1. Sorajja P, Gersh BJ, Cox DA, McLaughlin MG, Zimetbaum P, Costantini C, et al. Impact of multivessel disease on reperfusion success and clinical outcomes in patients undergoing primary percutaneous coronary intervention for acute myocardial infarction. Eur Heart J. 2007;28(14):1709–16.
2. Park DW, Clare RM, Schulte PJ, Pieper KS, Shaw LK, Califf RM, et al. Extent, location, and clinical significance of non-infarct-related coronary artery disease among patients with ST-elevation myocardial infarction. JAMA. 2014;312(19):2019–27.
3. Naghavi M, Libby P, Falk E, Casscells SW, Litovsky S, Rumberger J, et al. From vulnerable plaque to vulnerable patient: a call for new definitions and risk assessment strategies. Circulation. 2003;108(14):1664–72.
4. Kubo T, Imanishi T, Kashiwagi M, Ikejima H, Tsujioka H, Kuroi A, et al. Multiple coronary lesion instability in patients with acute myocardial infarction as determined by optical coherence tomography. Am J Cardiol. 2010;105(3):318–22.
5. O'Gara PT, Kushner FG, Ascheim DD, Casey Jr DE, Chung MK, de Lemos JA, et al. 2013 ACCF/AHA guideline for the management of ST-elevation myocardial infarction: a report of the American College of Cardiology Foundation/American Heart Association Task Force on Practice Guidelines. J Am Coll Cardiol. 2013; 61(4):e78–e140.
6. Levine GN, O'Gara PT, Bates ER, Blankenship JC, Kushner FG, Bailey SR, et al. 2015 ACC/AHA/SCAI Focused Update on Primary Percutaneous Coronary Intervention for Patients With ST-Elevation Myocardial Infarction: An Update of the 2011 ACCF/AHA/SCAI Guideline for Percutaneous Coronary Intervention and the 2013 ACCF/AHA Guideline for the Management of ST-Elevation Myocardial Infarction: A Report of the American College of Cardiology/American Heart Association Task Force on Clinical Practice Guidelines and the Society for Cardiovascular Angiography and Interventions. J Am Coll Cardiol. 2015. doi: 10.1016/j.jacc.2015.10.005. [Epub ahead of print].
7. Steg PG, James SK, Atar D, Badano LP, Blömstrom-Lundqvist C, Borger MA, et al. ESC Guidelines for the management of acute myocardial infarction in patients presenting with ST-segment elevation. Eur Heart J. 2012;33(20):2569–619.
8. Politi L, Sgura F, Rossi R, Monopoli D, Guerri E, Leuzzi C, et al. A randomised trial of target-vessel versus multi-vessel revascularisation in ST-elevation myocardial infarction: major adverse cardiac events during long-term follow-up. Heart. 2010;96(9):662–7.
9. Wald DS, Morris JK, Wald NJ, Chase AJ, Edwards RJ, Hughes LO, et al; PRAMI Investigators. Randomized trial of preventive angioplasty in myocardial infarction. N Engl J Med. 2013; 369(12):1115-1123
10. Gershlick AH, Khan JN, Kelly DJ, Greenwood JP, Sasikaran T, Curzen N, et al. Randomized trial of complete versus lesion-only revascularization in patients undergoing primary percutaneous coronary intervention for STEMI and multivessel disease: the CvLPRIT trial. J Am Coll Cardiol. 2015;65(10):963–72.
11. Engstrøm T, Kelbæk H, Helqvist S, Høfsten DE, Kløvgaard L, Holmvang L, et al; DANAMI-3—PRIMULTI Investigators. Complete revascularisation versus treatment of the culprit lesion only in patients with ST-segment elevation myocardial infarction and multivessel disease (DANAMI-3—PRIMULTI): an open-label, randomised controlled trial. Lancet. 2015; 386(9994):665-671
12. Hlinomaz O. Multivessel coronary disease diagnosed at the time of primary PCI for STEMI: complete revascularization versus conservative strategy, PRAGUE 13 trial. Available at: http://sbhci.org.br/wp-content/uploads/2015/05/PRAGUE-13-Trial.pdf.
13. Dambrink JH, Debrauwere JP, van 't Hof AW, Ottervanger JP, Gosselink AT, Hoorntje JC, et al. Non-culprit lesions detected during primary PCI: treat invasively or follow the guidelines? EuroIntervention. 2010;5(8):968–75.
14. Ghani A, Dambrink JH, van't Hof AW, Ottervanger JP, Gosselink AT, Hoorntje JC. Treatment of non-culprit lesions detected during primary PCI: long-term follow-up of a randomised clinical trial. Neth Heart J. 2012;20(9):347–53.
15. Kornowski R, Mehran R, Dangas G, Nikolsky E, Assali A, Claessen BE, et al; HORIZONS-AMI Trial Investigators. Prognostic impact of staged versus "one-time" multivessel percutaneous intervention in acute myocardial infarction: analysis from the HORIZONS-AMI (harmonizing outcomes with revascularization and stents in acute myocardial infarction) trial. J Am Coll Cardiol. 2011; 58(7):704-711
16. Manari A, Varani E, Guastaroba P, Menozzi M, Valgimigli M, Menozzi A, et al. Long-term outcome in patients with ST segment elevation myocardial infarction and multivessel disease treated with culprit-only, immediate, or staged multivessel percutaneous revascularization strategies: Insights from the REAL registry. Catheter Cardiovasc Interv. 2014;84(6):912–22.
17. Jensen LO, Terkelsen CJ, Horváth-Puhó E, Tilsted HH, Maeng M, Junker A, et al. Influence of multivessel disease with or without additional revascularization on mortality in patients with ST-segment elevation myocardial infarction. Am Heart J. 2015;170(1):70–8.
18. Lee HW, Hong TJ, Yang MJ, An SG, Oh JH, Choi JH, et al; Korea Acute Myocardial Infarction Registry Investigators. Comparison of infarct-related artery vs multivessel revascularization in ST-segment elevation myocardial infarction with multivessel disease: analysis from Korea Acute Myocardial Infarction Registry. Cardiol J. 2012; 19(3):256–66.
19. Toyota T, Shiomi H, Taniguchi T, Morimoto T, Furukawa Y, Nakagawa Y, et al; CREDO-Kyoto AMI Registry Investigators. Culprit Vessel-Only vs. Staged Multivessel Percutaneous Coronary Intervention Strategies in Patients With Multivessel Coronary Artery Disease Undergoing Primary Percutaneous Coronary Intervention for ST-Segment Elevation Myocardial Infarction. Circ J. 2015. doi: 10.1253/circj.CJ-15-0493. [Epub ahead of print].
20. Rodrigues G, de Araújo Gonçalves P, Madeira S, Rodrigues R, Borges Santos M, Brito J, et al. Impact of complete revascularization in patients with ST-elevation myocardial infarction: analysis of a 10-year all-comers prospective registry. Coron Artery Dis. 2015 Dec 18. doi: 10.1097/MCA.0000000000000334. [Epub ahead of print].

Culprit-only versus staged complete revascularization for patients with ST-segment elevation myocardial...

15

21. Jeger R, Jaguszewski M, Nallamothu BN, Lüscher TF, Urban P, Pedrazzini GB, et al ; AMIS Plus Investigators. Acute multivessel revascularization improves 1-year outcome in ST-elevation myocardial infarction: a nationwide study cohort from the AMIS Plus registry. Int J Cardiol. 2014; 172(1):76-81.

22. Bainey KR, Mehta SR, Lai T, Welsh RC. Complete vs culprit-only revascularization for patients with multivessel disease undergoing primary percutaneous coronary intervention for ST-segment elevation myocardial infarction: a systematic review and meta-analysis. Am Heart J. 2014;167(1):1–14. e2.

23. Spencer FA, Sekercioglu N, Prasad M, Lopes LC, Guyatt GH. Culprit vessel versus immediate complete revascularization in patients with ST-segment myocardial infarction-a systematic review. Am Heart J. 2015;170(6):1133–9.

24. Moretti C, D'Ascenzo F, Quadri G, Omedè P, Montefusco A, Taha S, et al. Management of multivessel coronary disease in STEMI patients: a systematic review and meta-analysis. Int J Cardiol. 2015;179:552–7.

25. Sheehan FH, Braunwald E, Canner P, Dodge HT, Gore J, Van Natta P, et al. The effect of intravenous thrombolytic therapy on left ventricular function: a report on tissue-type plasminogen activator and streptokinase from the Thrombolysis in Myocardial Infarction (TIMI Phase I) trial. Circulation. 1987; 75(4):817–29.

26. Mehran R, Rao SV, Bhatt DL, Gibson CM, Caixeta A, Eikelboom J, et al. Standardized bleeding definitions for cardiovascular clinical trials: a consensus report from the Bleeding Academic Research Consortium. Circulation. 2011;123(23):2736–47.

27. Cutlip DE, Windecker S, Mehran R, Boam A, Cohen DJ, van Es GA, et al. Academic Research Consortium. Clinical end points in coronary stent trials: a case for standardized definitions. Circulation. 2007;115(17):2344–51.

28. Ntalianis A, Sels JW, Davidavicius G, Tanaka N, Muller O, Trana C, et al. Fractional flow reserve for the assessment of nonculprit coronary artery stenoses in patients with acute myocardial infarction. JACC Cardiovasc Interv. 2010;3(12):1274–81.

29. Iannaccone M, Vadalà P, D'ascenzo F, Montefusco A, Moretti C, D'amico M, et al. Clinical perspective of optical coherence tomography and intravascular ultrasound in STEMI patients. J Thorac Dis. 2016;8(5):754–6.

30. Prasad A, Gersh BJ, Mehran R, Brodie BR, Brener SJ, Dizon JM, et al. Effect of Ischemia Duration and Door-to-Balloon Time on Myocardial Perfusion in ST-Segment Elevation Myocardial Infarction: An Analysis From HORIZONS-AMI Trial (Harmonizing Outcomes with Revascularization and Stents in Acute Myocardial Infarction). JACC Cardiovasc Interv. 2015;8(15):1966–74.

31. De Luca G, Suryapranata H, Zijlstra F, van 't Hof AW, Hoorntje JC, Gosselink AT, et al. Symptom-onset-to-balloon time and mortality in patients with acute myocardial infarction treated by primary angioplasty. J Am Coll Cardiol. 2003;42(6):991–7.

3

Root causes for delayed hospital discharge in patients with ST-segment Myocardial Infarction (STEMI)

Jeremy Adams[1,2], Brian Wong[2,3] and Harindra C. Wijeysundera[1,2,4,5,6]*

Abstract

Background: The majority of patients who suffer a ST-segment myocardial infarction (STEMI) are hospitalized for longer than 48 h. With the advent of reperfusion therapy, the benefits of such extended hospitalization has been questioned. The goal of this qualitative study was to identify the root causes for prolonged hospitalization in STEMI patients in order to refine future interventions to optimize the length of hospitalization.

Methods: Practitioners involved in the discharge process for STEMI patients at a single tertiary care STEMI center underwent semi-structured interviews focused on three fictional patient cases. Data were transcribed and analyzed for key themes by thematic analysis.

Results: Interviews were conducted with 17 practitioners (5 Attending Physicians, 4 Internal Medicine Residents, 4 Cardiology Residents, 4 Nursing Staff). The key themes were patient factors, provider factors, and transitions to outpatient care. Patient factors included concerns that early discharge would limit dose titration of medications, the educational experience of the patient, and prevent monitoring for complications. Provider factors included past clinical experience with STEMI complications, in turn impacting discharging behaviour. Transitions of care factors were difficulty in establishing reliable follow-up plans and home care services.

Conclusions: Several themes were identified that influence the timing of discharge post STEMI. The majority of these issues are not incorporated into currently available post STEMI risk stratification tools. Future quality improvement interventions to reduce STEMI length of stay should focus on in-patient and out-patient strategies to address these unique clinical situations.

Keywords: Zwolle Score, STEMI care, Qualitative analysis

Background

ST-segment myocardial infactions (STEMI) are caused by an acute total occlusion of an epicardial coronary vessel, and remain a significant cause of hospitalization in Canada [1, 2]. Published STEMI guidelines provide in-depth recommendations of pre-hospital, hospital-based, and post-hospital care and interventions for patients with STEMI [3]. Before the introduction of reperfusion therapy, length of stay was traditionally between 7–10 days [4]. This time in hospital was necessary for medication up titration, monitoring for arrhythmia, and patient education. With the development of modern reperfusion therapies, however, the benefit of an extended hospitalization has been questioned [5].

A study of 23,000 STEMI patients found that keeping patients beyond a third day in hospital was not cost effective [6]. This finding prompted the derivation of the Zwolle risk score to estimate early mortality risk, using data from 1794 patients who were treated with primary angioplasty from 1994 to 2001 [5]. The goal of this score was to identify patients who may be safe for early discharge after receiving contemporary STEMI care. The Zwolle score incorporates clinical variables such as presence of heart failure, location of the infarction, patient age, success of reperfusion therapy and the angiographic extent of

* Correspondence: harindra.wijeysundera@sunnybrook.ca
[1]Division of Cardiology, Schulich Heart Centre, Sunnybrook Health Sciences Centre, 2075 Bayview Avenue, Suite A202, Toronto, ON M4N3M5, Canada
[2]Department of Medicine, Sunnybrook Health Sciences Centre, University of Toronto, Toronto, ON, Canada
Full list of author information is available at the end of the article

underlying coronary disease (see Additional file 1: Appendix 1 for scoring details) to provide estimates for mortality at 0–2 days, 2–10 days, and 30 days. At a score of less than or equal to 3, mortality after 2 days was extremely small at 0.2 %. The Zwolle investigators argued these very low risk patients could be discharged from hospital between 48–72 h after STEMI and that substantial cost savings could be realized as a result.

Prior studies have investigated protocol-based interventions to reduce length of stay in hospital after STEMI. In 1988, Topol and colleagues randomized a group of 90 STEMI patients post reperfusion therapy to early discharge (within 3 days) or usual care [4]. These were patients with no obvious STEMI complications and a low risk exercise stress test. At 6 months of follow-up, there was no significant difference in hospital re-admissions or complications in the early discharge group. The second Primary Angioplasty in Myocardial Infarction (PAMI-II) trial randomized low risk patients (age < 70 years, left ventricular ejection fraction >45 %, one or two vessel disease, successful reperfusion, no persistent arrhythmias) to discharge on day 3 versus usual care with pre-discharge exercise testing [7]. The patients randomized to discharge on day 3 had similar rates of mortality, re-infarction, congestive heart failure, and stroke as patients randomized to usual care.

Despite such evidence, there has been minimal adoption of early discharge into routine clinical practice [8]. Pilot work from our institution showed that of the 1262 patients who were treated for STEMI at Sunnybrook Health Sciences Centre from 2007 to 2012, 1040 patients had low risk Zwolle scores. However, 75 % of these patients had lengths of stay greater than 48 h. These findings are consistent with those observed by other groups. A recent retrospective study of 255 STEMI patients at a Canadian academic hospital found that 72 % of low risk patients had lengths of stay that extended beyond 2 days [8]. Accordingly, the objective of this quality improvement project was to conduct a qualitative analysis to explore the root causes of prolonged post-STEMI at Sunnybrook to inform future interventions designed to reduce length of stay and subsequent hospitalization costs. The failure for risk scores to be successfully translated into changes in clinical practice extends beyond cardiology and the care of STEMI patients. As such, understanding the root causes of prolonged hospitalization and how these may or may not be potentially addressed by current risk scores will have broad implications on the development of new scores and how they are implemented in practice.

Methods

According to the policy activities that constitute research at Sunnybrook Health Sciences Center, this work met criteria for operational improvement activities exempt from institutional research board review.

Using the Model for Improvement as the theoretical basis for our study, our qualitative analysis intended to better characterize the nature of the QI problem at hand in order to answer the question: "What changes can we make that will result in improvement?" [9] Our goal was to have our results serve as the template for developing a quality intervention focused on increasing the proportion of low risk STEMI patients discharged within 72 h.

Our primary study was a qualitative analysis of discharge practices generated from semi-structured interviews with practitioners at Sunnybrook's Coronary Intensive Care Unit (CICU) and cardiology ward. [10] Qualitative data has previously been used to investigate processes of care in STEMI patients. Bradley and colleagues used qualitative methods to describe the characteristics of high performance hospitals in achieving optimal door to balloon times for primary PCI [11]. These investigators argued that qualitative data were essential for understanding variation in the complex clinical processes involved in providing primary PCI to a STEMI population. We believe that discharging STEMI patients from hospital represents a similar set of complex clinical processes and is well suited to a qualitative approach. We were interested in the clinical and system factors that influenced individual practitioner's discharging behaviour. We were particularly interested in understanding why a particular patient with a low risk Zwolle score (less than 3) might not be discharged early from hospital.

Qualitative data were generated using semi-structured interviews with practitioners involved in the front line care of STEMI patients. Interviews were structured around three fictional patient cases designed to illustrate a spectrum of risk according to the Zwolle score (see Additional file 1: Appendix 2 for list of cases). All study participants were asked to comment on the three clinical cases. Follow-up questions and discussion occurred around each case. The nature of the discussion around each clinical case was not scripted. Study participants were allowed to raise new themes and clinical scenarios related to STEMI care. A combination of convenience and purposive sampling was used to select interview participants [12, 13]. We attempted to include a representative sample of health care disciplines that are involved in the discharge process: attending physicians, medical and cardiology residents, and nursing staff involved in the discharge process (nurse practitioners and charge nurses). Staff were approached individually to participate. Given that this study was performed by a single investigator, it was not possible to approach all individuals at Sunnybrook Health Sciences centre who were involved in STEMI care.

Interviews were audio recorded and transcribed by a single investigator (JA). The same investigator carried out a thematic analysis of the data using a constant comparative approach to generate high-level themes. These themes or "codes" were used to analyze new data as they are required. As new data were analyzed, codes were adjusted and subcodes created [12, 13]. No major changes were made to the clinical cases of the semi-structured interviews during data collection and analysis. Themes were generated from the transcribed data with inductive reasoning. Data collection and analysis continued until no new themes are generated, at which point saturation was reached.

Results

Qualitative interviews were conducted with 17 practitioners connected with STEMI care at Sunnybrook. For a summary of disciplines represented, please see Table 1.

Thematic analysis of qualitative data

The themes generated from our qualitative data were organized into the following categories: patient factors, provider factors, and transitions to outpatient care (Table 2).

Patient factors

1. Medical Care

Most individuals interviewed discussed the specifics of providing medical care for patients post STEMI. Many practitioners expressed concern about not achieving maximal doses of medications in the post STEMI setting or the necessary diagnostic testing before sending a patient home. It was also acknowledged that a new medical diagnosis is occasionally uncovered post STEMI that requires an extended stay to investigate and treat.

Quotations

"...Depends when the echo [cardiogram] was done as well....If the echo wasn't done, then definitely not. I would wait for a formal echo. -Cardiology Resident

...so sometimes he's not as clean as you think he is... when the HbA1c comes back, you have to start him on a total new medical regimen -Nursing staff "

Table 1 Interview participants

Discipline	Number of participants
Attending physician	5
Medical residents	4
Cardiology residents	4
Nursing staff	4
Total	17

Table 2 Association between identified themes and category of interviewee

Theme	Category of participants who emphasized this theme
Medical Care	Attending physicians, residents
Post Myocardial Infarction Education	Nursing staff, residents
Post Myocardial Infarction Complications	Attending physicians, residents
Age/Functional Capacity	Attending physicians, nursing staff
Provider Factors (previous physician experience)	Attending physicians, nursing staff
Transitions to out patient care	Nursing staff, residents

2. Post MI Education

Many participants, especially the nursing staff and residents interviewed, emphasized the importance of post MI education. There was concern that reducing the length of stay in hospital may compromise the patient's understanding of their medical condition and compliance with medical and lifestyle therapy.

Quotations

"...how well do these patients know their meds and feel comfortable following it, is that preparation done well enough for that somewhat early discharge?...-Nursing Staff

To me if it is a patient that can be on top of his meds and everything and he gets his follow-up seriously...If he is a retired person who has no issues at home, I would say its fine (early discharge)- Nursing Staff"

3. Risk of Complications

It was widely acknowledged amongst the attending physicians and residents interviewed that the primary purpose for hospitalization after STEMI was for the detection and prompt treatment of complications. These complications could be related to the myocardial infarction or the subsequent treatment. When discussing stability for discharge, it was highlighted that lack of STEMI complications was a criteria for discharge. Larger infarctions generally made participants apprehensive about early discharge.

Quotations

"No clinical bleeding, no Right ventricular infarct, no mitral regurgitation, all the usual suspects that usually come with an inferior STEMI. And then no complications related to the PCI.- Attending Physician.

The one thing that I would want to know is how big his CK rise is. – Attending Physician
The only thing I would like to see would be his peak CK. Just to get an idea of how much muscle...In terms of his risk of mechanical complication afterwards.-Cardiology Resident"

The prevention of thromboembolic complications after STEMI garnered much discussion amongst the attending physicians ($n = 5$). The advent of dual antiplatelet therapy in post STEMI care has made the initiation and maintenance of anticoagulation in this setting a more nuanced and complicated process [3]. This primarily applies to patients at risk of left ventricular thrombus or a history of atrial fibrillation. While most study participants favoured anti-coagulation for prevention of LV thrombus and subsequent embolization after anterior infarction, there was significant variation in the enthusiasm for this intervention. Moreover, this was often cited as a reason to delay discharge in patients with anterior infarction. Kotowzcz et al. have demonstrated that patients started on anticoagulation have longer hospitalizations after STEMI [8]. According to the recent STEMI guidelines, anticoagulation with a vitamin K antagonist in patients with anteroapical akinesis or dyskinesis is a class IIb recommendation, indicating that evidence is uncertain and potentially harmful [3]. While there is no clear evidence of benefit in STEMI patients treated with PCI and modern antiplatelet agents, our qualitative data suggests the presence of significant practice variation when physicians are caring for patients with anterior infarctions.

Quotations

"Ant. STEMI (akinetic wall)...I would generally give them warfarin for the duration, although she is 88 years old. If it is an expanding akinetic apex, I would generally use triple therapy...-Attending Physician

She's not anti-coagulated. No, I wouldn't send her home today. She has an akinetic distal anterior wall and apex. She's on dual anti-platelet therapy. So her highest risk of embolization if she does develop a thrombus would be in the first week post MI, so I actually would have anticoagulated her and made sure she was actually stable on anticoagulation and not bleeding clinically. - Attending Physician
I would send her out on dual antiplatelet. If the CK rise was more than 2500 then I probably would end up getting an echo and then an echo a week after the

fact, just to make sure there is no suspected clot there. I'm assuming that it says here, grade 2 LV function, so I'm assuming that they did an echo at some point.... given that she is 88 years old (I prefer not to (anticoagulate).- Attending Physician
Do you anti-coagulate these guys? Grade 2 I don't. If its in the grade 3/4, then the contrast study can be very helpful if there is any clot there. If its grade 3 I'd prefer to not anticoagulate, grade 4 I would anticoagulate.- Attending Physician"

4. Age and functional capacity

Patient age played a role in participants' enthusiasm for early discharge. It was acknowledged that elderly patients were at higher risk for complications. Moreover, participants were concerned that some elements of post STEMI care, such as anticoagulation, were substantially more complicated in elderly patients. This often would increase the length of stay that participants would keep patients in hospital.

Quotations

"I would want to anticoagulate her and make sure she is not bleeding clinically, prior to assessing her falls risks. If she is a good 88 year old I would, if she is not a good 88 year old I wouldn't.- Attending Physicians
...they are 90 years old, they are not going to go out... most times, right?- Nursing Staff
There is no evidence of heart failure, but just given the fact that it is an anterior STEMI and she is 88.- Attending Physician
This one I'm holding because its anterior STEMI and old. - Attending Physician"

Provider factors
The influence of previous physician experience was discussed in a number of contexts by one of the attending physicians and members of the nursing staff. It was acknowledged that previous experience and personal beliefs play a significant role in clinical decision-making. As an example, a previous experience with a stroke complicating anterior myocardial infarction will make a physician more likely to recommend anticoagulation. Study participants hypothesized that older physicians may be more conservative in their discharging behaviour because of the era in which they trained and having witnessed a greater number of post discharge complications.

Quotations

"..the number of times that we have a post MI ventricular dysrythymia is pretty low, so I mean, my

tendency to keep them a little longer, I've seen more complications and I have started practicing in the era before primary angioplasty...people would keep infarcts in for a week.- Attending Physician
But it is all tempered by experience....when I was a medical student there was a patient at the counter of the nursing station being discharged after anterior infarct, and he had a big stroke in front of my eyes...I wish we had anti-coagulated that guy- Attending Physician
...or the physician, covering the ward...their preference, sometimes they feel comfortable that someone will stay an extra day, everyone is different- Nursing Staff "

Transitions to out-patient care

The ability to arrange timely support services for elderly patients with functional concerns was also discussed as a factor that would increase length of stay post STEMI. This issues was discussed primarily amongst the nursing staff interviewed. Practitioners, especially the nursing staff and residents, were concerned about the ability of to secure timely follow-up.

Quotations

"I think in this hospital a big issue is that we don't identify patients who may need help at home early enough, so we wait, wait...once a patient gets admitted, it should be identified this patient if they are going to go home, cannot live on its own...at least get social work or OT involved...our problems are that we wait, we wait, when you want to talk about it later, but that later...it causes at least 2–3 days...they is no guarantee there is a bed for this patient in rehab, there is not guarantee, so I think we really do poorly in that matter- Nursing Staff
...you're lucky to get follow-up in 6–8 weeks, its not 4 weeks any more.-Nursing staff
...maybe just one more day and then home. Because out there in the community they don't really change medications, so maybe we would want him on a higher target dose for his benefit.- Nursing Staff
I don't really expect them to have any follow-up for a month at least. The family doctors will not change anything. The next time it will be changed is when they see their cardiologist (whenever that is)-Internal Medicine Resident"

Discussion

This project was a locally based quality improvement initiative to understand the root causes of prolonged lengths of stay for post STEMI patients at a single tertiary care STEMI centre. Qualitative analysis was performed on interviews with 17 front line staff involved in STEMI care at Sunnybrook. Various themes were identified that influence a patient's length of stay and were organized into the following categories: patient factors, provider factors and transitions to outpatient care. Importantly, the majority of these themes identified issues that were not components of the Zwolle risk score used to identify potential patients for early discharge.

Despite published data supporting the safety of early discharge, the real world application of this strategy remains a challenge [8]. The goal of our qualitative analysis was to provide new insights into the discharge process of STEMI patients that will inform the development of further interventions to reduce length of stay and improve overall quality of care. Our data indicates that the reasons for increased length of stay are not likely a result of a knowledge gap regarding which patients are low risk after STEMI. While the Zwolle score may be effective at identifying patients at low risk of death, the score does not address many of the common concerns and clinical dilemmas faced by practitioners at the time of discharge. These concerns include the availability of adequate follow-up, medication compliance, and the safety of anti-coagulation in contemporary STEMI patients treated with PCI. Amongst practitioners at Sunnybrook, there was a general awareness of the impact of advanced age and frailty on the feasibility of early discharge. It was apparent that a low risk Zwolle score alone in these patients did not give practitioners enough re-assurance to aggressively pursue early discharge. Previous physician experience and personal experience with complications played a significant role in their discharging decisions. We infer from these observations that calculated risk scores alone may be insufficient to trump the powerful effect of witnessing a prior complication. Our research adds to the field by highlighting the potential shortcomings of using a risk score in isolation to promote practice change. Indeed our data suggest that in order for a risk score to be useful, it must address the factors that drive a practitioner's clinical decision. These findings suggest that work such as ours should be done, prior to the development of a risk score using traditional statistical methods.

We propose that systems of care be developed that address the clinical issues raised by our qualitative data. Concerns about medication adherence, patient education and length of time from discharge to follow-up may be mitigated by early visits to dedicated STEMI clinics. While potentially resource intensive, this approach may prove less costly than extra days in hospital. Improved systems of communication with primary care physicians, electronically or via telephone, should be trialed and evaluated. Targeted educational interventions focused on common clinical dilemmas in STEMI patients, such as anti-coagulation, may also be of benefit. Prompt referral to allied health practitioners may allow elderly patients to be discharged home with available supports. Each of these interventions could be evaluated in separate quality improvement initiatives.

Our work must be interpreted in the context of a number of limitations. First, ours was a single tertiary care center in Ontario, Canada. As such, the specific barriers we identified may not be generalizable to other practice locations. Second, we focused on a relatively narrow clinical area, that of discharge planning post reperfusion for acute STEMI patients. We feel however that the general principals identified by our work are broadly applicable.

Conclusions

This study was a quality improvement initiative designed to evaluate the prevalence and root causes of increased length of stay in STEMI patients. We identified patient factors, provider factors and factors related to transitions to outpatient care that influenced decisions regarding discharge. In particular, our data suggest that concerns about medication compliance, the adequacy of patient education and advanced patient age may make practitioners less likely to pursue early discharge. Future protocol based interventions to reduce length of stay post STEMI should focus on in-patient and out-patient strategies to address these unique clinical issues.

Competing interest
The authors declare they have no competing interests.

Author's contribution
JA – conception and design of study, acquired and analyzed data, interpreted results, drafted the manuscript and gave final approval of the version to be published. BW – interpreted the idea, revised the manuscript for important intellectual content and gave final approval of the version to be published. HW - conception and design of study, interpreted results, drafted the manuscript and gave final approval of the version to be published.

Authors' information
Not applicable.

Acknowledgment
Dr. Wijeysundera is supported by a Distinguished Clinician Scientist Award from the Heart and Stroke Foundation of Canada.

Author details
[1]Division of Cardiology, Schulich Heart Centre, Sunnybrook Health Sciences Centre, 2075 Bayview Avenue, Suite A202, Toronto, ON M4N3M5, Canada. [2]Department of Medicine, Sunnybrook Health Sciences Centre, University of Toronto, Toronto, ON, Canada. [3]Centre for Quality Improvement and Patient Safety, University of Toronto, Toronto, ON, Canada. [4]Institute of Health Policy, Management and Evaluation, University of Toronto, Toronto, ON, Canada. [5]Institute for Clinical Evaluative Sciences (ICES), Toronto, ON, Canada. [6]Li Ka Shing Knowledge Institute of St. Michael Hospital, University of Toronto, Toronto, ON, Canada.

References
1. Yeung DF, Boom NK, Guo H, Lee DS, Schultz SE, Tu JV. Trends in the incidence and outcomes of heart failure in Ontario, Canada: 1997 to 2007. CMAJ. 2012;184(14):E765–73.
2. Lloyd-Jones D, Adams R, Carnethon M, De Simone G, Ferguson TB, Flegal K, et al. Heart disease and stroke statistics–2009 update: a report from the American Heart Association Statistics Committee and Stroke Statistics Subcommittee. Circulation. 2009;119(3):480–6.
3. O'Gara PT, Kushner FG, Ascheim DD, Casey DE, Jr., Chung MK, de Lemos JA, et al. ACCF/AHA guideline for the management of ST-elevation myocardial infarction: executive summary: a report of the American College of Cardiology Foundation/American Heart Association Task Force on Practice Guidelines. Circulation. 2013;127(4):529–55.
4. Topol EJ, Burek K, O'Neill WW, Kewman DG, Kander NH, Shea MJ, et al. A randomized controlled trial of hospital discharge three days after myocardial infarction in the era of reperfusion. N Engl J Med. 1988;318(17):1083–8.
5. De Luca G, Suryapranata H, van 't Hof AW, de Boer MJ, Hoorntje JC, Dambrink JH, et al. Prognostic assessment of patients with acute myocardial infarction treated with primary angioplasty: implications for early discharge. Circulation. 2004;109(22):2737–43.
6. Newby LK, Eisenstein EL, Califf RM, Thompson TD, Nelson CL, Peterson ED, et al. Cost effectiveness of early discharge after uncomplicated acute myocardial infarction. N Engl J Med. 2000;342(11):749–55.
7. Grines CL, Marsalese DL, Brodie B, Griffin J, Donohue B, Costantini CR, et al. Safety and cost-effectiveness of early discharge after primary angioplasty in low risk patients with acute myocardial infarction. PAMI-II Investigators. Primary Angioplasty in Myocardial Infarction. J Am Coll Cardiol. 1998;31(5):967–72.
8. Kotowycz MA, Syal RP, Afzal R, Natarajan MK. Can we improve length of hospitalization in ST elevation myocardial infarction patients treated with primary percutaneous coronary intervention? Can J Cardiol. 2009;25(10):585–8.
9. Berwick DM. A primer on leading the improvement of systems. BMJ. 1996;312(7031):619–22.
10. Ring N, Jepson R, Hoskins G, Wilson C, Pinnock H, Sheikh A, et al. Understanding what helps or hinders asthma action plan use: a systematic review and synthesis of the qualitative literature. Patient Educ Couns. 2011;85(2):e131–43.
11. Bradley EH, Curry LA, Webster TR, Mattera JA, Roumanis SA, Radford MJ, et al. Achieving rapid door-to-balloon times: how top hospitals improve complex clinical systems. Circulation. 2006;113(8):1079–85.
12. Pope C, Mays N. Reaching the parts other methods cannot reach: an introduction to qualitative methods in health and health services research. BMJ. 1995;311(6996):42–5.
13. Creswell J. Research Design: Qualitative, Quantitative, and Mixed Methods Approaches. Thousand Oaks, California: Sage Publications; 2009. p. 145–73.

4

Rapid predictors for the occurrence of reduced left ventricular ejection fraction between LAD and non-LAD related ST-elevation myocardial infarction

Zhang-Wei Chen[1†], Zi-Qing Yu[1†], Hong-Bo Yang[1], Ying-Hua Chen[2], Ju-Ying Qian[1*], Xian-Hong Shu[1] and Jun-Bo Ge[1*]

Abstract

Backgrounds: Reduced left ventricular ejection fraction (LVEF) after acute myocardial infarction (AMI), which implies the occurrence of cardiac dysfunction, impacts cardiac prognosis, even after primary percutaneous coronary intervention (PCI). This study was designed to clarify the difference of clinical and angiographic predictors for reduced LVEF in ST-elevation myocardial infarction (STEMI) patients with left anterior descending artery (LAD) or non-LAD vessel as culprit artery.

Methods: This was a retrospective study to review a total of 553 patients of STEMI underwent primary PCI in our hospital. All patients underwent echocardiography. Univariate analysis, multivariate analysis and classification and regression tree (CART) were performed between LAD related AMI and non-LAD related STEMI. The primary outcome was the occurrence of reduced LVEF 4–6 days after PCI.

Results: In this study, culprit arteries of STEMI were 315 in LAD system (6 in left main artery, 309 in LAD) and 238 in non-LAD system (63 in left circumflex and 175 in right coronary artery). Compared with non-LAD group, post-MI LVEF was significantly reduced in LAD related STEMI group (52.4 ± 9.3 % vs. 57.1 ± 7.8 %, $P < 0.01$). Multivariate analysis indicated that elder (>65 years), time to hospital and proximal occlusion were associated with reduced LVEF (<55 %) in LAD related STEMI patients. However, in non-LAD patients, time to hospital, multivessel stenosis and post-PCI blood pressure predicted the occurrence of reduced LVEF. Furthermore, CART analysis also obtained similar findings.

Conclusions: Patients with LAD or non-LAD related STEMI could suffer reduced LVEF, while the clinical and angiographic predictors for the occurrence were different.

Keywords: ST-elevation myocardial infarction, Left ventricular ejection fraction, Primary percutaneous coronary intervention, Predictors

* Correspondence: Qian.juying@zs-hospital.sh.cn; Ge.junbo@hotmail.com
†Equal contributors
[1]Department of Cardiology, Shanghai Institute of Cardiovascular Diseases, Zhongshan Hospital, Fudan University, 180 Fenglin Road, Shanghai 200032, PR China
Full list of author information is available at the end of the article

Rapid predictors for the occurrence of reduced left ventricular ejection fraction between LAD...

23

Background

Reduced left ventricular ejection fraction (LVEF), which is significantly associated with cardiac dysfunction, occurs approximately in 30–40 % of patients who suffer ST-elevation myocardial infarction (STEMI). Although the incidence of reduced LVEF after STEMI declined significantly [1] because of great advancement in the treatment of anti-thrombotic therapy and primary percutaneous coronary intervention (PCI), it is still one of most critical complications after STEMI that carries a poor cardiac prognosis [2–7]. Reduced LVEF, which is common in STEMI patients with left main artery (LM) or left anterior descending artery (LAD) as culprit vessel. The occurrence was related to older ages, hypertension, diabetes [1], time to reperfusion [8], and higher prevalence of proximal occlusion [9]. The extent of acute myocardial damage in LAD occlusion is markedly larger than that in either left circumflex (LCX) or right coronary artery (RCA) occlusion. However, it has been also reported that reduced LVEF or cardiac dysfunction occurred in STEMI patients with RCA or LCX as culprit vessel [10, 11]. However, it was unclear whether there were predictors difference for reduced LVEF between LAD-related and non-LAD-related STEMI.

Given to the impact of new-onset cardiac dysfunction after STEMI on the cardiac prognosis, it is important to investigate the difference of clinical and angiographic predictors for reduced LVEF in STEMI patients with different culprit vessels. These findings will provide rapid prediction and beneficial effects on the early prevention of cardiac dysfunction after STEMI.

Methods

Study population

This was a retrospective clinical study to review the patients of acute STEMI underwent primary PCI ($n = 664$) in our hospital from Jul 2011 to Oct 2013. Baseline 12-lead electrocardiograms were performed at admission. A total of 553 patients were included in this study, while 111 patients were excluded according to follow exclusion criteria. The inclusion criteria were: (1) patients with 18 to 85 years of age; (2) diagnosed as acute STEMI; (3) underwent primary coronary intervention within 12 h after chest pain on-set. The exclusion criteria were as follows: (1) incomplete clinical history record ($n = 23$); (2) excluded the diagnosis of myocardial infarction by angiography, such as viral myocarditis, pericarditis or cardiomyopathy ($n = 26$); (3) not finish the detection of echocardiography in-hospitalization because of any reason ($n = 17$); (4) confirmed clinical heart failure before this admission, complicated with cardiomyopathy, congenital heart diseases and rheumatic heart disease ($n = 19$); (5) active chronic inflammation ($n = 14$); (6) dysfunction of hematological and immunological

system ($n = 4$); (7) carcinoma or a condition treated with immunosuppressive agents ($n = 8$). This study and consent procedure were approved by our local ethics committee (Ethics Committee of Zhongshan Hospital affiliated to Fudan University), and were carried out in accordance with the principles of the Declaration of Helsinki. Consent for publication of these data was obtained from each patient when they were admitted in our hospital.

Several important clinical variables were record, such as age, gender, hypertension, diabetes, stable angina history, Time to hospital (from chest pain on-set to diagnosis) and D-to-B time (door to balloon).

Primary percutaneous coronary intervention

Prior to primary PCI, all patients received adequate loading doses of aspirin (300 mg) and clopidogrel (300 mg) or ticagrelor (180 mg) immediately after diagnosed as STEMI. Procedure of PCI was performed immediately via the femoral or radial access route. The characteristics of coronary angiography were record, such as culprit artery, acute occlusive segment and multi-vessel disease (defined as having at least another vessel with 75 % or greater stenosis except the culprit occlusion artery, such as culprit vessel in LAD had LCX or RCA or LM stenosis, culprit vessel in LCX had RCA or LAD or LM stenosis, culprit vessel in RCA had LCX or LAD or LM stenosis). A lesion was considered proximal if it was located proximal to the first diagonal branch in the LAD, the first obtuse marginal branch in LCX, or the first acute marginal branch in RCA [12].

The usages of interventional techniques, thrombus aspiration and platelet glycoprotein IIb/IIIa receptor inhibitor were chosen at the operators' discretion. The phenomenon of no reflow or slow flow post-stenting was record. Post-PCI blood pressure, including systolic blood pressure (SBP) and diastolic blood pressure (DBP), was detected by invasive blood pressure monitor from radial or femoral vascular sheaths.

Echocardiography

Echocardiography was performed before discharge (4–6 days post-PCI) in all patients using a Philips IE33 instrument (Philips, Netherlands) with a 2–3.5 MHz transducer (X3-1), while left ventricular ejection fraction (LVEF) were detected by Simpson method. It was defined as reduced LVEF while LVEF less than 55 %. All exams were performed by one of three echocardiography operators. These three operators underwent standardized training before this study. Observers who detected LVEF were blinded to the results of coronary angiography and clinical record. The incidence of reduced LVEF after STEMI was compared between two different culprit artery systems, including LAD related STEMI

(LM occlusion and LAD occlusion, $n = 315$) and non-LAD related STEMI (LCX occlusion, $n = 63$; RCA occlusion, $n = 175$).

Statistical Analysis

All statistical analyses were performed with SPSS software 19.0. Data were presented as the percentage or mean ± standard deviation (SD). Chi-square analysis was used to compare the frequency for categorical variables, and Student's t or correction t tests were used to compare means for continuous variables. Multivariable logistic analysis was performed to identify the independent risk factors for reduced LVEF (LVEF < 55 %). Stratification according to different risk subsets was also made by classification and regression tree (CART) analysis. All P-values were two-sided, and $P < 0.05$ was considered to indicate statistical significance.

Results

Clinical and angiographic characteristics

A total of 553 STEMI patients enrolled with average age $64.0 ± 12.0$ years. There were 447 men (80.8 %) and 106 women (19.2 %). The prevalence of hypertension and diabetes were 60.4 % (334 patients) and 48.8 % (270 patients), respectively. Culprit arteries of STEMI were 6 in LM, 309 in LAD, 63 in LCX and 175 in RCA, respectively. Baseline clinical and angiographic characteristics of patients with different culprit arteries were shown in Table 1. Compared with the non-LAD related STEMI (culprit arteries were RCA and LCX), patients of LAD related STEMI (culprit arteries were LM and LAD) had lower LVEF ($52.4 ± 9.3$ % vs. $57.1 ± 7.8$ %, $P < 0.01$) and higher incidence of reduced LVEF (LVEF < 55 %: 53.7 and 26.9 %, $P < 0.01$).

Reduced LVEF and predictor analysis

In order to clarify the predictor difference for reduced LVEF in LAD system and non-LAD system groups, several clinical and angiographic predictors were analyzed by univariate analysis, shown in Table 1 and Fig. 1. It was demonstrated that elder (more than 65 years), time to hospital (from chest pain on-set to diagnosis), acute occlusion in proximal segment and post-PCI blood pressure significantly increased the risk of reduced in LAD system. However, in non-LAD related STEMI patients, beside the factors of age and time to hospital,

Table 1 Comparison of clinical and angiographic characteristics among STEMI patients with different culprit vessel

	LAD system ($n = 315$)			Non-LAD system ($n = 238$)		
	EF < 55 % $n = 169$	EF ≥ 55 % $n = 146$	P	EF < 55 % $n = 64$	EF ≥ 55 % $n = 174$	P
(1) Clinical characteristics						
Male (%)	133 (78.7 %)	121 (82.9 %)	0.349	54 (84.4 %)	139 (79.9 %)	0.433
Age (years)	65.4 ± 11.4	60.7 ± 12.7	<0.01	67.4 ± 11.9	63.9 ± 11.3	0.034
Hypertension (%)	98 (58.7 %)	82 (56.6 %)	0.704	40 (62.5 %)	114 (65.9 %)	0.627
Diabetes (%)	94 (55.6 %)	68 (46.6 %)	0.098	29 (45.3 %)	79 (45.7 %)	0.961
Stable angina history (%)	58 (34.3)	59 (40.4 %)	0.265	25 (39.1 %)	62 (35.6 %)	0.626
Time to hospital (hours)	6.0 ± 2.5	5.3 ± 2.7	<0.01	6.6 ± 2.7	5.3 ± 2.4	<0.01
D-to-B time (minutes)	76.2 ± 27.4	74.6 ± 25.6	0.675	71.2 ± 21.3	74.3 ± 22.7	0.304
(2) Angiographic characteristics						
Number of disease vessels	1.8 ± 0.8	1.6 ± 0.8	0.197	2.2 ± 0.8	1.9 ± 0.8	0.061
Multi-vessel stenosis (%)	94 (55.6 %)	66 (45.2 %)	0.065	47 (73.4 %)	100 (57.5 %)	0.025
–two vessels disease (including culprit vessel)	56	35		19	51	
–three vessels disease (including culprit vessel)	38	31		28	49	
–LAD AMI complicated with LCX stenosis	64	46		–	–	
–LAD AMI complicated with RCA stenosis	68	51		–	–	
–non-LAD AMI complicated with LAD stenosis	–	–		24	48	
Occlusion in proximal segment (%)	101 (59.8 %)	70 (47.9 %)	0.036	21 (32.8 %)	57 (32.8)	0.994
Slow or no reflow (%)	34 (20.1 %)	26 (17.8 %)	0.603	12 (18.8 %)	20 (11.5 %)	0.146
Post-PCI SBP (mmHg)	114.5 ± 16.8	119.2 ± 16.7	0.014	110.7 ± 18.7	113.1 ± 16.5	0.368
Post-PCI DBP (mmHg)	70.7 ± 9.1	72.9 ± 7.7	0.027	68.5 ± 11.0	70.9 ± 9.0	0.123

LAD system STEMI in left main or left main artery or left anterior descending artery; Non-LAD system STEMI in left circumflex or right coronary artery;
DBP diastolic blood pressure; D-to-B door to balloon; SBP systolic blood pressure;
STEMI ST-Elevation Myocardial Infarction; Time to hospital: from chest pain on-set to diagnosis;

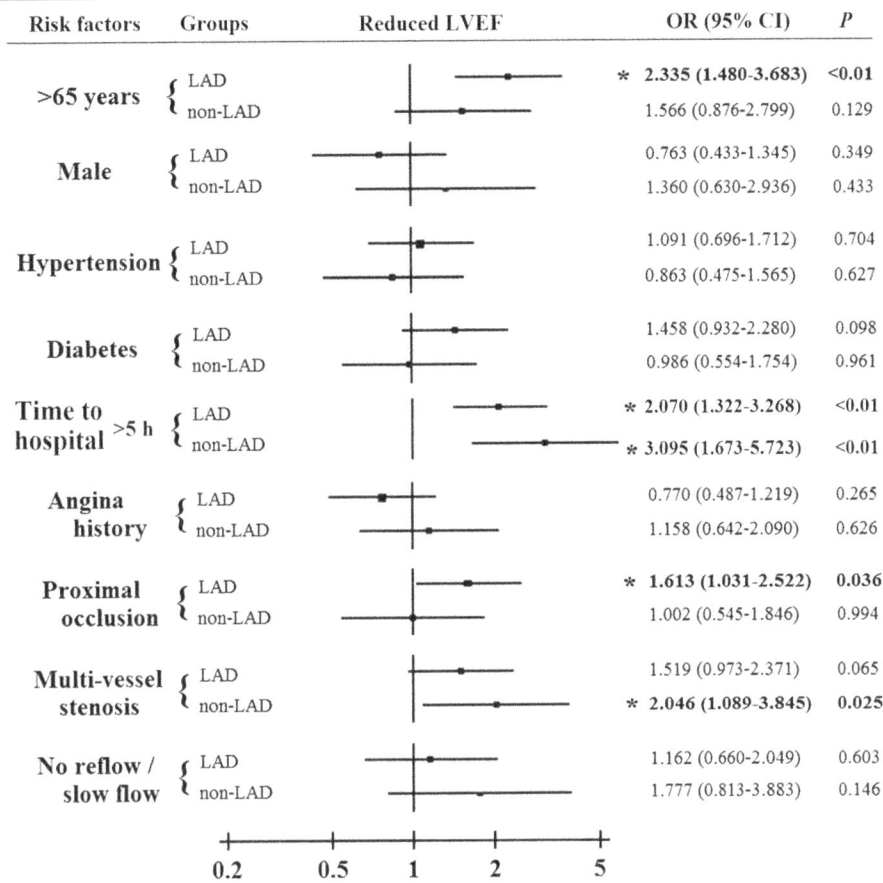

Risk factors	Groups	Reduced LVEF	OR (95% CI)	P
>65 years	LAD		* 2.335 (1.480-3.683)	<0.01
	non-LAD		1.566 (0.876-2.799)	0.129
Male	LAD		0.763 (0.433-1.345)	0.349
	non-LAD		1.360 (0.630-2.936)	0.433
Hypertension	LAD		1.091 (0.696-1.712)	0.704
	non-LAD		0.863 (0.475-1.565)	0.627
Diabetes	LAD		1.458 (0.932-2.280)	0.098
	non-LAD		0.986 (0.554-1.754)	0.961
Time to hospital >5 h	LAD		* 2.070 (1.322-3.268)	<0.01
	non-LAD		* 3.095 (1.673-5.723)	<0.01
Angina history	LAD		0.770 (0.487-1.219)	0.265
	non-LAD		1.158 (0.642-2.090)	0.626
Proximal occlusion	LAD		* 1.613 (1.031-2.522)	0.036
	non-LAD		1.002 (0.545-1.846)	0.994
Multi-vessel stenosis	LAD		1.519 (0.973-2.371)	0.065
	non-LAD		* 2.046 (1.089-3.845)	0.025
No reflow / slow flow	LAD		1.162 (0.660-2.049)	0.603
	non-LAD		1.777 (0.813-3.883)	0.146

0.2 0.5 1 2 5

Fig. 1 Subgroups analysis of clinical and angiographic factors for the increasing risk of reduced LVEF (LVEF < 55 %) in LAD and non-LAD related STEMI groups

multivessel stenosis significantly increased the risk of reduced LVEF. In order to further clarify the influence of post-PCI blood pressure, the occurrence of reduced LVEF was analyzed among four groups classified by the quartile of post-PCI blood pressure in patients with LAD system or non-LAD system STEMI, shown in Fig. 2. We found that lower SBP and DBP after primary PCI predicted the higher risk of reduced LVEF.

Multivariate analysis

Multivariate logistic analysis was performed to demonstrate the independent effect of these predictors (confirmed statistic difference in univariate analysis) on the occurrence of reduced LVEF after STEMI, In this analysis, reduced LVEF (LVEF < 55 %) was employed as a dependent variable in both LAD and non-LAD system subgroups, while age > 65 years, multi-vessel stenosis, acute occlusion in proximal segment, time to hospital, post-PCI SBP <100 mmHg and post DBP <65 mmHg were set as independent variables, shown in Table 2. These results demonstrated that elder (OR = 1.984, 95 % CI = 1.205–3.266, P < 0.01), proximal occlusion (OR = 1.681, 95 % CI = 1.042–2.713, P = 0.033) and time to

hospital (OR = 1.106, 95 % CI = 1.010–1.210, P = 0.029) were major independent predictors for reduced LVEF in LAD system, while time to hospital (OR = 1.246, 95 % CI = 1.097–1.414, P < 0.01), multi-vessel stenosis (OR = 2.394, 95 % CI = 1.185–4.836, P = 0.015) and post-PCI SBP < 100 mmHg (OR = 2.927, 95 % CI = 1.052121–7.643, P = 0.028) in non-LAD system.

CART analysis

In order to confirm the impact of predictors on reduced LVEF and simply the prediction process, CART analysis was also applied to assess the incidence of reduced LVEF after STEMI in multivariate subgroups. Reduced LVEF was employed as a dependent variable, while age > 65 years, male gender, stable angina history, diabetes, hypertension, culprit vessel (LAD system or non-LAD system), time to hospital >5 h, multi-vessel stenosis, occlusion in proximal segment, slow or no reflow, post-PCI SBP <100 mmHg and post DBP < 65 mmHg were set as independent variables. CART analysis results were shown in Fig. 3. We found that LAD system was the major determinant of reduced LVEF after STEMI. Beside culprit artery, elder, time to hospital > 5 h and proximal

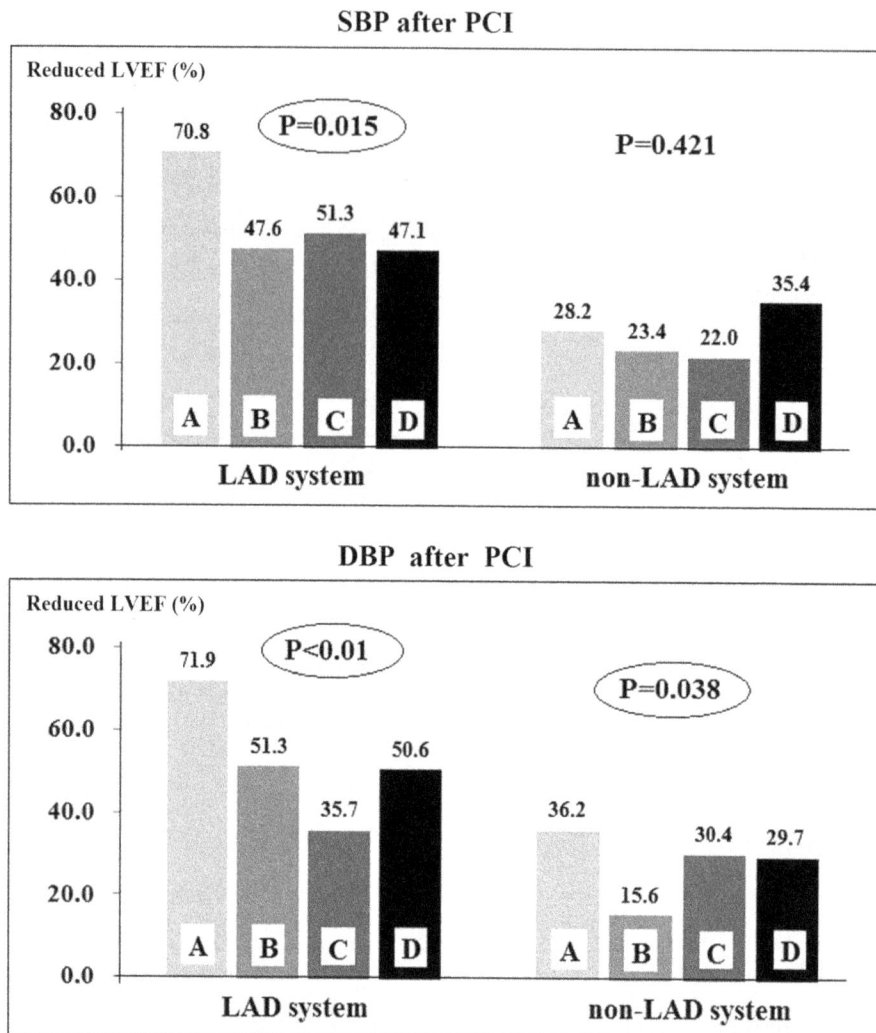

Fig. 2 LAD system: STEMI in left main or left main artery or left anterior descending artery; Non-LAD system: STEMI in left circumflex or right coronary artery; DBP: diastolic blood pressure; SBP: systolic blood pressure; Groups A to D indicated four groups classified by the quartile of post-PCI blood pressure SBP: group A: <102mmHg; Group B: 103-110mmHg; Group C: 111-120mmHg; Group D: >120mmHg DBP: group A: <65mmHg; Group B: 66-70mmHg; Group C: 71-78mmHg; Group D: >79mmHg. The incidence of reduced LVEF in different post-PCI blood pressure subgroups

occlusion were most critical three steps in risk stratification for reduced LVEF in LAD system, while time to hospital and post-PCI diastolic blood pressure < 60 mmHg in non-LAD system.

Discussion

Acute myocardial infarction (AMI), which is mostly caused by coronary plaque rupture or erosion, could result in several clinical complications and impact cardiac prognosis [4, 13]. Reduce LVEF or cardiac dysfunction occurs approximately in 30–40 % of patients who suffer STEMI, and the mortality of patients with post-MI cardiac dysfunction is 20 to 30 % [7]. As we know, reduced LVEF was common in STEMI patients with LM or LAD as culprit vessel. It has also been reported that reduced LVEF could occurred in patients with RCA or

LCX as culprit vessel [10, 11, 14]. However, there were few studies focused on the risk factors or clinical predictors for reduced LVEF caused by RCA or LCX-related MI. Furthermore, it was unclear whether there were different clinical and angiographic characteristics between LAD and non-LAD-related STEMI with reduced LVEF.

In this study, we confirmed the occurrence of reduced LVEF (LVEF < 55 %) in non-LAD related MI patients, although this prevalence was lower than that in LAD related MI group (26.9 vs. 53.7 %, $P < 0.01$). In order to clarify the difference of predictors between these two different culprit vessels, sub-group analyses and multivariate logistic analysis were also performed. We found that elder age, Time to hospital and proximal occlusion were critical for reduced LVEF in LAD related STEMI, while multi-vessel stenosis, Time to hospital

Table 2 Odds ratios of independent predictors for reduced LVEF after STEMI in LAD and non-LAD system (multivariate logistic analysis)

Predictors	OR	95 % confidence intervals	P
LAD system			
Elder (>65 years)	1.984	1.205–3.266	<0.01
Proximal occlusion	1.681	1.042–2.713	0.033
Time to hospital	1.106	1.010–1.210	0.029
Multi-vessel stenosis	1.395	0.848–2.296	0.190
Post-PCI SBP < 100 mmHg	1.563	0.540–4.521	0.410
Post-PCI DBP < 60 mmHg	1.677	0.778–3.613	0.187
Non-LAD system			
Elder (>65 years)	1.167	0.616–2.209	0.635
Proximal occlusion	1.108	0.569–2.159	0.762
Time to hospital	1.246	1.097–1.414	<0.01
Multi-vessel stenosis	2.394	1.185–4.836	0.015
Post-PCI SBP < 100 mmHg	2.927	1.121–7.643	0.028
Post-PCI DBP < 60 mmHg	1.778	0.792–3.988	0.163

LAD system STEMI in left main or left main artery or left anterior descending artery;
Non-LAD system STEMI in left circumflex or right coronary artery;
DBP diastolic blood pressure; *SBP* systolic blood pressure;
STEMI ST-Elevation Myocardial Infarction;
Time to hospital: from chest pain on-set to diagnosis

and post-PCI blood pressure contributed most to reduce LVEF in non-LAD related STEMI.

De Luca G reported [15] that elderly patients complicated with higher incidence of hypertension and diabetes, more advanced Killip class at presentation, longer time to treatment, higher prevalence of distal embolization and significantly impaired myocardial perfusion, which resulted in

worse coronary microcirculation and higher mortality after STEMI [16], even undergoing primary angioplasty. Previously, few studies reported the different impact of older age on cardiac dysfunction between LAD and non-LAD related STEMI. In the LAD related MI, significantly impaired microcirculation and proximal occlusion directly resulted in more severe ischemia and large area of infarction, which

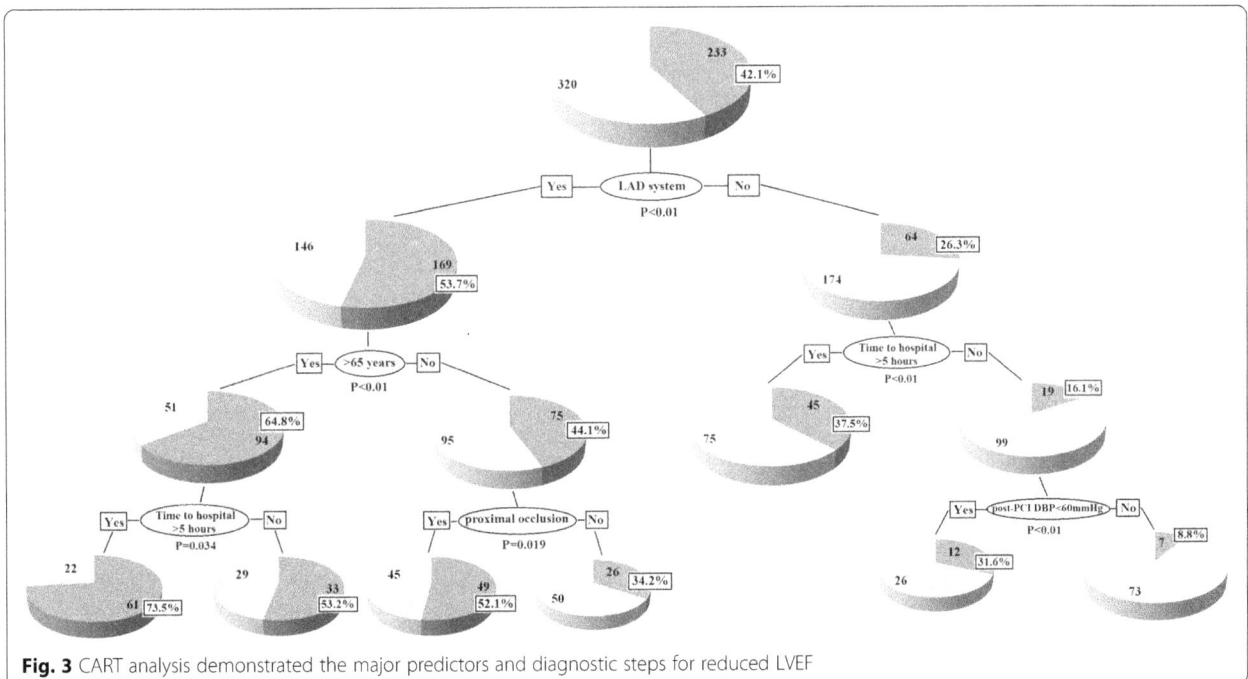

Fig. 3 CART analysis demonstrated the major predictors and diagnostic steps for reduced LVEF

exacerbated left ventricular systolic dysfunction. However, on the contrary, the extent of myocardial perfusion injury in non-LAD vessels contributes less to the left ventricular systolic function. In the non-LAD related MI, multivessel stenosis, which contained LAD stenosis, was more important for left ventricular function.

Hypertension has also been one of well-established factors for increasing risk of cardiovascular diseases, such as acute myocardial infarction and heart failure [17]. Meanwhile, low admission blood pressure in MI patients has been suggested as a predictor for cardiac mortality [18]. However, it was unclear about the predictive value of post-PCI blood pressure on the risk of reduced LVEF between different culprit arteries. In our study, we found that lower post-PCI systolic (<100 mmHg) or diastolic (<60 mmHg) blood pressure indicated the higher incidence of reduced LVEF (Fig. 2). After adjusted by other factors, post-PCI systolic blood pressure was also independently associated with cardiac dysfunction in non-LAD related MI.

As we know, reperfusion time to STEMI is one of the most important factors for short- and long-term cardiac prognosis [19]. In our study, there was no significant difference of D-to-B time between cardiac dysfunction and preserved function groups. However, time from chest pain on-set to diagnosis, defined as Time to hospital, was quite different between these two groups. As demonstrated in multivariable analysis, STEMI patients with Time to hospital more than 5 h had less LVEF no matter in LAD or non-LAD related STEMI groups, which could be resulted in more injured cardiomyocytes and higher risk of cardiac complications. CART analysis, which was analyzed based different risk factors' subgroups, indicated rapid prediction for the occurrence of reduced LVEF.

We should note some of our study's limitations. First, the number of included patients was small size. Second, its retrospective nature limited its potency to clarify the cause relation between predictions and reduced LVEF. Third, the inclusion of LVEF in this study was only short-term data, therefore, long-term data will be needed to document the association between predictors and post-PCI LVEF. These limitations will be taken into account in our further clinical researches and prospective studies.

Conclusions

Patients with LAD or non-LAD related STEMI could suffer reduced LVEF, while the clinical and angiographic predictors for the occurrence were quite different.

Abbreviations

AMI: Acute myocardial infarction; CAD: Coronary artery disease; CART: Classification and regression tree; LAD: Left anterior descending artery; LCX: Left circumflex; LVEF: Left ventricular ejection fraction; PCI: Percutaneous

coronary intervention; RCA: Right coronary artery; STEMI: ST-elevation myocardial infarction.

Competing interests

There are no conflicts of interest pertained to this submission.

Authors' contributions

Z-WC participated in conception and design, acquisition of data and drafting the manuscript; Z-qY took part in acquisition of data and analysis of data; H-BY carried out acquisition of data and statistical analysis; Y-HC took part in acquisition of data; J-YQ participated in design, have given final approval of the version to be published; X-HS took part in interpretation of data; J-BG carried out design, have given final approval of the version to be published. All authors read and approved the final manuscript.

Acknowledgement

This study was supported by the National Natural Science Foundation of China (Grant No: 81200146, 81570314 and 81370322), Zhongshan hospital Youth Science Funding (Grant No: 2012ZSQN12), New Teacher Foundation of Ministry of Education (Grant No: 20120071120061), Scientific research for Young teacher of Fudan University (Grant No: 20520133477), Grant of Shanghai municipal commission of health and family planning (Grant No: XBR2013071, 15XD1501100, 20134001 and 20144Y0240) and Grant of Shanghai Pudong New District of health and family planning (Grant No: PW2014A-13).

Author details

[1]Department of Cardiology, Shanghai Institute of Cardiovascular Diseases, Zhongshan Hospital, Fudan University, 180 Fenglin Road, Shanghai 200032, PR China. [2]Department of Endocrinology Medicine, East Hospital, Tongji University School of Medicine, Shanghai 200120, China.

References

1. Hung J, Teng TH, Finn J, Knuiman M, Briffa T, Stewart S, et al. Trends from 1996 to 2007 in incidence and mortality outcomes of heart failure after acute myocardial infarction: a population-based study of 20,812 patients with first acute myocardial infarction in Western Australia. J Am Heart Assoc. 2013 Oct 8;2(5):e000172.
2. Thomas KL, Velazquez EJ. Therapies to prevent heart failure post-myocardial infarction. Curr Heart Fail Rep. 2005;2(4):174–82.
3. Zaret BL, Wackers FJ, Terrin ML, Forman SA, Williams DO, Knatterud GL, et al. Value of radionuclide rest and exercise left ventricular ejection fraction in assessing survival of patients after thrombolytic therapy for acute myocardial infarction: results of Thrombolysis in Myocardial Infarction (TIMI) phase II study. The TIMI Study Group. J Am Coll Cardiol. 1995;26:73–9.
4. Møller JE, Egstrup K, Køber L, Poulsen SH, Nyvad O, Torp-Pedersen C. Prognostic importance of systolic and diastolic function after acute myocardial infarction. Am Heart J. 2003;145:147–53.
5. van der Vleuten PA, Rasoul S, Huurnink W, van der Horst IC, Slart RH, Reiffers S, et al. The importance of left ventricular function for long-term outcome after primary percutaneous coronary intervention. BMC Cardiovasc Disord. 2008;8:4.
6. Ng VG, Lansky AJ, Meller S, Witzenbichler B, Guagliumi G, Peruga JZ, et al. The prognostic importance of left ventricular function in patients with ST-segment elevation myocardial infarction: the HORIZONS-AMI trial. Eur Heart J Acute Cardiovasc Care. 2014 Mar;3(1):67–77.
7. Campo G, Saia F, Guastaroba P, Marchesini J, Varani E, Manari A, et al. Prognostic impact of hospital readmissions after primary percutaneous coronary intervention. Arch Intern Med. 2011;171:1948–9.
8. Goel K, Pinto DS, Gibson CM. Association of time to reperfusion with left ventricular function and heart failure in patients with acute myocardial infarction treated with primary percutaneous coronary intervention: a systematic review. Am Heart J. 2013;165(4):451–67.
9. Karha J, Murphy SA, Kirtane AJ, de Lemos JA, Aroesty JM, Cannon CP, et al. Evaluation of the association of proximal coronary culprit artery lesion location with clinical outcomes in acute myocardial infarction. Am J Cardiol. 2003 Oct 15;92(8):913–8.
10. Sohrabi B, Separham A, Madadi R, Toufan M, Mohammadi N, Aslanabadi N, et al. Difference between Outcome of Left Circumflex Artery and Right

Coronary Artery Related Acute Inferior Wall Myocardial Infarction in Patients Undergoing Adjunctive Angioplasty after Fibrinolysis. J Cardiovasc Thorac Res. 2014;6(2):101–4.

11. Rasoul S, de Boer MJ, Suryapranata H, Hoorntje JC, Gosselink AT, Zijlstra F, et al. Circumflex artery-related acute myocardial infarction: limited ECG abnormalities but poor outcome. Neth Heart J. 2007;15(9):286–90.

12. Gibson CM, Ryan K, Sparano A, Moynihan JL, Rizzo M, Kelley M, et al. Angiographic methods to assess human coronary angiogenesis. Am Heart J. 1999;137:169–79.

13. Sinnaeve PR, Armstrong PW, Gershlick AH, Goldstein P, Wilcox R, Lambert Y, et al. ST-segment-elevation myocardial infarction patients randomized to a pharmaco-invasive strategy or primary percutaneous coronary intervention: Strategic Reperfusion Early After Myocardial Infarction (STREAM) 1-year mortality follow-up. Circulation. 2014;130(14):1139–45.

14. Kim SS, Choi HS, Jeong MH, Cho JG, Ahn YK, Kim JH, et al. Korea Acute Myocardial Infarction Registry Investigators. Clinical outcomes of acute myocardial infarction with occluded left circumflex artery. J Cardiol. 2011; 57(3):290–6.

15. De Luca G, van't Hof AW, Huber K, Gibson CM, Bellandi F, Arntz HR, et al. Impact of advanced age on myocardial perfusion, distal embolization, and mortality patients with ST-segment elevation myocardial infarction treated by primary angioplasty and glycoprotein IIb-IIIa inhibitors. Heart Vessels. 2014;29(1):15–20.

16. Gharacholou SM, Lopes RD, Alexander KP, Mehta RH, Stebbins AL, Pieper KS, et al. Age and outcomes in ST-segment elevation myocardial infarction treated with primary percutaneous coronary intervention: findings from the APEX-AMI trial. Arch Intern Med. 2011;171(6):559–67.

17. Park JS, Cha KS, Shin D, Lee DS, Lee HW, Oh JH, et al. Korea Working Group on Myocardial Infarction Investigators. Prognostic Significance of Presenting Blood Pressure in Patients With ST-Elevation Myocardial Infarction Undergoing Percutaneous Coronary Intervention. Am J Hypertens. 2015. On press

18. Roth D, Van Tulder R, Heidinger B, Herkner H, Schreiber W, Havel C. Admission blood pressure and 1-year mortality in acute myocardial infarction. Int J Clin Pract. 2015. On press.

19. Thygesen K, Alpert JS, Jaffe AS, Simoons ML, Chaitman BR, White HD, et al. Third universal definition of myocardial infarction. Eur Heart J. 2012;33:2551–67.

5

Prostatic abscess in a patient with ST-elevation myocardial infarction

Yoshito Kadoya[1]* [iD] and Tsuneaki Kenzaka[2]

Abstract

Background: In patients with ST-elevation myocardial infarction (STEMI), urinary tract infection is the most common infection-related complication. Prostatic abscess in a patient with STEMI is very rare.

Case presentation: We report the case of a 49-year-old Japanese man who developed fever and shaking chills during hospitalization for STEMI. We initially diagnosed catheter-associated urinary tract infection. However, subsequent contrast-enhanced computed tomography revealed multiple large abscesses in his prostate. We decided to treat with antimicrobial agents alone because the patient was receiving dual-antiplatelet therapy and discontinuation is very high risk for in-stent thrombosis. The patient recovered remarkably after treatment without drainage or surgery.

Conclusions: Here, we described the world's first reported case of prostatic abscess in an immunocompetent patient with STEMI. Early removal of indwelling bladder catheters in patients with STEMI receiving dual-antiplatelet therapy is important to avoid development of prostatic abscess. Furthermore, unnecessary invasive instrumentation should be avoided or limited to diminish the risk of infections.

Keywords: Prostatic abscess, ST-elevation myocardial infarction, Catheter-associated urinary tract infection, Urinary tract infection, Indwelling bladder catheter

Background

The infection-related complication rate in patients hospitalized for ST-elevation myocardial infarction (STEMI) has been reported to be 16.6 % [1]. Urinary tract infection (UTI) is the most common infection-related complication, reported in approximately 6 % of patients with STEMI [1]. Risk factors associated with UTI in such patients include urinary tract catheterization and several comorbidities, such as diabetes mellitus and chronic kidney disease [1]. Here, we report a rare case of prostatic abscess in an immunocompetent patient hospitalized for STEMI.

Case presentation

A 49-year-old Japanese man complaining of chest pain was taken by ambulance to our hospital. His medical

* Correspondence: m03020kdy@gmail.com
[1]Department of Internal Medicine, Kyotambacho Hospital, Kyotambacho, Kyoto, Japan
Full list of author information is available at the end of the article

history included surgery for inguinal hernia at 45 years of age. He also had a history of smoking with a Brinkman index score of 300. Electrocardiography showed ST elevation in leads V2-5. Cardiac biomarkers were also elevated as following: high sensitive Troponin I, 0.067 ng/ml (standard value: 0.00–0.03 ng/ml). Based on these findings, we diagnosed STEMI, and performed emergent coronary angiography, which showed occlusion of the left anterior descending artery (Fig. 1a, b). Thus, we performed emergent percutaneous coronary intervention (PCI) (Fig. 1c). After surgery, the patient was moved to the intensive care unit with an indwelling bladder catheter, where he recovered without any acute complications.

Three days after PCI, the patient developed fever and shaking chills. He had a body temperature of 39.2 °C, blood pressure of 103/68 mmHg, regular pulse rate of 103 beats/min, respiratory rate of 18 breaths/min, and oxygen saturation of 97 % (without oxygen administration). His heart and breath sounds were normal, and his abdomen was soft and flat with no tenderness. There was no skin rash, and joint findings were normal.

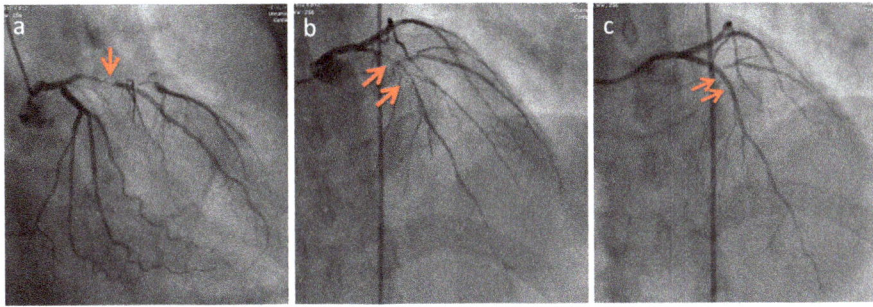

Fig. 1 Coronary angiogram of left coronary artery. **a** Right anterior oblique (RAO)-Caudal view, pre-percutaneous coronary intervention (PCI), (**b**) Anteroposterior (AP)-Cranial view, pre-PCI, (**c**) AP-Cranial view, post-PCI. Red arrows are culprit lesion

Laboratory data at onset of fever and shaking chills are shown in Table 1. Notably, he had a white blood cell count of 13,760 cells/mm^3, hemoglobin level of 12.4 g/dL, and C-reactive protein level of 8.29 mg/dL. Cardiac enzymes were still elevated due to the STEMI, but were returning toward normal. Chest radiography showed no infiltrative shadows (Fig. 2). Urinary Gram staining revealed middle-sized gram-negative rods that were phagocytized by leukocytes. We initially diagnosed catheter-associated UTI. Blood and urine cultures were performed, his indwelling bladder catheter was removed, and he was initially administered intravenous (IV) cefmetazole (1 g every 8 h). The fever was brought down temporarily, but fever developed again at 4 days after starting the antimicrobial agent. In addition, micturition and pain while urinating persisted. Blood and urine cultures were both positive for *Pseudomonas aeruginosa*. We suspected abscess formation, and performed contrast-enhanced computed tomography, which showed multiple large abscesses in his prostate (Fig. 3).

After consulting a urology specialist about drainage or surgical treatment, we decided to treat with antimicrobial agents alone because the patient was receiving dual-antiplatelet therapy and discontinuation is very high risk for in-stent thrombosis. We administered IV meropenem (1 g every 12 h) and amikacin (200 mg every 12 h) for 2 days, and then changed to levofloxacin (750 mg per day) based on drug sensitivity. Blood cultures were negative on the 10th day

Table 1 Laboratory data at onset of fever and shaking chills

Parameter	Recorded value	Standard value
White blood cell count	13.76 × 10^9 /L	4.00–7.50 × 10^9 /L
Hemoglobin	12.4 g/dL	11.3–15.2 g/dL
Hematocrit	37 %	36–45 %
Platelet	184 × 10^9 /L	130–350 × 10^9 /L
C-reactive protein	8.29 mg/dL	≦0.14 mg/dL
Total protein	6.2 g/dL	6.9–8.4 g/dL
Albumin	3.4 g/dL	3.9–5.1 g/dL
Total bilirubin	0.8 mg/dL	0.4–1.5 mg/dL
Aspartate aminotransferase	72 U/L	11–30 U/L
Alanine aminotransferase	41 U/L	4–30 U/L
Lactate dehydrogenase	402 U/L	109–216 U/L
Alkaline phosphatase	192 U/L	107–330 U/L
γ-glutamyltranspeptidase	19 U/L	<70 IU/L
Creatinine	0.79 mg/dL	0.63–1.03 mg/dL
Sodium	137 mEq/L	136–148 mEq/L
Potassium	4.1 mEq/L	3.6–5.0 mEq/L
Glucose	113 mg/dl	70–109 mg/dl
B-type natriuretic peptide	107 pg/mL	<20 pg/mL
Urinary protein	+	-
Urinary occult blood	+++	-
Urinary nitrite	+	-
Urinary white blood cell	20–29/high-power field	-
Urinary red blood cell	50–99/high-power field	-

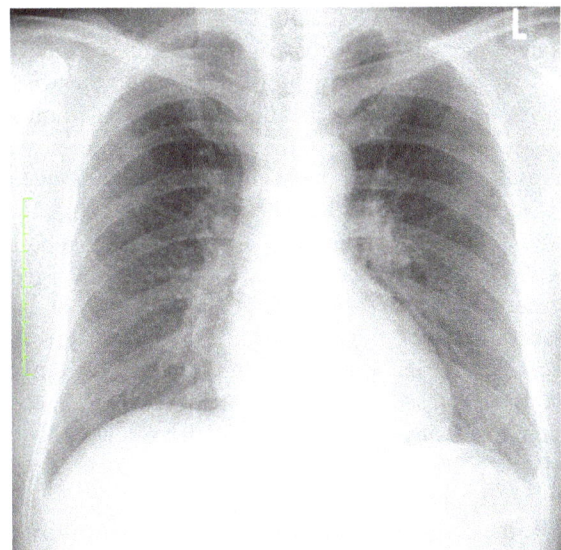

Fig. 2 Chest radiograph, showing no infiltrative shadows

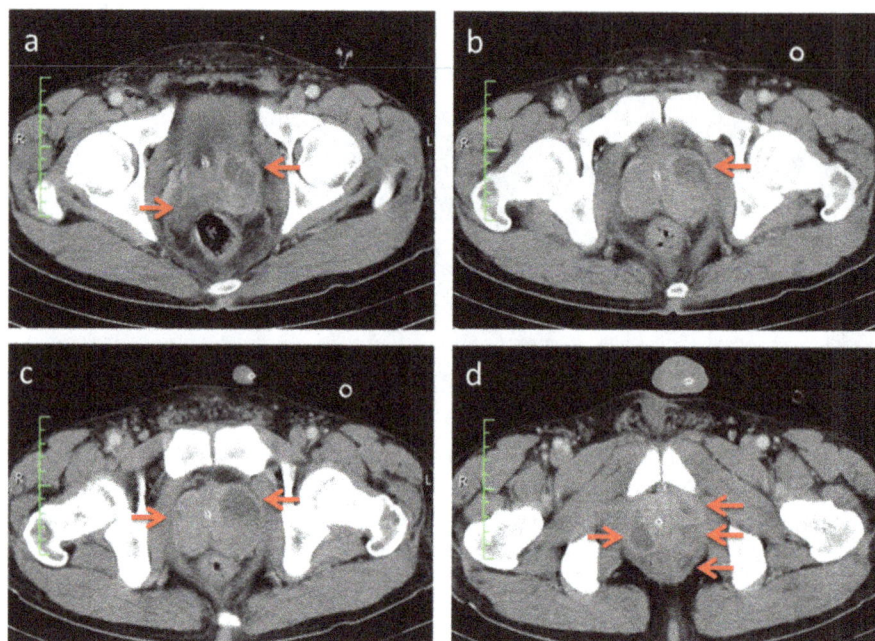

Fig. 3 Contrast-enhanced computed tomography scan, revealing multiple large prostatic abscesses (red arrows). In sequence from (**a**) to (**d**), the images are sliced from the head side to the foot side

after onset of fever and shaking chills, while contrast-enhanced computed tomography showed the abscess was decreasing on the 17th day. The patient was discharged on the 27th day of hospitalization. He had in total 6 weeks of antimicrobial therapy, and showed remarkable recovery. We continue to see this patient regularly at our clinic, and he has been in good health for more than 3 years.

Discussion

We experienced a case of prostatic abscess in a patient hospitalized for STEMI. In such patients, UTI is a frequent complication, whereas prostatic abscess is very rare. To the best of our knowledge, this is the world's first reported case of prostatic abscess in an immuno-competent patient with STEMI.

Prostatic abscess is thought to occur as a consequence of inadequately treated acute bacterial prostatitis [2]. In recent years, prostatic abscess has rarely been reported due to the widespread use of antibacterial agents. Furthermore, it has been noted that only 2.7 % of cases of acute bacterial prostatitis will develop into prostatic abscess [3]. Based on the fact that acute bacterial prostatitis is diagnosed in approximately 0.5 to 2.5 % of patients with prostate symptoms [4], we can assume that prostatic abscess accounts for a very small percentage of all UTIs.

The most common pathogen associated with prostatic abscess is *Escherichia coli*. However, unusual pathogens, such as *Staphylococcus aureus*, *Pseudomonas aeruginosa*,

Mycobacterium tuberculosis, and *Candida*, also have been reported [5, 6]. Prostatic abscess usually occurs in immunosuppressed patients with such conditions as diabetes mellitus, chronic renal failure, hemodialysis, cancer, cirrhosis, or human immunodeficiency virus infection [7–10]. Other predisposing factors include indwelling bladder catheter, instrumentation of the lower urinary tract, bladder outlet obstruction, and biopsy of the prostate [7–10]. In the present case, the patient was not immunosuppressed. Therefore, the indwelling bladder catheter at the time of emergent PCI for STEMI was recognized as the main cause of his prostatic abscesses.

Currently, drug-eluting stents are commonly used in PCI for acute myocardial infarction. Such patients should receive dual-antiplatelet therapy after drug-eluting stent implantation. In the present case, prostatic abscess drainage, which should be done in many cases, was not performed because the patient was receiving dual-antiplatelet therapy. Because patients who undergo PCI usually receive dual-antiplatelet therapy, they have a higher risk of hemorrhagic complications with drainage or surgical treatment for an abscess. Thus, it is important to avoid unnecessary indwelling bladder catheters, or to promptly remove those that are no longer required, so that patients can avoid development of prostatic abscess. Furthermore, for all the patients, unnecessary invasive instrumentation should be avoided or limited as much as possible to diminish the risk of infections.

Conclusions

In conclusion, we described the world's first reported case of prostatic abscess in an immunocompetent patient STEMI. Such patients usually have a higher risk with drainage due to receiving dual-antiplatelet therapy. Early removal of indwelling bladder catheters is important to avoid development of prostatic abscess. Unnecessary invasive instrumentation should be avoided or limited to diminish the risk of infections.

Consent

Written informed consent was obtained from the patient for publication of this Case report and any accompanying images. A copy of the written consent is available for review by the Editor of this journal.

Abbreviations

IV: intravenous; PCI: percutaneous coronary intervention; STEMI: ST-elevation myocardial infarction; UTI: urinary tract infection.

Competing interests

Both authors have no financial interests to disclose and no competing interest to declare.

Authors' contributions

YK: Clinical management of the case, manuscript redaction and correction. TK: Manuscript redaction and correction. Both authors read and approved the final manuscript.

Acknowledgments

None.

Author details

[1]Department of Internal Medicine, Kyotambacho Hospital, Kyotambacho, Kyoto, Japan. [2]Division of Community Medicine and Career Development, Kobe University Graduate School of Medicine, Kobe, Japan.

References

1. Nash MC, Strom JA, Pathak EB. Prevalence of major infections and adverse outcomes among hospitalized ST-elevation myocardial infarction patients in Florida, 2006. BMC Cardiovac Disord. 2011;11:69.
2. Kravchick S, Cytron S, Agulansky L, Ben-Dor D. Acute prostatitis in middle-aged men: a prospective study. BJU Int. 2004;93:93–6.
3. Millan-Rodriguez F, Palou J, Bujons-Tur A, Musquera-Felip M, Sevilla-Cecilia C, Serrallach-Orejas M, et al. Acute bacterial prostatitis: two different sub-categories according to a previous manipulation of the lower urinary tract. World J Urol. 2006;24:45–50.
4. Granados EA, Riley G, Salvador J, Vincente J. Prostatic abscess: diagnosis and treatment. J Urol. 1992;148:80–2.
5. Weinberger M, Cytron S, Servadio C, Block C, Rosenfeld JB, Pitlik SD. Prostatic abscess in the antibiotic era. Rev Infect Dis. 1988;10:239–49.
6. Vandover JC, Patel N, Dalawari P. Prostatic abscess. J Emerg Med. 2011;40:e83–5.
7. Oliveira P, Andrade JA, Porto HC, Filho JE, Vinhaes AF. Diagnosis and treatment of prostatic abscess. Int Braz J Urol. 2003;29:30–4.
8. Trauzzi SJ, Kay CJ, Kaufman DG, Lowe FC. Management of prostatic abscess in patients with human immunodeficiency syndrome. Urology. 1994;43:629–33.
9. Park SC, Lee JW, Rim JS. Prostatic abscess caused by community-acquired methicillin-resistant Staphylococcus aureus. Int J Urol. 2011;18:536–8.
10. Lim JW, Ko YT, Lee DH, Park SJ, Oh JH, Yoon Y, et al. Treatment of prostatic abscess: value of transrectal ultrasonographically guided needle aspiration. J Ultrasound Med. 2000;19:609–17.

6

Management and outcomes of acute ST-segment-elevation myocardial infarction at a tertiary-care hospital in Sri Lanka

Ruwanthi Bandara[1], Arjuna Medagama[2*], Ruwan Munasinghe[1], Nandana Dinamithra[1], Amila Subasinghe[1], Jayantha Herath[1], Mahesh Ratnayake[1], Buddhini Imbulpitiya[1] and Ameena Sulaiman[2]

Abstract

Background: Sri Lanka is a developing country with a high rate of cardiovascular mortality. It is still largely dependent on thrombolysis for primary management of acute myocardial infarction. The aim of this study was to present current data on the presentation, management, and outcomes of acute ST-segment-elevation myocardial infarction (STEMI) at a tertiary-care hospital in Sri Lanka.

Methods: Eighty-one patients with acute STEMI presenting to a teaching hospital in Peradeniya, Sri Lanka, were included in this observational study.

Results: Median interval between symptom onset and hospital presentation was 60 min (mean 212 min). Thrombolysis was performed in 73% of patients. The most common single reason for not performing thrombolysis was delayed presentation. Median door-to-needle time was 64 min (mean, 98 min). Only 16.9% of patients received thrombolysis within 30 min, and none underwent primary PCI. Over 98% of patients received aspirin, clopidogrel, and a statin on admission. Intravenous and oral beta blockers were rarely used. Follow-up data were available for 93.8% of patients at 1 year. One-year mortality rate was 12.3%. Coronary intervention was performed in only 7.3% of patients post infarction.

Conclusion: Late presentation to hospital remains a critical factor in thrombolysis of STEMI patients in Sri Lanka. Thrombolysis was not performed within 30 min of admission in the majority of patients. First-contact physicians should receive further training on effective thrombolysis, and there is an urgent need to explore the ways in which PCI and post-infarction interventions can be incorporated into treatment protocols.

Keywords: ST-segment-elevation myocardial infarction, STEMI, Thrombolysis, Door-to-needle time, Survival, 1-year mortality, Sri Lanka

Background

Sri Lanka is a developing country with a population of 21 million and a rapidly increasing burden of non-communicable diseases.

In 2005, the prevalences of hypertension, diabetes, and dysglycemia were 20%, 11%, and 20%, respectively [1].

* Correspondence: arjuna.medagama@gmail.com
[2]Department of Medicine, Faculty of Medicine, University of Peradeniya, Peradeniya, Sri Lanka
Full list of author information is available at the end of the article

Mortality from cardiovascular disease is recognized to be one of the highest worldwide [2]. Ischemic heart disease (IHD) is the leading cause of death in Sri Lanka and accounts for 27.6 deaths per 100,000 people. Data from 2004 to 2012 show a steady increase in hospital mortality from IHD; in 2012 it accounted for 14.4% all hospital deaths [3]. This high mortality remains unexplained but may be attributable in part to the clustering of modifiable and non-modifiable cardiovascular risk factors.

Acute coronary syndrome (ACS) encompasses a spectrum of coronary artery diseases, including unstable angina, ST-segment-elevation myocardial infarction (STEMI), and non-STEMI.

There has recently been a worldwide transition in the acute management of ACS. Primary percutaneous coronary intervention (PCI) is steadily being introduced in most parts of the developed world and middle-income countries. However, in Sri Lanka, ACS is still managed primarily medically and, in most instances, in non-specialized general medical units. Rates of secondary prevention of cardiovascular disease are low in middle-income countries like Sri Lanka, but offer substantial oppurtunties for further development [4].

Clinical trials have provided clinicians with many evidence-based interventions and medications. These are augmented by observational studies, which provide useful information about patients hospitalized for acute coronary events [5]. Observational studies have revealed differences and shortcomings in management practices among countries as well as within different regions of the same country [6,7]. The development of patient registries is an important step toward increased awareness of cardiovascular disease and establishment of appropriate management strategies. Although developed countries already have such registries, these need to be established in developing countries so that current preventive and management strategies can be audited.

At present, there is little information on the management and outcomes of acute myocardial infarction (AMI) [8] in Sri Lanka. The aim of this study was to examine current data on the presentation, management, and outcomes of acute STEMI at a tertiary-care hospital in Sri Lanka.

Methods

This prospective observational study was carried out at the Professorial Medical Unit of Peradeniya Teaching Hospital, Sri Lanka, over a 6-month period beginning November 2011. This is a busy state-run tertiary-care institution with a nonselective intake of acute patients.

To be eligible for enrollment, patients had to present within 24 h of onset of symptoms likely to be of myocardial origin. In addition, they had to have electrocardiographic (ECG) changes fulfilling current ECG criteria in the diagnosis of acute STEMI or new-onset left bundle-branch block, and an increase in a biochemical marker of myocardial necrosis where results were available. All patients presenting with chest pain within the preceding 24 h who fulfilled ECG criteria for acute STEMI were included in the study. A diagnosis of STEMI was made by a senior house officer or registrar on admission and later confirmed by a consultant physician. Troponin level is not checked at most government hospitals; when required, the test is performed in a private laboratory at the patient's expense.

Cardiac troponin levels were therefore not routinely available to us and were requested only in instances where diagnosis was uncertain. Assessment with history, physical examination, and ECG was performed for every patient presenting with chest pain, and those patients fulfilling the criteria for STEMI were included in the present study. Patients provided written informed consent prior to collection of management data, which were extracted from interviews conducted by the authors and from hospital records.

Following hospital discharge, patients were allowed to be followed up at their usual clinics. One year from the onset of STEMI, patients were invited for another interview with the authors. At this visit, patients' current symptoms and examination findings were recorded and data from clinic records regarding management during the previous year was obtained. An echocardiogram was performed to assess left ventricular function and to detect new onset of regional wall-motion abnormalities and other structural abnormalities.

The study did not alter the standard care given to the patients. Ethical clearance for this study was obtained from the ethics review committee of the faculty of medicine at University of Peradeniya, Sri Lanka (2011/EC/22).

Binary logistic regression was used to assess the association of mortality at 1 year with history of smoking, hypertension, dyslipidemia, time taken for presentation, door-to-needle time, ejection fraction, and hypotension during the index admission and the mode (direct vs. redirected) of admission to the hospital. A P value less than 0.05 was considered to be statistically significant.

Results

There were 81 admissions with confirmed STEMI during the study period. There were 21 (26%) females and 60 (74%) males and the mean age was 61.7 (SD 10.7) years. The majority of patients (59.5%) belonged to the age group of 50–69 years, and a further 20% were from the 70–79 year group.

Seventeen (21%) were current smokers, 47 (58%) had smoked at some time during their lives and 34 (42%) patients had never smoked. None of the females had ever smoked. Seven patients (8.6%) had previous history of ischaemic heart disease. Twenty two (27%) had a history of hypertension, 25 (30.8%) diabetes mellitus and 6 (7%) isolated dyslipidaemia. Socio-demographic profile, co-morbidities and risk factors are gven in Table 1.

There were 45 (58%) direct admissions to Teaching Hospital Peradeniya (THP), 23 (27%) were referred from the regional hospitals and 11 (12.5%) referred by the general practitioner (GP).

Time to presentation by direct or redirected admission is presented in Table 2. Of the patients presenting directly to our facility, median time from symptom onset to admission was 60 min, the mean was 212 min. Patients who had been seen at a peripheral hospital or by a general

Table 1 Patients' socio-demographic variables and risk factors

Gender		No	(%)
	Males	21	26
	Females	60	74
Age		Mean (years)	SD (years)
	Males	59.38	10.62
	Females	70.70	8.67
BMI (kg/m^2)		Mean	SD
	Males	25.12	6.64
	Females	23.59	3.73
Ethnicity		No	(%)
	Sinhalese	59	73
	Muslim	14	17
	Tamil	08	10
Comorbidities and risk factors		Frequency	(%)
	Hypertension	22	27
	Diabetes mellitus	25	30.8
	Dyslipidemia	6	7
	Ischemic Heart Disease	7	8.6
	Smoking	Males (n)	Females (n)
	Current	17	0
	Ex	30	0
	Never	34	0

BMI, body mass index.

practitioner took longer to present (median, 75 min; mean, 281 min). The difference did not reach statistical significance (P = 0.45).

Seventy seven patients (95%) presented with chest pain and four patients had symptoms other than chest pain. Forty three patients (53%) had anterior STEMI or new-onset left bundle-branch block, 32 (40%) had inferior STEMI, and six (7%) had lateral STEMI. Of the 81 patients studied, 10 (12.3%) were not eligible for thrombolysis because of late presentation; thus, 71 patients (87%) were eligible for thrombolytic therapy, and 59 (72.8%) underwent thrombolysis with streptokinase.

Twelve patients were therefore eligible on the basis of arrival time, but three of these (3.7%) had absolute or relative contraindications to thrombolysis and nine (11.1%)

Table 2 Comparison of time to presentation between direct and redirected admission

	Time taken for admission to tertiary care center (minutes)	
	Median	Mean
Direct admission (n = 45)	60	212
Re-directed admissions (n = 36)	75	281

P = 0.45.

eligible patients did not undergo thrombolysis for unknown reasons. The 12 patients who were eligible for, but did not undergo, thrombolysis and those who presented late were treated with either low-molecular-weight heparin or unfractionated heparin.

Median door-to-needle time was 64 min (mean, 98 min). Ten patients (16.9%) underwent thrombolysis within 30 min, 28 (47.4%) within 60 min and 39 (66%) within 90 min. Twenty (33.9%) underwent thrombolysis more than 90 min after arriving at the hospital. Time to thrombolytic therapy is shown in Table 3.

Of the 81 patients presenting to our facility, 99% received aspirin, 97% received clopidogrel, and 95% received a statin on admission. Oxygen was given to 79%, analgesics to 61%, and oral beta blockers to 35%. Only 16% of patients presenting to either a peripheral hospital or a general practitioner received aspirin.

During hospitalization, patients were administered aspirin (91%), clopidogrel (95%), statin (91%), angiotensin-converting-enzyme inhibitor (ACEI) or angiotensin-receptor blocker (ARB) (95%), and nitrates (60%). At discharge, over 88% received a combination of aspirin, clopidogrel, statin, and ACEI or ARB. At discharge, only 59% of patients were prescribed nitrates and only 34% were prescribed beta blockers.

Following thrombolysis, four patients (5%) were managed in the intensive care unit, 38 (47%) in the high-dependency unit, and remainder in the general medical unit. One patient developed gastrointestinal bleeding following thrombolysis.

Mean duration of hospital stay following acute STEMI was 5.5 days. There was no difference in duration of stay between patients who experienced anterior STEMI and those who experienced STEMI located elsewhere. During hospitalization, one patient developed bleeding while on low-molecular-weight heparin, four had reversible arrhythmias, seven developed heart failure, four had heart failure with reversible cardiogenic shock, and two developed pneumonia.

A pre-discharge echocardiogram was performed in 72 patients (88%), of whom 10 (12.3%) had an ejection fraction < 40%. Mean ejection fraction of the study population during the index admission was 48.4% (range, 20–68%).

Follow-up data were available for 93.8% of patients. At the end of 1 year, 66 (81.5%) of the 81 patients with

Table 3 Door-to-needle times of patients receiving streptokinase

	Number	Cumulative percentage (%)
≤30 minutes	10	16.9
>30 ≤ 60 minutes	18	47.4
>60 ≤ 90 minutes	11	66
>90 minutes	20	100

STEMI were reassessed, five (6.1%) were lost to follow-up, and 10 (12.3%) had died. Thirty-seven patients (45.6%) had been referred to a specialized cardiology unit, 22 (27%) underwent exercise ECG testing, 10 (12.3%) underwent coronary angiography, five (6%) underwent percutaneous transluminal coronary angiography, and two (2.3%) underwent coronary artery bypass grafting. Six patients had been readmitted for cardiac-related problems, four for heart failure associated with ACS, and two for ACS. Outcomes of patients at 1-year is tabulated in Table 4.

At the end of 1 year, six patients (7%) were still smoking; mean systolic and diastolic blood pressures were 128 mmHg and 79 mmHg, respectively; and medications being used were aspirin (83%), clopidogrel (82%), statin (90%), and ACEI or ARB (85%).

Echocardiography at 1-year follow-up revealed new-onset regional wall-motion abnormalities in six patients (9%), of whom five demonstrated new-onset left ventricular dysfunction (ejection fraction <40%). Mean ejection fraction at 1 year was 49%.

Of the ten patients who died, four had anterior STEMI and six had inferior myocardial infarction during the index admission. The immediate cause of death is not known. Thrombolysis was not received by one patient. There was no significant difference in mean door-to-needle time between patients who died within the first year (129 min) and those who were alive at 1-year follow-up (92 min) ($P = 0.3$). Mean time to hospital presentation was 61.8 min in those who died and 247 min in those who survived. Mean ejection fraction at the index admission did not differ significantly between non-surviving patients (49%) and surviving patients (49%). Only one patient had post-infarction heart failure during the index admission. Two patients were referred to a cardiologist. The deceased patients had received aspirin, clopidogrel, and a statin at admission and at discharge. The presence of diabetes mellitus ($P = 0.01$) and previous IHD ($P = 0.05$) were associated with death at 1 year.

Table 4 One-year outcomes

	Number	Percentage (%)
1 year follow up	66	81.5
Lost to follow up	5	6
Deceased at 1 year	10	12.3
Referral done to specialized cardiology center	37	45.6
Underwent Exercise ECG	22	27
Underwent Coronary angiogram	10	12.3
Underwent Revascularization	7	7.3
Re-admitted with Coronary events	6	7.4

ECG, electrocardiogram.

No significant association was found between death at 1 year and history of smoking, hypertension, dyslipidaemia, time taken for presentation, door to needle time, ejection fraction and hypotension during the index admission and the mode of admission to hospital.

Discussion

STEMI was diagnosed with reasonable accuracy in our study by clinical and ECG criteria. Troponin levels were obtained in a minority of patients because of the unavailability of the test in the state sector and the high cost in private-sector laboratories.

Despite coronary vascular disease being the largest cause of mortality among Sri Lankan adults, no study has described the presentation, management, and outcomes of STEMI; likely because of lack of resources and funding. Peradeniya Teaching Hospital is one of the two largest tertiary-care institutions in the area, and many smaller hospitals redirect patients with ACS to this unit; the sample can thus be considered representative. Percutaneous Coronary Interventions (PCI) or CABG is not performed at this hospital and specialized cardiology services are available only at the Teaching Hospital Kandy situated 4 km away. At the time of the study Primary PCI was not routinely performed at this instituttion either.

The prevalences of smoking (58%) and diabetes (30.8%) in this study are comparable with data from regional and global studies [5,9]. The prevalences of hypertension, dyslipidemia, and preexisting coronary heart disease (Table 1) were considerably lower than in other studies. Mohanan et al. reported the prevalence of hypertension and previous IHD among patients in Kerala, India, presenting with ACS to be 48% and 14% [9]; the Access study investigators reported higher prevalences of 65% and 26%, respectively [5]. The prevalences of hypertension and diabetes among adult Sri Lankans are 23% and 10.8%, respectively [10,11], but they seem to be underreported in the current study. In Sri Lanka, the first recognition of risk factors for cardiovascular disease is often at presentation for STEMI and may explain the low prevalence of risk factors reported in the current study.

Late presentation; contraindications; and other factors that are undocumented and therefore unknown rendered 27% of patients ineligible for thrombolysis following STEMI. Better training of staff can facilitate recognition of the need for thrombolysis at presentation. Better record keeping is also essential.

Delayed presentation resulting in ineligibility for thrombolysis was mainly pre-hospital, and similar delays have been observed in other studies carried out in Sri Lanka. Constantine et al. reported median pre-hospital delays of 130 min in 1997 and 720 min in 1999, and the delay was longer in patients who sought pre-hospitalization medical advice than in those who presented directly [12,13]. In our study, median delay was 60 min (mean, 212 min) in patients presenting directly to our center and 75 min (mean 281 min) in those presenting through another hospital or general practitioner, a trend similar to those reported previously [13]. However it did not reach statistical significance. The longer mean than median time to presentation is the result of several patients presenting more than 12 hours following onset of pain. Mohanan et al. recently reported time from ACS symptom onset to ER presentation of over 6 hours in India [9].

While time to presentation has greatly improved, there is still considerable delay at peripheral hospitals and clinics, and while we did not identify an association between time to presentation and 1-year mortality, this could have been because of our relatively small sample size.

In the present study, 83% of eligible patients underwent thrombolysis, a result consistent with that of Rajapakse et al., who reported that thrombolysis was performed in 84.6% of a cohort of AMI patients at another tertiary-care institution in Sri Lanka, the National Hospital Colombo, in 2008 [8]. Both figures show a tremendous improvement from the 17% reported in 1999 [13]. However a large proportion of patients with STEMI (27%) did not receive thrombolysis or PCI in our study. Access investigators who studied the outcomes of ACS patients in the developing countries of Latin America, the Middle East, and Africa reported that 39% of STEMI patients did not receive thrombolysis or PCI [5]. However, in this multi-national survey, which included 11,731 patients, the overall rates for angiography and PCI were 58 and 35%, respectively.

Our data suggest that time delay to presentation to a tertiary-care center is a critical factor that reduced patients' eligibility for thrombolysis. Reasons for this delay are likely 1) the absence of organized emergency medical transport [9] and cardiac response teams, requiring patients to provide their own transportation to the hospital; and 2) lack of patient awareness regarding ACS.

The benefits of early thrombolytic therapy are well established. Mean absolute reduction in mortality per hour of delay is 1.6 (standard deviation, 0.6) per 1,000 patients [12]. Median door-to-needle time in our study was 64 min; the mean of 96 min was due to late thrombolysis in some patients because of difficulty making a definitive diagnosis of STEMI. Guidelines recommend a door-to-needle time of less than 30 min. This was achieved in only 16.9% of our patients, but thrombolysis was performed within 60 min of admission in 47% and within 90 min of admission in 66%. In a previous study, a median door-to-needle time of 70 min was reported [12]. In Malaysia the median door-to-needle time was 48–54 min in a prospective study in which medical and emergency department doctors administered thrombolysis [14]. Mohanan et al. reported that less than one-third

of patients undergoing thrombolysis had door-to-needle times of more than 30 min in India [9]. Door-to-needle time is a critical factor in the management of STEMI and first-contact doctors at all hospitals should be educated in early diagnosis and immediate thrombolysis.

More than 95% of STEMI patients received aspirin, clopidogrel, and a statin on presentation to our unit. However, a considerable proportion (84%) of STEMI patients who presented initially to another hospital or a general practitioner did not receive aspirin prior to being referred for thrombolysis. In 2010, Rajapakse et al. reported that aspirin and clopidogrel loading was performed in only 69% and 61% of patients, respectively [8]. Our use of aspirin and clopidogrel on admission seems to be satisfactory and compares well with other studies of the region [9] and of the developing world in general [5]. Continued therapy with aspirin, clopidogrel, and statin medication was observed in more than 88% of participants during hospitalization and on discharge. Aspirin was the medication most likely to be withheld, mostly for reasons of epigastric pain or presumed gastrointestinal hemorrhage. An ACEI or ARB was administered to over 90% of patients during hospitalization and to over 88% on discharge. At the end of 1 year, the use of the above medications remained over 82%. Access investigators who studied over 11,000 patients with ACS in the developing world reported the use of ACEIs to be 68% [5]. The World Health Organization considers the use of aspirin, statin and blood pressure-lowering agents post discharge in ACS patients to be cost-effective strategies and are considered *best buys* [15]. Nitrates were prescribed to more than 59% of patients during hospitalization and on discharge.

Intravenous beta blockers were not used in the acute management of STEMI in the present study or in previous Sri Lankan studies. However 35% of patients received oral beta blockers during the initial assessment. Intravenous beta blockers followed by oral beta blockers should be administered immediately, in the absence of contraindications, to all patients with STEMI [16]. Underutilization of intravenous beta blockers persists and should be analyzed in future studies. Oral beta blockers were prescribed at discharge to 34% of our study patients, compared with 78% in other developing countries [5].

Eighteen (22%) of our patients had complications during the post-infarction period, the majority of which were from cardiac causes. Only one patient developed a major gastrointestinal hemorrhage following thrombolytic therapy. Seventy six (85%) of our patients had pre-discharge echocardiography performed and 14% had evidence of left ventricular dysfunction, defined as an ejection fraction <40%, at the time of discharge. Rajapakse et al. also reported a complication rate of 25% in their ACS patients [8]. Both studies show an improvement from the previously reported incidence of 37% [13] that may be due to the higher adherence to guidelines and wider use of thrombolysis. There were no in-hospital deaths during the index admission in the present study, which probably reflects our small sample size. Mohanan et al. reported an in-hospital mortality of 4.3–8.6% among various cardiac registries globally [9].

This study examined 1-year survival of post-STEMI patients in Sri Lanka. Ten of the initial 81 STEMI patients were deceased at 1-year follow-up. The 1-year mortality of 12.3% in our study was slightly greater than the observed value of 8–10% in the major thrombolysis trials [17]. Similarly, an all-cause death rate of 7.3% at 1 year was observed by the Access investigators [5]. The higher 1-year mortality observed in the present study is probably the result of late presentation at the index admission, underutilization of thrombolysis, a longer-than-recommended door-to-needle time, and a very low rate of coronary intervention in the post-infarction period. However, there were no significant associations of mortality at 1 year with either time to presentation or the door-to-needle time, probably because of our small study sample.

Meta-analysis has shown primary PCI to be superior to thrombolysis in the treatment of STEMI and to benefit long term survival and reduce strokes, recurrent ischemia, and reinfarction [18]. Unfortunately, only a minority of Sri Lankan patients have the opportunity to undergo primary PCI at present. Only 27% of patients from the current study went onto have a cardiac stress test, only 12.3% underwent coronary angiography, and only 7.3% underwent revascularization within 1 year of STEMI. Regionally, in India 7.5–12% of patients presenting with ACS undergo primary PCI and 20% undergo angiography [9,19]. By comparison, western countries report rates of 56.3% for angiography, 40.4% for percutaneous intervention, and 3.4% for coronary artery bypass grafting for patients presenting with acute STEMI [20,21]. Cardiac care infrastructure, personnel, and protocols in Sri Lanka need to keep pace with expanding facilities globally to confer the benefits of new developments to patients.

Limitations
Limitations of this study were its relatively small sample size, that it was a single-center investigation, and that it included only patients in the acute-care setting, which may have led to underestimation of the event rates, since patients who were dead on admission would not have been included in our analysis. Absence of the causes of death for those who died during the first year after STEMI is another notable limitation.

Conclusions
Sri Lanka still relies heavily on thrombolysis for the acute management of STEMI. Pre-hospital delays remain a critical factor in underutilization of thrombolysis, and recommended door-to-needle time is achieved in only a minority. Primary PCI and use of coronary intervention in the post-infarction period remain underutilized. In an environment that still relies heavily on thrombolysis as the primary treatment option for STEMI, more streamlined services, strict adherence to guidelines, and training of first-contact physicians is paramount in reducing mortality from myocardial infarction.

Competing interests
The authors declare that they have no competing interests.

Authors' contributions
RB and AM conceptualized the study, collected and analyzed the data, and wrote the manuscript. RW, ND, AS, A Sulaiman, BI, and JH collected and analyzed the data. MR collected the data and performed echocardiography. All authors read and approved the final manuscript.

Acknowledgments
The authors received no financial sponsorship, grants, or funding.

Author details
[1]Professorial Medical Unit, Teaching Hospital Peradeniya, Peradeniya, Sri Lanka. [2]Department of Medicine, Faculty of Medicine, University of Peradeniya, Peradeniya, Sri Lanka.

References
1. Wijewardene K, Mohideen MR, Mendis S, Fernando DS, Kulathilaka T, Weerasekara D, et al. Prevalence of hypertension, diabetes and obesity: baseline findings of a population based survey in four provinces in Sri Lanka. Ceylon Med J. 2005;50(2):62–70.
2. Abeywardena MY. Dietary fats, carbohydrates and vascular disease: Sri Lankan perspectives. Atherosclerosis. 2003;171(2):157–61.
3. Medical statistics Unit Ministry of Health. Annual Health Bulletin 2012. Colombo: Ministry of Health Sri Lanka; 2012.
4. Mendis S, Abegunde D, Yusuf S, Ebrahim S, Shaper G, Ghannem H, et al. WHO study on Prevention of REcurrences of Myocardial Infarction and StrokE (WHO-PREMISE). Bull World Health Organ. 2005;83(11):820–9.
5. Investigators A. Management of acute coronary syndromes in developing countries: acute coronary events-a multinational survey of current management strategies. Am Heart J. 2011;162(5):852–9. e22.
6. Eagle KA, Goodman SG, Avezum A, Budaj A, Sullivan CM, Lopez-Sendon J, et al. Practice variation and missed opportunities for reperfusion in ST-segment-elevation myocardial infarction: findings from the Global Registry of Acute Coronary Events (GRACE). Lancet. 2002;359(9304):373–7.
7. Fox KA, Goodman SG, Anderson Jr FA, Granger CB, Moscucci M, Flather MD, et al. From guidelines to clinical practice: the impact of hospital and geographical characteristics on temporal trends in the management of acute coronary syndromes. The Global Registry of Acute Coronary Events (GRACE). Eur Heart J. 2003;24(15):1414–24.
8. Rajapakse S, Rodrigo PC, Selvachandran J. Management of acute coronary syndrome in a tertiary care general medical unit in Sri Lanka: how closely do we follow the guidelines? J Clin Pharm Ther. 2010;35(4):421–7.
9. Mohanan PP, Mathew R, Harikrishnan S, Krishnan MN, Zachariah G, Joseph J, et al. Presentation, management, and outcomes of 25 748 acute coronary syndrome admissions in Kerala, India: results from the Kerala ACS Registry. Eur Heart J. 2013;34(2):121–9.
10. Katulanda P, Ranasinghe P, Jayawardena R, Constantine GR, Rezvi Sheriff MH, Matthews DR. The prevalence, predictors and associations of hypertension in Sri Lanka: a cross-sectional population based national survey. Clin Exp Hypertens. 2014;36(7):484–91.
11. Katulanda P, Constantine GR, Mahesh JG, Sheriff R, Seneviratne RD, Wijeratne S, et al. Prevalence and projections of diabetes and pre-diabetes in adults in Sri Lanka–Sri Lanka Diabetes, Cardiovascular Study (SLDCS). Diabet Med. 2008;25(9):1062–9.

12. Constantine GR, Thenabadu PN. Time delay to thrombolytic therapy—a Sri Lankan perspective. Postgrad Med J. 1998;74(873):405–7.

13. Constantine GR, Herath JI, Chang AA, Suganthan P, Hewamane BS, Thenabadu PN. Management of acute myocardial infarction in general medical wards in Sri Lanka. Postgrad Med J. 1999;75(890):718–20.

14. Loch A, Lwin T, Zakaria IM, Abidin IZ, Wan Ahmad WA, Hautmann O. Failure to improve door-to-needle time by switching to emergency physician-initiated thrombolysis for ST elevation myocardial infarction. Postgrad Med J. 2013;89(1052):335–9.

15. World Health Organization. Global status report on noncommunicable diseases 2010. Geneva: Switzerland; 2011.

16. Chen ZM, Pan HC, Chen YP, Peto R, Collins R, Jiang LX, et al. Early intravenous then oral metoprolol in 45,852 patients with acute myocardial infarction: randomised placebo-controlled trial. Lancet. 2005;366(9497):1622–32.

17. Sikri N, Bardia A. A history of streptokinase use in acute myocardial infarction. Tex Heart Inst J. 2007;34(3):318–27.

18. Keeley FC, Boura JA, Grines CL. Primary angioplasty versus intravenous thrombolytic therapy for acute myocardial infarction: a quantitative review of 23 randomised trials. Lancet. 2003;361(9351):13–20.

19. Xavier D, Pais P, Devereaux PJ, Xie C, Prabhakaran D, Reddy KS, et al. Treatment and outcomes of acute coronary syndromes in India (CREATE): a prospective analysis of registry data. Lancet. 2008;371(9622):1435–42.

20. Hasdai D, Behar S, Wallentin L, Danchin N, Gitt AK, Boersma E, et al. A prospective survey of the characteristics, treatments and outcomes of patients with acute coronary syndromes in Europe and the Mediterranean basin; the Euro Heart Survey of Acute Coronary Syndromes (Euro Heart Survey ACS). Eur Heart J. 2002;23(15):1190–201.

21. Fox KA, Goodman SG, Klein W, Brieger D, Steg PG, Dabbous O, et al. Management of acute coronary syndromes. Variations in practice and outcome; findings from the Global Registry of Acute Coronary Events (GRACE). Eur Heart J. 2002;23(15):1177–89.

7

The prognostic utility of GRACE risk score in predictive cardiovascular event rate in STEMI patients with successful fibrinolysis and delay intervention in non PCI-capable hospital

Yotsawee Chotechuang[1,2], Arintaya Phrommintikul[3*], Roungtiva Muenpa[4], Jayanton Patumanond[5], Tuanchai Chaichuen[6], Srun Kuanprasert[3], Noparat Thanachikun[3], Thanawat Benjanuwatra[3] and Apichard Sukonthasarn[3]

Abstract

Background: Fibrinolytic therapy is the main reperfusion therapy for most STEMI patients in several countries. Current practice guidelines recommended routine early pharmacoinvasive (within 3–24 h after successful fibrinolysis, however it cannot be performed in timely fashion due to limitation of PCI-capable hospitals. This study aimed to evaluate the prognostic utility of the GRACE score in patients receiving delayed intervention after successful fibrinolysis in non PCI-capable hospital.

Methods: We retrospectively analysed the data from the Maharaj Nakorn Chiang Mai Hospital acute ST-elevation myocardial infarction (STEMI) registry during the period 2007–2012. The STEMI patients who had successfully fibrionolysis in non PCI-capable hospital and received delayed PCI (during 24 h to 14 days after successful fibrinolytic therapy) at Maharaj Nakorn Chiang Mai hospital were included. The primary end point for this analysis was the composite outcomes, which included all-cause mortality, re-hospitalization with acute coronary syndrome (ACS), re-hospitalization with heart failure (HF) and stroke at 1 and 6-month.

Results: A total of 152 patients were included. 88 patients and 64 patients were in low GRACE group (GRACE risk score ≤ 125) and intermediate to high GRACE group (GRACE risk score above 126), respectively. The median time from fibrinolysis to coronary intervention in low GRACE group was 8.5 days (interquartile range, 4.6–10.9) and 7.9 days (interquartile range,3.2,12.0) in intermediate to high GRACE group ($p = 0.482$). At 1 month, the composite cardiovascular outcome at 1 month occurred in 2 patients (2.3 %) in low GRACE group and 10 patients (15.6 %) in intermediate to high GRACE group ($P = 0.003$). During 6 months, the composite cardiovascular outcomes occurred in 6 patients (6.8 %) in low GRACE group and 12 patients (18.7 %) in intermediate to high GRACE group ($P = 0.024$). The cumulative of composite cardiovascular outcome was significant higher in intermediate to high GRACE group than in low GRACE group (Hazard ratio: 2.97, 95 % CI 1.11–7.90; $p = 0.030$).

(Continued on next page)

* Correspondence: arintaya.p@cmu.ac.th
[3]Cardiology Division, Department of Internal Medicine, Faculty of Medicine, Chiang Mai University, Chiang Mai 50200, Thailand
Full list of author information is available at the end of the article

(Continued from previous page)

Conclusion: The long delay pharmacoinvasive strategy in intermediate to high GRACE score after successful fibrinolysis in non PCI-capable facilities were associated with worse cardiovascular outcomes than the patients with low GRACE score at 1 and 6 months. GRACE risk score may be helpful and guided the clinicians in non PCI-capable center in early transferred to early intervention in STEMI patients after fibrinolytic therapy.

Keywords: GRACE risk score, STEMI patients with successfully fibrinolysis, Delay pharmacoinvasive strategy

Background

Primary percutaneous coronary intervention (PPCI) is preferred reperfusion therapy for acute ST-elevation myocardial infarction (STEMI). However, the PCI-capable center is still limited in several countries including Thailand. Therefore, fibrinolytic therapy is the main reperfusion therapy for most STEMI patients in our country. Current practice guidelines recommended routine coronary angiogram (CAG) after successful fibrinolysis, the so called pharmacoinvasive strategy [1–5]. However, early pharmacoinvasive (within 3–24 h after successful fibrinolysis) cannot be performed in a timely fashion due to limitation of PCI-capable hospitals. Previous acute coronary syndrome (ACS) registries, Thailand Registry in Acute Coronary Syndrome (TRACS) showed a low rate of coronary angiography and intervention during index admission and referral centers for early pharmacoinvasive strategy are still limited [6]. Therefore, risk stratification and identify risk of the patients are important in non PCI-capable hospital. Patients with intermediate to high risk for adverse cardiovascular event should be transferred for coronary angiogram as soon as possible. Although several risk scores for acute coronary syndrome (ACS) have been developed for stratified risk of ACS patients, GRACE (Global Registry of Acute Coronary Events) score is developed to focus on clinical risk assessment and to improve the selection of patients for clinical and interventional procedures following an ACS episode [7]. Many studies and meta-analysis demonstrated the accuracy and the usefulness of the GRACE score on the mortality of ACS patients in hospital and follow-up after hospital discharged [8–13]. This study aimed to evaluate the prognostic utility of the GRACE score in patients receiving delayed intervention after successful fibrinolysis.

Methods

Study design and population

We retrospectively analysed the data from the Maharaj Nakorn Chiang Mai Hospital STEMI registry during the period 2007–2012. The STEMI patients who had successfully fibrinolysis in non PCI-capable hospital and received delayed coronary intervention (during 24 h to 14 days after successful fibrinolytic therapy) at Maharaj Nakorn Chiang Mai hospital were included for analysis in the study. The exclusion criteria were the patients who unsuccessfully fibrinolysis (ST-segment decrease in

elevation less than 50 % at 90 min after fibrinolysis), received early coronary intervention (<24 h after fibrinolytic therapy), received very delayed coronary intervention (>2 weeks after fibrinolytic therapy), the patients who denied for further interventions after fibrinolysis, the patients who received primary PCI or rescue PCI and the patients who had the previous history of coronary-artery bypass surgery. The protocol design was approved by the local institutional Research Ethics Committees of Faculty of Medicine, Chiang Mai University and Lampang hospital.

The data were collected from the medical recorded by the researcher. Demographic characteristics, medical history, presenting symptoms, baseline GRACE score time from symptom onset to administration fibrinolytic therapy, time from fibrinolysis to percutaneous coronary intervention, coronary intervention procedure and clinical outcomes were collected for analysis. In the patients who did not visit to the hospital to follow up, the telephone call was used to interview for evaluating the clinical outcomes.

Definitions and end points

The STEMI was defined as the presence of at least 0.1-mV ST-segment elevation or new or presumably new left bundle branch block with elevation of cardiac enzyme levels above the reference range. Successfully fibrinolysis means the ST-segment decrease in elevation ≥ 50 % (partial resolution) and ≥ 70 % (complete resolution) at 90 min after fibrinolysis. Delayed coronary intervention means coronary intervention, including coronary angiogram and percutaneous coronary intervention performed during 24 h to 14 days after successfully fibrinolysis. The GRACE score composed of medical history (age, history of congestive heart failure, and history of myocardial infarction), findings at initial presentation (resting heart rate, systolic blood pressure, and ST-segment depression), and findings during hospitalization (initial serum creatinine, elevation of cardiac enzyme, and no in-hospital PCI), the total score range from 0–258 points. The patients were stratified into low (GRACE risk score <126), intermediate to high risk group (GRACE risk score ≥ 126). The primary end point for this analysis was composite outcomes, which included all-cause mortality, re-hospitalization with

ACS, re-hospitalization with heart failure (HF) and stroke at 1 and 6-month. Re-hospitalized with ACS was defined as re-admission after discharge from hospital with ACS composed with clinical chest pain, rising of cardiac enzymes and dynamic ST-segment change. Re-hospitalized with heart failure was defined as re--admission after discharge from hospital with clinical de-compensated heart failure or received intravenous diuretic. Culprit vessel PCI was defined as PCI confined to culprit vessel lesion only. The multivessel PCI was defined as PCI in which lesions in the culprit vessel as well as ≥1 non-culprit vessel lesions.

Statistical analysis

Baseline demographics, procedural and angiographic characteristics presented with continuous measures and are expressed as mean ± standard deviation (SD) or me-dian and interquartile range (IQR) wherever appropriate. The categorical data are expressed as number (percent-ages), except where indicated. Differences in continuous variables were analyzed with the Student's t test or Wilcoxon rank-sum tests. The categorical variables were analyzed with Chi-square test and Fisher's exact test. A P-value <0.05 was considered statistically significant. Composite endpoints and other clinical outcomes will be expressed as number (percentages). The prognostic utility of GRACE score on clinical outcomes was analyzed by logistic regression analysis and presented as odd ratio and area under the ROC curve (AuROC). The composite outcome was analyzed by use time to event analysis and presented with Kaplan-Meier curve. We conducted statistical analyses using Stata version 13 (Stata corporation, College Station, TX). The sample size was calculated by base on the data of the previous study of Yan et al. [14] reported death/myocardial re-infarction at 30 days in the standard treatment was 8.1 % and estimated 5 % loss of follow-up. To achieve a power of 80 %, with a type-1 error probability of 5 % (two-sided), allowable of estimated error (margin error) was 5 %, 120 patients were needed in this study.

Results

Baseline clinical characteristics

Among 3171 STEMI patients during study period, 2045 STEMI patients received fibrinolytic therapy and a total of 152 patients met inclusion criteria, as shown in Fig. 1. Eighty-eight patients and 64 patients were in low GRACE group (GRACE risk score ≤ 125) and intermedi-ate to high GRACE group (GRACE risk score above 126), respectively. The 6-month follow-up was available in 97 % of the patients in both groups. The clinical characteristics were shown in Table 1. The median time from fibrinolysis to coronary intervention in low GRACE group was 8.5 days (interquartile range, 4.6–10.9) and

7.9 days (interquartile range,3.2,12.0) in intermediate to high GRACE group ($p = 0.482$) (Additional file 1).

Angiographic findings, procedural details and complications of the procedure

Angiographic findings and procedural details were presented in Table 2. Double vessel disease and triple vessel disease presented in 45.5 and 65.6 % in low GRACE group and intermediate to high GRACE group respectively. Lesion type B2 and C presented in 44.6 and 53.8 % in low GRACE group and intermediate to high GRACE group respectively. Sixty-three percent ($N = 56$) of the patients in low GRACE group and 61 % ($N = 39$) of the patients in intermediate to high GRACE group underwent PCI ($P = 0.738$) while 36 % of the patients in low GRACE group ($N = 32$) and 39 % of the patients in intermediate to high GRACE group ($N = 25$) had only coronary angiography ($p = 0.738$). Culprit vessel PCI was performed in 89 % ($N = 50$) of the patients in low GRACE group and 92 % ($N = 36$) of the patients in intermediate to high GRACE group (=0.733). Among the patients underwent PCI, 76.8 % ($N = 43$) of the patients in low GRACE group and 76.3 % ($N = 29$) of the patients in intermediate to high GRACE group received drug-eluting stent (DES). The complications during and post procedure were shown in Table 3.

Clinical outcomes

At 1 month, the composite cardiovascular outcome at 1 month occurred in 2 patients (2.3 %) in low GRACE group and 10 patients (15.6 %) in intermediate to high GRACE group ($P = 0.003$). During 6 months, the com-posite cardiovascular outcomes occurred in 6 patients (6.8 %) in low GRACE group and 12 patients (18.7 %) in intermediate to high GRACE group ($p = 0.024$) (Table 4). There was no death in hospital in low GRACE group when 2 patients (3.1 %) in intermediate to high GRACE group died ($P = 0.176$). Rate of re-hospitalized with HF at 1 and 6 months were significantly higher in inter-mediate to high GRACE group than low GRACE group (9.4 % vs 1.1 %, $p = 0.022$ and 10.9 % vs 2.3 %, $p = 0.036$, respectively).

The GRACE score and clinical outcomes

The composite cardiovascular outcome and re-hospitalized with HF at 6 months were higher in intermediate to high GRACE group than in the low GRACE group (OR: 3.20, 95 % CI: 1.13–9.06; $P = 0.029$ and OR: 5.34, 95 % CI: 1.07–26.68; $P = 0.041$ respectively). The cumulative of composite cardiovascular outcome was significant higher in intermediate to high GRACE group than in low GRACE group (Hazard ratio: 2.97, 95 % CI 1.11–7.90; $P = 0.030$), as shown in Fig. 2. We analysed the prognostic utility of GRACE score on clinical outcomes by the evidence from

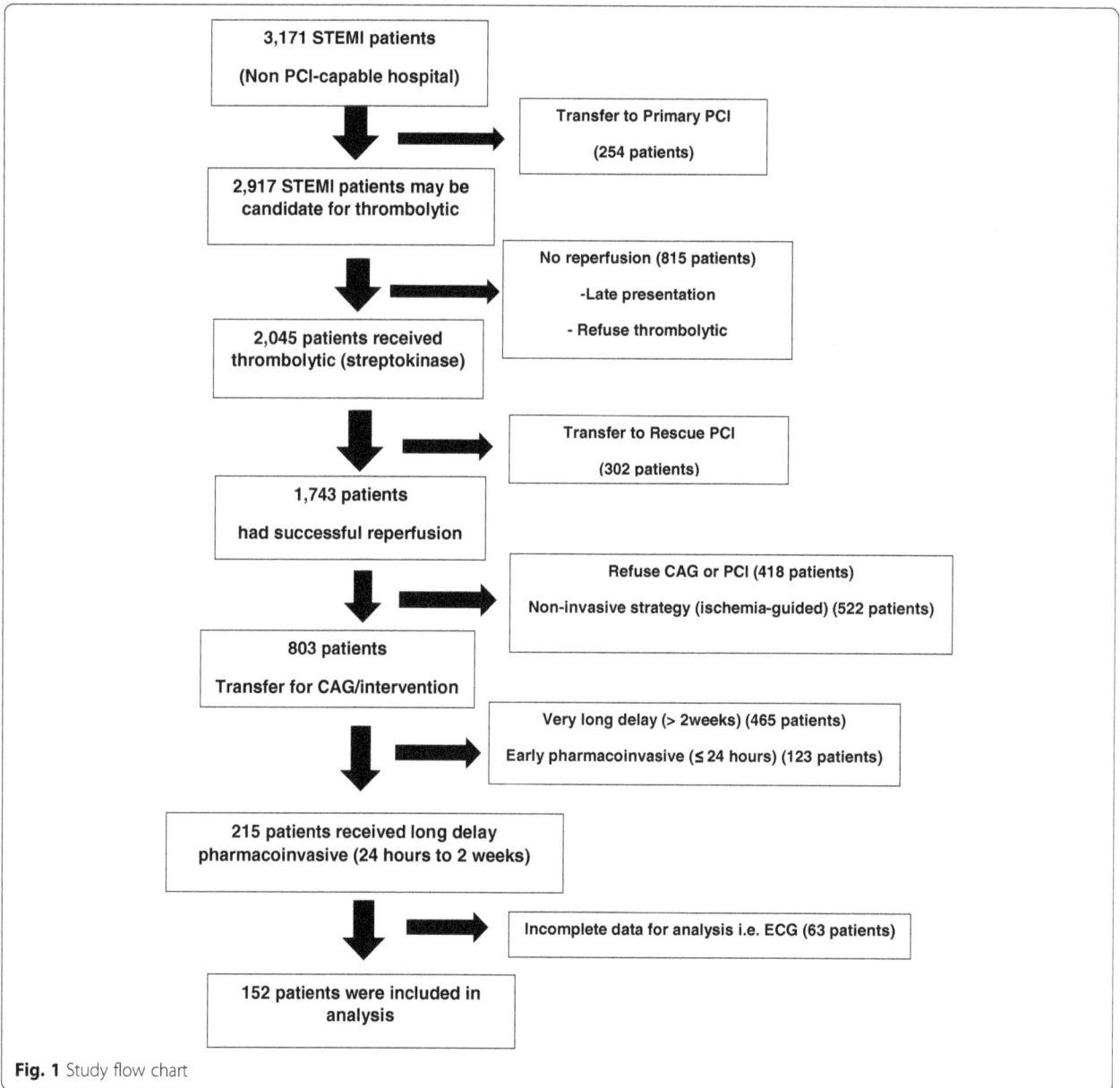

Fig. 1 Study flow chart

the area under the ROC curve. The area under the ROC (AuROC) of GRACE score for 6-month cardiovascular death was 0.794 (95 % CI 0.75–0.83). The AuROC of composite cardiovascular outcomes was 0.641 (95 % CI 0.52–0.76), as shown in Fig. 3.

Discussion

Although early pharmacoinvasive strategy (within 3–24 h) after successful reperfusion are recommended by several guidelines [1–5], timely fashion CAG is not widely available in countries with limited PCI capable hospitals including Thailand. Several randomized trials and meta-analysis have shown that early routine post-thrombolysis angiography with subsequent PCI reduced the rates of re-infarction and recurrent ischemia

compared with a watchful waiting strategy, in which angiography and revascularization were indicated only in the patients with spontaneous or induced severe ischemia or left ventricular (LV) dysfunction [15, 16]. The benefits of early routine PCI after thrombolysis were seen in the absence of increased risk of adverse events in many studies [15, 16]. The data from TRACS showed only half (50 %) of STEMI patients performed CAG on index admission. Fibrinolysis (especially streptokinase), is the first choice for treatment in low risk STEMI patients (42.6 % of STEMI patients received streptokinase and 1 % received Tenecteptase) [6]. Because of only one cardiac catheterization (during the period 2007–2012) in Northern Thailand (Maharaj Nakorn Chiang Mai Catheterization laboratory), the

Table 1 Baseline clinical characteristics of patients according to GRACE risk score (n = 152)

Clinical characteristics	Low GRACE group (N = 88)	Intermediate to high GRACE group (N = 64)	P-value
Age (years), mean ± SD	55.3 ± 8.5	67.7 ± 3.2	< 0.001
Gender, (%)			0.696
Male	55(62.5)	38(59.4)	
Female	33(37.5)	26 (40.6)	
Time from symptoms onset to fibrinolysis, median (hours) (IQR:25th,75th percentile)	2.7 (IQR: 2,3.8)	2.8 (IQR: 2,4.5)	0.347
Time from fibrinolysis to CAG or PCI median (days) (IQR:25th,75th percentile)	8.5 (IQR:4.6,10.9)	7.9 (IQR: 3.2,12.0)	0.482
GRACE score, mean ± SD	100.2 ± 15.7	142.2 ± 13.4	< 0.001
LVEF (%)	54.9 ± 10.6	52.5 ± 13.6	0.239
Preexisting medical conditions, n (%)			
Diabetes	18 (20.4)	10.6 (15.6)	0.448
Hypertension	39 (44.3)	27 (42.2)	0.794
Dyslipidemia	30 (34.1)	16 (25.0)	0.228
Smoking	50 (56.8)	34 (53.1)	0.651
Chronic kidney disease	3 (3.4)	3 (4.7)	0.681

Table 2 Angiographic findings and procedural details (n = 152)

Angiographic findings and procedural details	Low GRACE group (N = 88)	Intermediate to high GRACE group (N = 64)	P-value
Angiographic findings, n (%)			
Mild disease	9 (10.2)	1 (1.6)	0.045
Single vessel disease	39 (44.3)	21 (32.8)	0.180
Double vessel disease	24 (27.3)	22 (34.4)	0.375
Triple vessel disease	16 (18.2)	20 (31.2)	0.082
Lesions (according to ACC/AHA), n (%)			
Type A	14 (25.0)	7 (18.0)	0.461
Type B1	17 (30.4)	11 (28.2)	0.503
Type B2	17 (30.4)	10 (25.6)	0.651
Type C	8 (14.2)	11 (28.2)	0.120
Procedural performed			
CAG without PCI, n (%)	32 (36.4)	25 (39.1)	0.738
Medical treatment	26 (81.2)	15 (60.0)	0.136
CABG	6 (18.8)	10 (40.0)	0.136
PCI, n (%)	56 (63.6)	39 (60.9)	0.738
Culprit vessel PCI	50 (89.3)	36 (92.3)	0.733
Multivessel PCI	6 (10.7)	3 (7.7)	0.733
Procedural details, n (%)			
POBA	1 (1.8)	6 (15.4)	0.018
Thrombus aspiration	0 (0)	3 (7.7)	0.066
Bare metal stent	13 (23.2)	5 (13.2)	0.290
Drug eluting stent	43 (76.8)	29 (76.3)	0.574

Table 3 Complications during and post-procedure (n = 152)

Complications	Low GRACE group (N = 88)	Intermediate to high GRACE group (N = 64)	P-value
During procedure, n (%)			
Abrupt vessel closure	0 (0)	0 (0)	NS
New thrombus formation	2 (3.57)	0 (0)	0.511
Side branch occlusion	0 (0)	0 (0)	NS
No reflow	2 (3.57)	0 (0)	0.511
Dissection	1 (1.8)	0 (0)	0.589
Emergency unplanned CABG	0 (0)	0 (0)	NS
Post procedure, n (%)			
Hematoma	0 (0)	0 (0)	NS
Hematuria	1 (1.1)	0 (0)	0.579
Gastrointestinal bleeding	0 (0)	0 (0)	NS
Required blood transfusion	0 (0)	0 (0)	NS
Contrast-induced nephropathy	0 (0)	0 (0)	NS

geographic and long distance of transfer and few of number of interventional cardiologists, primary PCI and early routine PCI after successful fibrinolysis were very difficult for this situation. Rescue PCI or primary PCI were performed in the patients who failed fibrinolytic therapy or cardiogenic shock at presentation. Hence, most of the STEMI patients in Thailand, especially in Northern of Thailand who successfully fibrinolytic therapy received the long delay coronary intervention (more than 24 h after fibrinolysis) and some of them received elective PCI or very long delayed intervention or elective PCI (after 2 weeks from successful fibrinolytic therapy) [6]. Several studies demonstrated the worst cardiovascular outcomes in the patients who received delay coronary intervention after thrombolysis [15–21]. The Southwest German Interventional Study in Acute Myocardial infarction (SIAM III) evaluated the effects of transfer early PCI (within 6 h after fibrinolysis) compared with delay PCI strategy (elective PCI 2 weeks after fibrinolysis) [17]. The early PCI showed significant reduction of primary end point (death, re-infarction, target lesion revascularization (TLR) and ischemic events) (HR: 0.61; 95 % CI 0.42–0.88, p = 0.008) and higher long term survival than delayed PCI (p = 0.057) [17]. Similarly to The Trial of Routine Angioplasty and Stenting after Fibrinolysis to Enhance Reperfusion in Acute Myocardial Infarction (TRANSFER-AMI) trial, showed that the patients who transfer from non-PCI

Table 4 Clinical outcomes at 1 and 6 months of follow-up ($n = 152$)

Clinical outcomes	Low GRACE group ($N = 88$)	Intermediate to high GRACE group ($N = 64$)	P-value
In-hospital mortality, n (%)	0 (0)	2 (3.1)	0.095
At 1 month			
Composite outcomes	2 (2.3)	10 (15.6)	0.003
ACS	1 (1.1)	1 (1.6)	0.666
Heart failure	1 (1.1)	6 (9.4)	0.022
Stroke	0 (0)	1 (1.6)	0.421
CV death	0 (0)	2 (3.1)	0.180
Non-CV death	0 (0)	0 (0)	NS
Loss to follow-up	2 (2.3)	2 (3.1)	0.562
At 6 month (cumulative)			
Composite outcomes	6 (6.8)	12 (18.7)	0.024
ACS	4 (4.5)	1 (1.6)	0.298
Heart failure	2 (2.3)	7 (10.9)	0.036
Stroke	0 (0)	2 (3.1)	0.421
CV death	0 (0)	2 (3.1)	0.175
Non-CV death	0 (0)	0(0)	NS
Loss to follow-up	2 (2.3)	2 (3.1)	0.562

center within 6 h after thrombolysis had fewer ischemic complications than standard treatment (delayed PCI) without increasing of major bleeding [18]. A meta-analysis showed mortality benefit at 30-day and 1 year of the STEMI patients with early transfer PCI after fibrinolysis as compared with ischemic-guided intervention (delayed PCI) [15, 16]. The NORwegian study on District treatment of ST-Elevation Myocardial infarction (NORDISTEMI) study also demonstrated a significant reduction in the composite cardiovascular outcome (death, re-infarction, stroke, or recurrent ischemia) at 1 year in the patients with immediate transferred to PCI following with thrombolysis as compared with the patients in conservative arm treatment (6 % vs 16 %, $p = 0.01$) [19]. Similarly to The Combined Abciximab RE-teplase Stent Study in Acute Myocardial Infarction (CARESS-AMI) study, a more conservative strategy (i.e. angiogram only in cases of failed thrombolysis) was associated with a worse clinical outcome than the strategy of angiogram and intervention (if indicated) in all cases following thrombolysis (composite of death, re-infarction and refractory ischemia at 30-day, 11 % vs 4 %, $p = 0.004$) [20]. From the previous data, no studies demonstrated of the benefit in the cardiovascular outcomes of the early and/or delay pharmacoinvasive strategies in STEMI patients who received streptokinase for treatment similar to our study. On the data from CARESS-AMI [20] and TRANSFER-AMI [18], The American College of Cardiology (ACC) and the American heart association (AHA) give a class IIa

recommendations for high risk features (such as Kilip class >2, extensive ST-elevation, left ventricular ejection fraction (LVEF) <35 %, or hypotension) should be immediate transferred to PCI-capable facilities [3, 4]. The transfer of low and moderate risk STEMI patients to PCI-capable center received a class IIb recommendation. No available data showed the benefit outcome of early transferred for PCI in low and moderate risk patients.

Risk stratification of the STEMI patients were very important for the clinicians in non-PCI capable hospital to use to guide for judged and selected the STEMI patients for early invasive strategy. GRACE risk score, one of clinical risk score, has been shown to be a good risk stratification score in population with STEMI and NSTE-ACS. Several studies demonstrated the validation and the usefulness of GRACE score in stratified the STEMI patients for an early invasive management (AUC = 0.81; 95 % CI 0.80–0.82 for STEMI and AUC = 0.80; 95 % CI 0.74–0.89 for NSTE-ACS) [12]. The AuROC of 6-month mortality and the composite cardiovascular outcome of our study were 0.794 (95 % CI 0.75–0.83) and 0.641 (95 % CI 0.52–0.76). From our study, the GRACE score seem to be better performance in the cardiovascular mortality rather than the composite cardiovascular outcome of the patients with long delay pharmacoinvasive as similar as the previous study [12]. But the usefulness of GRACE score for predict the composite cardiovascular outcome is still unclear. A subgroup analysis of TRANSFER-AMI trial revealed the beneficial outcome of early pharmacoinvasive strategy only in patient with a low to intermediate GRACE risk score (<155), while the early invasive strategy was associated with worse outcome in high-risk patients (≥155) [14]. The pharmacoinvasive strategy was associated with a lower risk of death/re-MI in the low-intermediate GRACE risk group (HR = 0.52, 95 % CI 0.32–0.86, $p = 0.010$), but a higher risk of death/re-MI in the GRACE high-risk group (HR = 1.98, 95 % CI 1.06–3.67, $p = 0.031$) [14]. From this subgroup analysis from TRANSFER-AMI, risk score may also guide the best strategy to achieve and maintain myocardial reperfusion after administration of fibrinolytic therapy [14]. Similar to our study, the longer delay pharmacoinvasive strategy (24 h to 2 weeks after successful fibrinolysis) in non PCI-capable facilities may associate with the worst of composite cardiovascular outcome (death, re-hospitalized with ACS, re-hospitalized with HF and stroke) at 30-day and 6-month when compared with the patients with low GRACE score (15.6 % vs 2.3 % at 30 days, $p = 0.003$ and 16.7 % vs 6.8 % at 6 months, $p = 0.024$). Therefore, the patients with intermediate to high GRACE risk score should be early transferred to PCI-capable center after fibrinolytic therapy.

The in-hospital mortality and 6-month mortality of our study was lower than the previous registry (TRACS) because the difference in baseline patient characteristics, the severity of the patients and the number of the

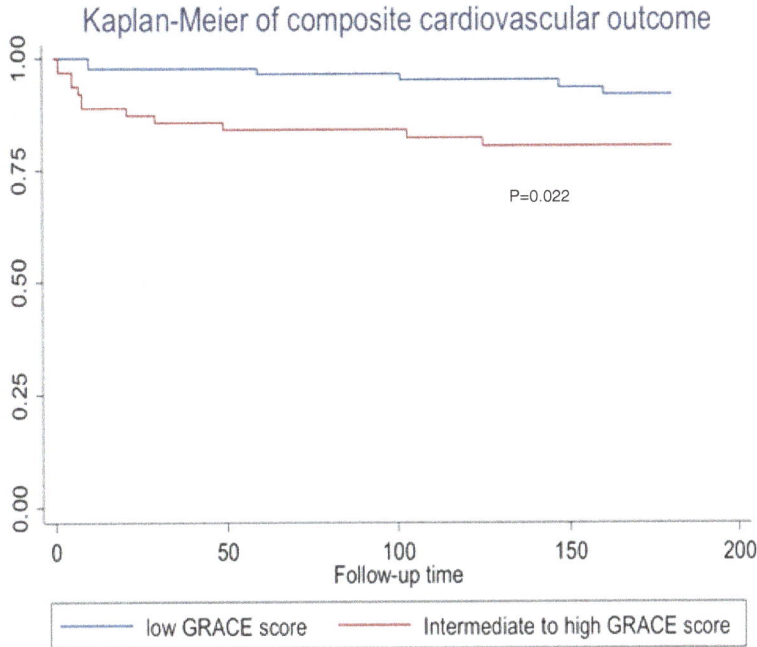

Fig. 2 Kaplan-Meier of composite cardiovascular outcome

patients received of the percutaneous coronary intervention on admission (in-hospital mortality 5.3 % vs 3.1 % and 6-month mortality 12.1 % vs 3.1 %) [6]. Most of the patients in our study had multivessel disease but underwent culprit vessel PCI only in significant proportion of patients. A small number of the patients underwent multivessel PCI during index hospitalization (10.7 % in low GRACE group vs 7.7 % in intermediate to high GRACE group). The meta-analysis and systematic review of Moretti et al. [22] in management multivessel coronary disease in STEMI patients, 5855 patients from 6 studies (1 RCT) compared between only culprilt vessel PCI vs complete PCI performed during index hospitalization. No difference in major adverse cardio-vascular events (MACE) at short-term (90 days) and long term outcome at 1 year but significant reduced the repeat revascularization at 1 year similar to culprit vessel PCI vs complete revascularization during PCI. The rate of CABG was high especially in intermediate

to high GRACE group because of high prevalence of multivessel disease and complex coronary artery disease (Type B2 and C) which may suitable for CABG after acute phase of STEMI. Previous ACS registry in Thailand (TRACS) showed the lower rate of CABG but the revascularization data was collected only in hospital-phase of STEMI [6]. The selective biased in enrolled patients who survived during index admission may contribute to low cardiovascular event in our study. We showed the performance of GRACE score for mortality of in-hospital, short term (30 days) and 6-month Therefore, the GRACE risk score is useful for prediction in short- and long-term mortality of the STEMI patients with successful fibrinolysis and delay intervention in non PCI-capable hospital.

There are some limitations in our study that may compromise clinical implication. Our study was a retrospective observational study (non-randomized). The large number of excluded patients reflected the limited

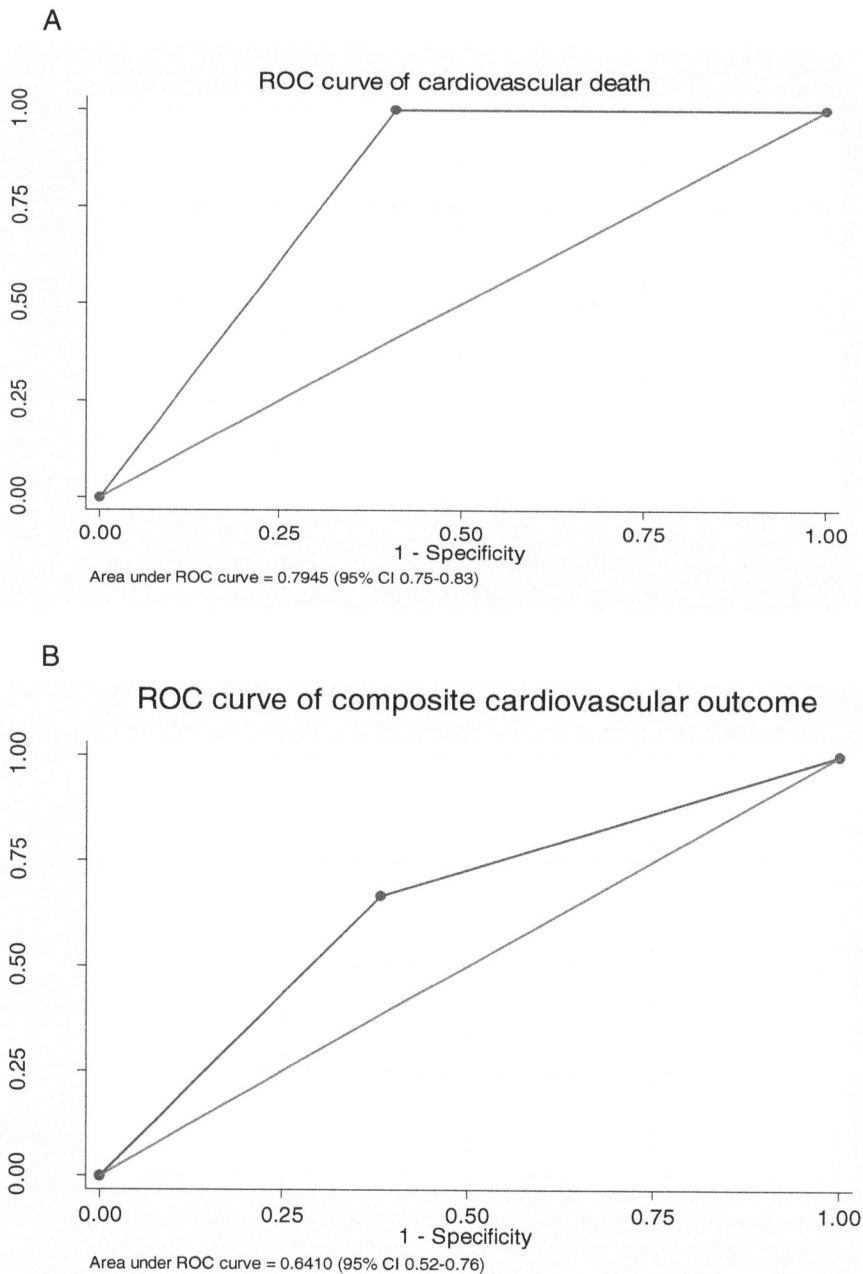

Fig. 3 The Area under the Curve (AuROC) for the performance of GRACE score in predicting cardiovascular event. **a** 6-month cardiovascular death 6-month cardiovascular death (AuROC =0.794, 95 % CI 0.75–0.83). **b** Composite cardiovascular outcome (AuROC = 0.641, 95% CI 0.52–0.76)

accessibility to coronary intervention within 2 weeks. The mortality was lower than the previous study because the small number of patients with high GRACE risk were included in our study.

Conclusion

The long delay pharmacoinvasive strategy in intermediate to high GRACE score after successful fibrinolysis in non PCI-capable facilities were associated with worse cardiovascular outcomes (death, re-hospitalized with ACS, re-hospitalized with HF and stroke) than the patients with low GRACE score at 30 days and 6 months. GRACE risk score may be helpful and guided the clinicians in non PCI-capable center in early transferred to early intervention in STEMI patients after fibrinolytic therapy.

Abbreviations
ACC: The American College of Cardiology; ACS: Acute coronary syndrome; AHA: The American heart association; AuROC: Area under receiver operating characteristic; BMI: Body mass index; CAG: Coronary angiography; CARESS-AMI: The combined abciximab RE-teplase stent study in acute myocardial infarction study; CV: Cardiovascular; GRACE score: The Global Registry for Acute Coronary Events score; HF: Heart failure; IQR: Interquartile range; LVEF: Left ventricular ejection fraction; MACE: Major adverse cardiovascular events; NORDISTEMI: The NORwegian study on District treatment of ST-Elevation Myocardial infarction study; NS: No statistical significant; NSTE-ACS: Non ST-elevation acute coronary syndrome; PCI: Percutaneous coronary intervention; PPCI: Primary percutaneous coronary intervention; RCT: Randomized control trial; ROC: Receiver operating characteristic; SD: Standard deviation; SIAM III: Southwest German Interventional Study in Acute Myocardial infarction study group; STEMI: ST- elevation myocardial infarction; TLR: Target lesion revascularization; TRACS: Thailand Registry in Acute Coronary Syndrome; TRANSFER-MAI trial: The trial of routine angioplasty and stenting after fibrinolysis to enhance reperfusion in acute myocardial infarction

Acknowledgments
I would like to special thank all staffs from Cardiology Division, Department of Internal Medicine, Chiang Mai University. I also thank nurses and all administers in Northern Cardiac Center, who always helpful and supported me in data collection.

Funding
No source of funding were used to conducted this study or prepare this manuscript.

Authors' contributions
All authors made substantial contributions to conception, design, and drafting the manuscript. YC design study, conducted the data collection, analysis and prepared the manuscript. AP, RM, JP, TC, SK, NT, TB and AS conducted a critical review of the manuscript and provided final editing to the manuscript. All authors read and approved the final manuscript.

Competing interests
The authors declare that they have no competing interests.

Author details
[1]Clinical Epidemiology Program, Faculty of Medicine, Chiang Mai University, Chiang Mai 50200, Thailand. [2]Cardiology Division, Internal Medicine Department, Lampang Hospital, Lampang 52000, Thailand. [3]Cardiology Division, Department of Internal Medicine, Faculty of Medicine, Chiang Mai University, Chiang Mai 50200, Thailand. [4]Pharmaceutical Care Unit, Pharmacy Department, Lampang Hospital, Lampang 52000, Thailand. [5]Center of Excellence in Applied Epidemiology, Faculty of Medicine, Thammasat University, Bangkok 12121, Thailand. [6]Cardiac catheterization laboratory Unit, Maharaj Nakorn Chiang Mai Hospital, Chiang Mai, Thailand50200.

References
1. Wijns W, Kolh P, Danchin N, Di Mario C, Falk V, Folliguet T, Garg S, Huber K, James S, Knuuti J, Lopez-Sendon J, Marco J, Menicanti L, Ostojic M, Piepoli MF, Pirlet C, Pomar JL, Reifart N, Ribichini FL, Schalij MJ, Sergeant P, Serruys PW, Silber S, Uva MS, Taggart D. Guidelines on myocardial revascularization. The Task Force on Myocardial Revascularization of the European Society of Cardiology (ESC) and the European Association for Cardio-Thoracic Surgery (EACTS). Developed with the special contribution of the European Association for Percutaneous Cardiovascular Interventions (EAPCI). Eur Heart J. 2010;31:2501–55.

2. Steg PG, James SK, Atar D, Badano LP, Blomstrom-Lundqvist C, Borger MA, Di Mario C, Dickstein K, Ducrocq G, Fernandez-Aviles F, Gershlick AH, Giannuzzi P, Halvorsen S, Huber K, Juni P, Kastrati A, Knuuti J, Lenzen MJ, Mahaffey KW, Valgimigli M, van't Hof A, Widimsky P, Zahger D. ESC

guidelines for the management of acute myocardial infarction in patients presenting with ST-segment elevation. Eur Heart J. 2012;33:2569–619.

3. Levine GN, Bates ER, Blankenship JC, Bailey SR, Bittl JA, Cercek B, Chambers CE, Ellis SG, Guyton RA, Hollenberg SM, Khot UN, Lange RA, Mauri L, Mehran R, Moussa ID, Mukherjee D, Nallamothu BK, Ting HH. 2011 ACCF/AHA/SCAI guideline for percutaneous coronary intervention: a report of the American College of Cardiology Foundation/American Heart Association Task Force on Practice Guidelines and the Society for Cardiovascular Angiography and Interventions. J Am Coll Cardiol. 2011;58(24):e44–122.

4. O'Gara PT, Kushner FG, Ascheim DD, Casey Jr DE, Chung MK, de Lemos JA, Ettinger SM, Fang JC, Fesmire FM, Franklin BA, Granger CB, Krumholz HM, Linderbaum JA, Morrow DA, Newby LK, Ornato JP, Ou N, Radford MJ, Tamis-Holland JE, Tommaso CL, Tracy CM, Woo YJ, Zhao DX, Anderson JL, Jacobs AK, Halperin JL, Albert NM, Brindis RG, Creager MA, DeMets D, Guyton RA, Hochman JS, Kovacs RJ, Ohman EM, Stevenson WG, Yancy CW. 2013 ACCF/AHA guideline for the management of ST-elevation myocardial infarction: a report of the American College of Cardiology Foundation/American Heart Association Task Force on Practice Guidelines. Circulation. 2013;127(4):e362–425.

5. Windecker S, Kolh P, Alfonso F, Collet JP, Cremer J, Falk V, Filippatos G, Hamm C, Head SJ, Juani P, Kappetein AP, Kastrati A, Knuuti J, Landmesser U, Laufer G, Neumann FJ, Richter DJ, Schauerte P, Uva MS, Stefanini GG, Taggart DP, Torracca L, Valgimigli M, Wijns W, Witkowski A. 2014 ESC/EACTS Guidelines on myocardial revascularization: The Task Force on Myocardial Revascularization of the European Society of Cardiology (ESC) and the European Association for Cardio-Thoracic Surgery (EACTS)Developed with the special contribution of the European Association of Percutaneous Cardiovascular Interventions (EAPCI). Eur Heart J. 2014;35(37):2541–619.

6. Srimahachota S, Boonyaratavej S, Kanjanavanit R, Sritara P, Krittayaphong R, Kunjara-Na-ayudhya R, Tatsanavivat P, TRACS Group. Thai Registry in Acute Coronary Syndrome (TRACS)-An Extension of Thai Acute Coronary Syndrome Registry (TACS) Group: Lower In-hospital but still high mortality at one-year. J Med Assoc Thai. 2012;95(4):508–18.

7. The GRACE Investigators. Rationale and design of the GRACE (Global Registry of Acute Coronary Events) project: a multinational registry of patients hospitalized with acute coronary syndromes. Am Heart J. 2001;141:190–9.

8. Eagle KA, Lim MJ, Dabbous OH, GRACE Investigators, et al. A validated prediction model for all forms of acute coronary syndromes in an international registry. JAMA. 2004;291:2727–33.

9. Granger CB, Goldberg RJ, Dabbous O, Pieper KS, Eagle KA, Cannon CP, Van de Werf F, Avezum A, Goodman SG, Flather MD, Fox KAA, for the GRACE Investigators. Predictors of hospital mortality in the global registry of acute coronary events. Arch Intern Med. 2003;163:2345–53.

10. Fox KAA, Carruthers KF, Dunba DR, Graham C, Manning JR, Raedt HD, Buysschaert I, Lambrechts D, Van de Werf F. Underestimated and under-recognized: the late consequences of acute coronary syndrome (GRACE UK–Belgian study). Eur Heart J. 2010;31:2755–64.

11. Tang EW, Wong CK, Herbison P. Global Registry of Acute Coronary Events (GRACE) hospital discharge risk score accurately predicts long term mortality post acute coronary syndrome. Am Heart J. 2007;153(1):29–35.

12. Ascenzo FD, Biondi-Zoccai G, Moretti C, Bollati M, Omedè P, Sciuto F, Presutti DG, Modena MG, Gasparini M, Reed MJ, Sheiban I, Gaita F. TIMI, GRACE and alternative risk scores in acute coronary syndromes: a meta-analysis of 40 derivation studies on 216,552 patients and of 42 validation studies on 31,625 patients. Contemp Clin Trials. 2012;33:507–14.

13. Elbarouni B, Goodman SG, Yan RT, Welsh RC, Kornder JM, Deyoung JP, et al. Validation of the Global Registry of Acute Coronary Event (GRACE) risk score for in-hospital mortality in patients with acute coronary syndrome in Canada. Canadian Global Registry of Acute Coronary Events (GRACE/GRACE (2)) investigators. Am Heart J. 2009;158:392–9.

14. Yan AT, Yan RT, Cantor WJ, Borgundvaag B, Cohen EA, Fitchett DH, Dzavik V, Ducas J, Tan M, Casanova A, Goodman SG, for the TRANSFER-AMI Investigators. Relationship between risk stratification at admission and treatment effects of early invasive management following fibrinolysis: insights from the Trial of Routine ANgioplasty and Stenting after Fibrinolysis to Enhance Reperfusion in Acute Myocardial Infarction (TRANSFER-AMI). Eur Heart J. 2011;32:1994–2002.

15. Borgia F, Goodman SG, Halvorsen S, Cantor WJ, Piscione F, Le May MR, Fernandez-Aviles F, Sanchez PL, Dimopoulos K, Scheller B, Armstrong PW, Di Mario C. Early routine percutaneous coronary intervention after fibrinolysis

vs. standard therapy in ST-segment elevation myocardial infarction: a meta-analysis. Eur Heart J. 2010;31:2156–69.

16. D'Souza SP, Mamas MA, Fraser DG, Fath-Ordoubadi F. Routine early coronary angioplasty vs. ischaemia-guided angioplasty after thrombolysis in acute ST-elevation myocardial infarction: a meta-analysis. Eur Heart J. 2011;32(8):972–82.

17. Scheller B, Hennen B, Hammer B, Walle J, Hofer C, Hilpert V, Winter H, Nickenig G, Böhm M, SIAM III Study Group. Beneficial effects of immediate stenting after thrombolysis in acute myocardial infarction. J Am Coll Cardiol. 2003;42:634–41.

18. Cantor WJ, Fitchett D, Borgundvaag B, Ducas J, Heffernan M, Cohen EA, Morrison LJ, Langer A, Dzavik V, Mehta SR, Lazzam C, Schwartz B, Casanova A, Goodman SG, TRANSFER-AMI Trial Investigators. Routine early angioplasty after fibrinolysis for acute myocardial infarction. N Engl J Med. 2009;360:2705–18.

19. Bohmer E, Hoffmann P, Abdelnoor M, Arnesen H, Halvorsen S. Efficacy and safety of immediate angioplasty versus ischemia-guided management after thrombolysis in acute myocardial infarction in areas with very long transfer distances results of the NORDISTEMI (NORwegian study on DIstrict treatment of ST-elevation myocardial infarction). J Am Coll Cardiol. 2010;55:102–10.

20. Di Mario C, Dudek D, Piscione F, Mielecki W, Savonitto S, Murena E, Dimopoulos K, Manari A, Gaspardone A, Ochala A, Zmudka K, Bolognese L, Steg PG, Flather M, CARESS-in-AMI (Combined Abciximab RE-teplase Stent Study in Acute Myocardial Infarction) Investigators. Immediate angioplasty versus standard therapy with rescue angioplasty after thrombolysis in the combined Abciximab REteplase Stent Study in Acute Myocardial Infarction (CARESS-in-AMI): an open, prospective, randomised, multicentre trial. Lancet. 2008;371:559–68.

21. Clever YP, Cremers B, Link A, Böhm M, Scheller B. Long-term follow-up of early versus delayed invasive approach after fibrinolysis in acute myocardial infarction. Circ Cardiovasc Interv. 2011;4:342–8.

22. Moretti C, Ascenzo FD, Quadri G, Omedè P, Montefusco A, Taha S, Cerrato E, Colaci C, Chen SL, Biondi-Zoccai G, Gaita F. Management of multivessel coronary disease in STEMI patients: a systematic review and meta-analysis. Int J Cardiol. 2015;179:552–7.

8

A novel model for evaluating thrombolytic therapy in dogs with ST-elevation myocardial infarction

Hong Zhang[1†], Yong-chun Cui[1†], Yi Tian[1], Wei-min Yuan[1], Jian-zhong Yang[1], Peng Peng[1], Kai Li[1], Xiao-peng Liu[1], Dong Zhang[1], Ai-li Wu[1], Zhou Zhou[2*] and Yue Tang[1*]

Abstract

Background: There is still no standard large animal model for evaluating the effectiveness of potential thrombolytic therapies. Here, we aimed to develop a new beagle model with ST-elevation myocardial infarction (STEMI) by injecting autologous emboli with similar components of coronary thrombus.

Methods: 18 male beagles were included and divided into three groups: red embolus group ($n = 6$), white embolus group ($n = 6$) or white embolus + rt-PA group ($n = 6$). Autologous emboli were infused into the mid-distal region of the left anterior descending coronary artery. The composition of embolus was examined by scanning electron microscope (SEM). Coronary angiography was performed to verify the status of embolism. Myocardial infarct size was measured by 2, 3, 5- triphenyltetrazolium chloride (TTC) staining.

Results: Red thrombus was characteristic of loose reticular structure of erythrocytes under SEM, while the white embolus had compacted structure that mainly consisted of a dense mass of fibrin. Coronary angiography showed the recanalization rate was 2/6 in the red embolus group versus 0/6 in the white embolus group in three hours after occlusion. Arrhythmia, resolution of ST-segment elevation and lower T wave on the electrocardiogram appeared in the red embolus group but not in the white embolus group. Another six dogs with white thrombi were treated with rt-PA. Five out of six dogs exhibited coronary recanalization after two hours of therapy, compared to zero dogs without rt-PA treatment. The size of myocardial infarction in rt-PA group reduced significantly compared with white embolus group using TTC staining method.

Conclusions: The white embolism model was more convenient experimentally and had a higher uniformity, stability and success rate. The major innovation of our study is that we applied fibrin-rich white thrombi to establish beagle model possessing features of clinically observed coronary thrombi in time window of intravenous thrombolysis of STEMI. This model can be used to evaluate new thrombolytic drugs for the treatment of STEMI.

Keywords: Thrombolytic therapy, White thrombus, Coronary artery occlusion

Background

Thrombolytic therapies are critical in salvaging ST-segment elevation (STEMI), which accounted for 25 % to 40 % of cases in myocardial infarction [1]. When percutaneous coronary intervention (PCI) cannot be administered in a timely manner [anticipated first medical contact (FMC) to device time > 120 min], thrombolytic therapies were recommended for STEMI according to the most recent ACCF/ AHA and ESC guidelines [1, 2]. Pre-hospital fibrinolysis is an important intervention to salvage ischemic myocardium, improve prognosis and offer additional time for clinical treatment [3]. Most patients can benefit from thrombolysis, however, the specificity, effectiveness and safety of thrombolytic drugs are still required to be

* Correspondence: fwcomd@126.com; tangyue1226@vip.sina.com
†Equal contributors
²Center of Clinical Laboratory, State Key Laboratory of Cardiovascular Disease, Fu Wai Hospital, National Center for Cardiovascular Diseases, Chinese Academy of Medical Sciences and Peking Union Medical College, Beijing 100037, China
¹Animal Experiment Center & Beijing Key Laboratory of Pre-clinical Research and Evaluation for Cardiovascular Implant Materials, Beijing 100037, People's Republic of China

improved [4, 5]. To develop new drugs with faster effects and fewer side effects, it is essential to establish an animal model of the coronary artery embolism mimicking clinical status, especially the thrombus composition, good uniformity and repeatability. However, the coronary thrombi in previous animal models mostly were red or mixed emboli, which were different from that of clinical settings. The composition of the coronary thrombi in time window of thrombolysis was not clarified until the coronary thrombus suction technique was used. Recently, we understood the coronary thrombi in STEMI patients are mainly composed of fibrin with a small portion of platelets that decrease over time, a few erythrocytes, cholesterol crystals and leukocytes [6]. This kind of fibrin-rich thrombi is similar to those in cerebrovascular thrombosis. Kirchhof et al. used white embolus to make rabbit model of cerebral embolism to evaluate thrombolytic drugs [7], which has not been applied to the heart. The aim of present work was to set up an ideal arterial thrombus model that reflected the clinical syndrome in patients with STEMI. Therefore, we compared red and white embolism models via catheter injection into coronary arteries in animal models and investigated the effectiveness of thrombolytic drugs.

Methods
Animals
Twenty-one adult male beagles (12 to 17 kg) were used in this study, which was approved by the animal welfare and the ethical review committee of Fuwai Hospital, Chinese Academy of Medical Sciences (permission number 2013-2-30-BJK02). The animal procedures of this experiment were performed according to the guidelines from Directive 2010/63/EU of the European Parliament on the protection of animals used for scientific purposes.

Preparation of emboli
Based on previous methods [7], we do some modification. Four hours before the operation, 3 ml autologous venous blood was collected from each experimental animal to prepare the individual matched emboli. For white embolus: the venous blood without anticoagulant was centrifuged at 1500 rpm, for 5 min at 4 °C. After extracting the supernatant and injecting it into a silicone tube (2.5 mm in diameter), the blood clots were put into a 37 °C water bath for 0.5 h. The blood clots were extruded into a sterile plate by needle tubing for automatic retraction for 3 h (about 1.2 mm in diameter) and were cut into 5 mm long cylinders. For the red embolus: the blood in the syringe was directly injected into a silicone tube, followed by incubation at 37 °C for 0.5 h. The subsequent processes were identical to those used to make the white embolus. We also measured the concentrations of fibrin, platelets and erythrocytes in whole blood or supernatant. Fibrin

parameters were determined by an automatic coagulation analyzer (STA-Revolution, Stago), platelets and erythrocytes were measured by an automated hematology analyzer (XE-2100, Sysmex).

Coronary artery thrombosis embolism model
Animals were anesthesied with ketamine (35 mg/kg) and diazepam (15 mg/kg) and maintained with the same drugs (dose = 1/2 of induction) administered once every hour. Fentanyl (0.03 mg/kg) was used for analgesia during the operation and post-operation. After anesthesia, animals were affixed to the operation table in the supine position and given endotracheal intubation for assisted respiration in synchronized intermittent mandatory ventilation (SIMV) mode (Savina, Draeger Medical AG&Co.KG, Germany). The parameters include tidal volume (10 ml/kg), breathing rate (20 times/min), expiration/inspiration (E/I) ratio (1:1.5–2) and oxygen saturation (55 %). The arrhythmias were also monitored (M8005A, Philips Medizin Systeme Boeblingen GmbH, Germany). The branchiocephalic vein of the left forelimb was used for heparin and rt-PA injection. An artery sheath catheter was inserted in the axillary artery branch of right forelimb. Under fluroscopic guidance of C arm X-ray (9800–12, Beijing Tongyong Medical Equipment Co., Ltd, China), a 5 F catheter was inserted into the left coronary artery to obtain a coronary angiogram. Keeping the 5 F catheter positioned at the left anterior descending artery near the first diagonal branch, one embolus were injected to occlude blood flow through the mid-distal region of the LAD. Because the catheter cannot be inserted too deeply, the embolus might reach the diagonal branch. So, the operator must carefully handle and avoid the embolus flowing into the vessels with lower pressure.

Thrombolysis treatment
After LAD occlusion for 60 min, 1000 U heparin sodium injection was henceforth given once every two hours. The rt-PA infusion (0.4 mg/kg) was given as a loading dose, and the thrombolytic agent was continuously infused over 30 min (1.2 mg/kg) afterwards. The remainder of the rt-PA was continuously infused over 60 min (0.8 mg/kg). This protocol was according with drug specification and the dose used in dogs was based on the equivalence of clinical safe dosage [8].

Measurements of coronary perfusion
The animals received electrocardiogram (ECG) examination before embolus injection, at the moment of injection and every 15 min for three hours after injection to record the changes of ST-segment, T wave and other variations to estimate the statuses of embolism. For coronary angiogram, animals received right anterior oblique, anteroposterior and left anterior oblique coronary angiography before injection

of the embolus, at the moment of injection and every 30 min for three hours after injection to evaluate the degree of occlusion and/or autolysis. Coronary angiogram was also carried out at 10, 20, 30, 60, 90 and 120 min after using rt-PA or at the time of occurrence of arrhythmia or electrocardiographic changes to evaluate the thrombolytic effects. Reperfusion time was defined as the time when recanalization was verified by coronary angiogram [9].

Pathological studies

Autologous emboli were analyzed by scanning electron microscope (SEM). After three hours automatic retraction, specimens were washed three times with phosphate buffer, fixed for 120 min in 2 % glutaraldehyde and rinsed three times with phosphate buffer. Samples were then fixed for 120 min with osmic acid, rinsed, and dehydrated in a graded series of ethanol concentrations (50 %, 70 %, 90 % and 100 %) over a period of 40 min and further dehydrated in a graded series of concentrations (50 %, 70 %, 90 %, 100 %) of isoamyl acetate-ethanol solvent. The clots were dried with hexamethyldisilazane for 10 min and fractured naturally through pulling to obtain a fracture surface for analysis. Finally, clots were coated with gold-palladium prior to examination in a scanning electron microscope (TM-1000, HITACHI).

The infarct size was determined by 2,3,5-triphenyltetrazolium chloride (TTC) staining. The animals were anesthetized by intravenously injecting Ketamine (35 mg/kg) combined with diazepam (1.5 mg/kg) and euthanized through injecting 10 % potassium chloride (15-20 ml) after that. The hearts were excised and cut cross-sectionally into plates with 10 mm thick and stained with 2,3,5-triphenyltetrazolium chloride (TTC) [10]. The infarct size was identified as the non-TTC-stained area and the infarct ratio (%) is the ratio of area of infarction size to area of left ventricular. We also dissected LAD to observe the situation of thrombolysis. The skin, mucosa, hearts, brains, lungs, livers, spleens and kidneys were subjected for microscopic examination to estimate the bleeding risk according to the previous study [11].

Statistical analysis

Data were analyzed by SPSS 10.0 software (Chicago, IL: SPSS Inc.) and presented as mean $\pm$ SEM. The frequency of recanalization was statistically analysed with Fisher's exact, 2-tailed test. Infarct size ratio was evaluated by unpaired Student's t-Test. $P < 0.05$ indicated a significant difference.

Results

A total of twenty-one dogs were used in the experiment. One animal died of ventricular fibrillation due to the extended duration of the catheter in the LAD. Two animals had diagonal branch embolisms. These three animals were excluded from the study. Finally, eighteen animals were divided into three groups, including red embolus group ($n = 6$), white embolus group ($n = 6$) and white embolus + rt-PA group ($n = 6$).

ECG

The ECG of all animals was normal before the operation. Transient premature ventricular fibrillation occurred in two cases in the red embolus group and four cases in the rt-PA group and was reversed to sinus rhythm after defibrillation. Furthermore, these six animals were present coronary recanalization (reperfusion) according to coronary angiogram as described below. ST-segment and T wave of lead V1-V4 elevated after injection of autologous emboli. ST-segment resolution and lower T wave appeared on the ECG in the red embolus group at 120 min, indicating that the embolism autolyzed. Neither of these was observed in the white embolus group. ST-segment resolution and a lower T wave were observed after the administration of rt-PA to dissolve the white embolus (Fig. 1).

Coronary angiogram

The preoperative coronary angiograms showed that all coronary arteries in the experimental animals were normal. Three hours after LAD occlusion, two animals in red embolus group appeared to have recanalization and the embolism position in white embolus group was still in the mid-distal LAD. These results indicated the white embolus might be better for subsequent experiments. In addition, five out of six animals (5/6) received rt-PA had recanalization flow compared with none in control group (0/6; $p = 0.015$) after two hours (Fig. 2). The average time to reperfusion was 43.2 ± 7.4 min in the rt-PA group (Table 1).

Pathological studies

SEM examination was carried out to identify the characteristics of different autologous emboli (Fig. 3). Blood parameters of whole blood and supernatant after emboli preparation were shown in Table 2. White emboli were more rigid than whole blood emboli because the white emboli contained more fibrin and less erythrocytes under same volume.

After autopsy, no obvious signs of bleeding were seen in the skin, mucosa, heart, brain, lungs, liver, spleen, kidneys or other important organs (data not shown).

For infarct size measurement, individual slices were photographed in color using Image J, and the extent of myocardial necrosis was determined by quantifying the unstained sections of the heart. Infarct size ratios were 11.61 ± 0.64 % and 4.48 ± 0.52 % in the white embolus group and rt-PA group respectively (Fig. 4). The situations of thrombolysis detected through

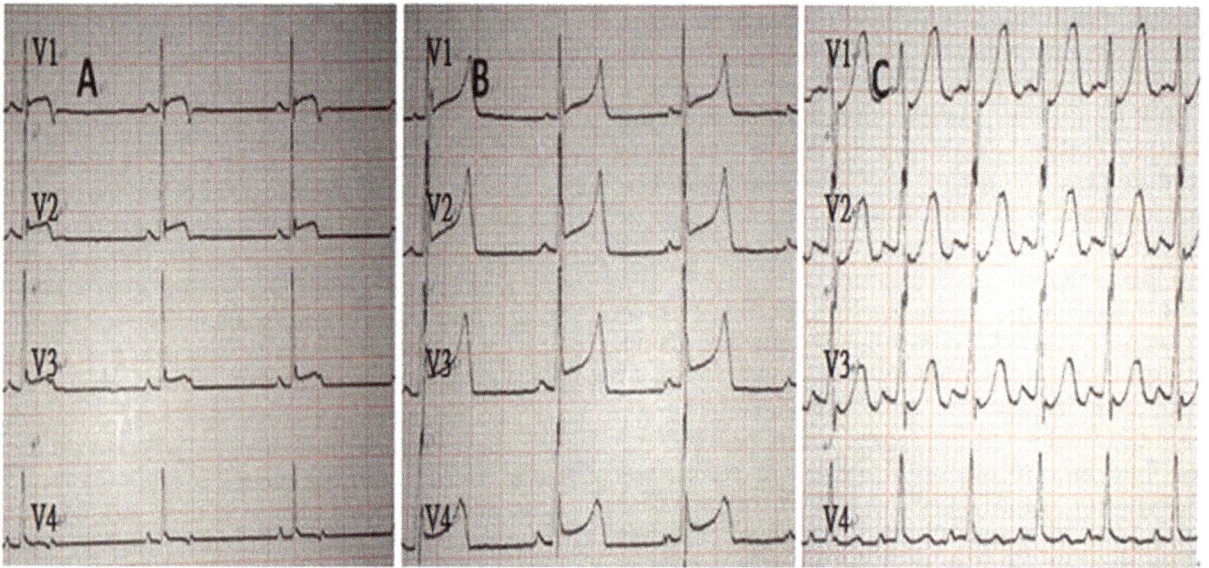

Fig. 1 Example of lead V1-V4 of white embolus + rt-PA group. **a** Baseline ECG. **b** Acute ECG injury pattern of LAD occlusion following white embolus injection, exhibiting marked ST segment elevation. **c** ECG of the dog after using rt-PA; note the relative normalization of the ST segment and elevated heart rate

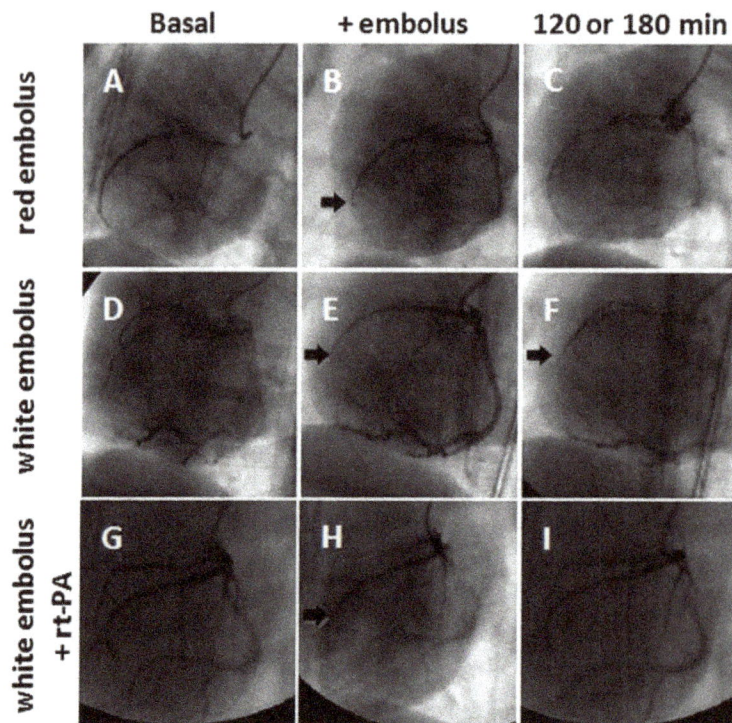

Fig. 2 Coronary embolism changes at different time points were revealed by coronary angiography. The up-panel images represented respectively: before (**a**), 60 min (**b**) or 120 min (**c**) after occlusion with red embolus; mid-panel images represented respectively before (**d**), 60 min (**e**) or 180 min (**f**) after occlusion with white embolus; bottom-panel images represented respectively before occlusion (**g**) by white embolus in the rt-PA group; 60 min after injection of the white embolus (**h**) and 120 min after rt-PA treatment (**i**). Arrows in (**b**), (**e**), (**f**) and (**h**) indicate the location of embolus

Table 1 Effects of rt-PA on thrombolysis

	rt-PA group	white embolus group	P value
Thrombolytic effect			
Reperfusion rate	5/6	0/6	0.015
Reperfusion time (min)	43.2 ± 7.4	–	–

In the rt-PA group, coronary recanalization was achieved in 5 of 6 animals. The reperfusion time was 43.2 ± 7.4 min. There was no coronary recanalization observed in the white embolus group

Table 2 Blood parameters of whole blood and supernatant for emboli preparation

Blood parameters	Mean ± SD	n
Erythrocytes in whole blood, ×10^{12}/L	7.45 ± 0.37	12
Platelets in whole blood, ×10^9/L	319.00 ± 45.80	12
Platelets in supernatant[a], ×10^9/L	456.00 ± 51.50*	6
Fibrinogen in whole blood, g/L	2.21 ± 0.04	6
Fibrinogen in supernatant[a], g/L	4.09 ± 0.25*	6

[a]The supernatant was extracted from the venous blood and centrifuged at 4 °C and 1500 rpm for 5 min
*$p < 0.05$ compare with whole blood

coronary artery dissection were in accordance with the results of coronary angiogram.

Discussion

About 70 % of cases of acute coronary thrombosis are associated with a disrupted atherosclerotic plaque and about 30 % of them are only with superficial intimal injury [12]. In case of plaque rupture or endothelial damage, the exposure of collagen and tissue factor triggers the activation of platelets and coagulation factors, which result in thrombus formation [13, 14]. The different components of thrombus in coronary artery can affect the pathological process of STEMI and the thrombolytic effect directly. In recent years, the pathological analysis of aspirated intracoronary thrombi demonstrated that about 65 % of patients had platelet-rich (white) thrombi, particularly in the early hours of AMI, the remaining 35 % of cases had erythrocyte-rich (red) thrombi with low thrombolysis in myocardial infarction (TIMI) flow [15]. Silvain et al. found that intracoronary thrombi were mainly composed of fibrin with the median ischemic time of 175 min. The fibrin content increased with the ischemic time, whereas the platelet content decreased and the erythrocyte content had no changes [6]. The results showed that there were fibrin-rich thrombi in the early time (<3 h) after onset of STEMI. The white thrombi in our experiments are similar to the fibrin-rich thrombi in patients with STEMI. Erythrocytes may contribute more to thrombus

composition at later stages but not in the time window of acute reperfusion of STEMI. Red thrombus are composed of fewer massed platelets and more erythrocytes [16]. As previously reported, the ratio of erythrocytes determines the size of the pores between cellulose meshes. The softer thrombi with larger pores [7] are easier to be penetrated by fibrinogenase to dissolve. In this study, after injecting of red thrombi into coronary artery of dogs, the fibrinolytic system was activated, and the thrombi started dissolved through coronary angiogram, ECG and occurrence of arrhythmia. Whereas white thrombus with compacted structure has strong ability to resist fibrinolysis and no thrombolytic phenomenon occurred obviously. Recent experiments have reported the high stability of white emboli used in animal models in agreement with our observations [7, 17]. Overall, the white thrombus is more stable in animal model and has similar components of STEMI patients in early time of onset of this disease. These results made the animal model suitable for subsequent application in evaluating thrombolytic therapy.

The new model has better uniformity not only in embolus preparation but also in animal model establishment. Firstly, the white thrombi have identical components. To mimic this kind of fibrin-rich white thrombus, centrifugation conditions of 1500 rpm at 4 °C for 5 min were

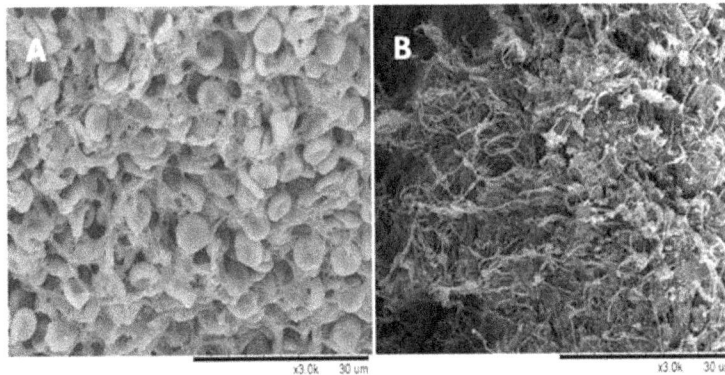

Fig. 3 The characteristics of different thrombi were evaluated by SEM. **a** The structure of whole blood thrombus was incompact and sparse cellulose meshes were full of erythrocytes. **b** White thrombus with compacted structure that mainly consisted of a dense mass of fibrin

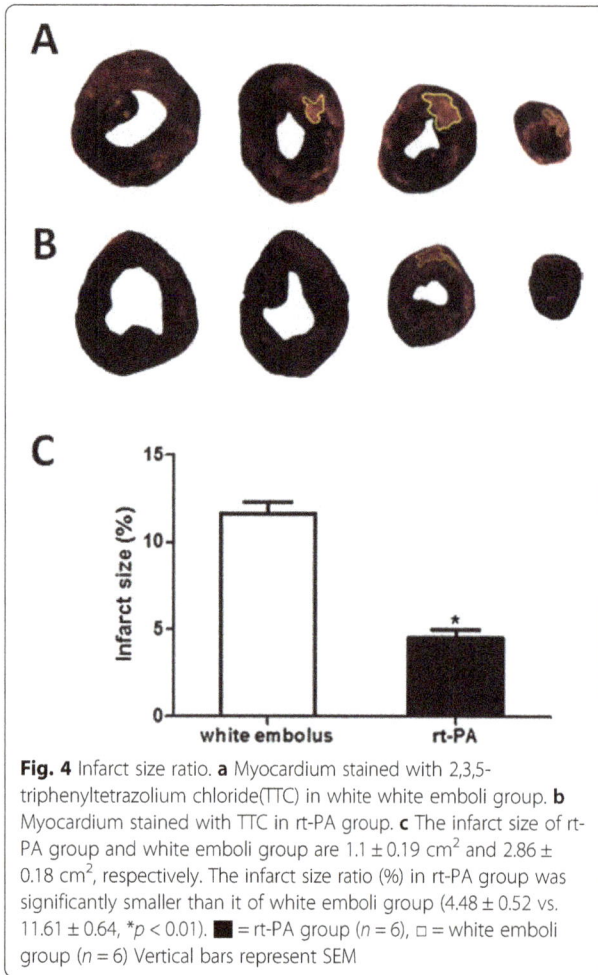

Fig. 4 Infarct size ratio. **a** Myocardium stained with 2,3,5-triphenyltetrazolium chloride(TTC) in white white emboli group. **b** Myocardium stained with TTC in rt-PA group. **c** The infarct size of rt-PA group and white emboli group are 1.1 ± 0.19 cm^2 and 2.86 ± 0.18 cm^2, respectively. The infarct size ratio (%) in rt-PA group was significantly smaller than it of white emboli group (4.48 ± 0.52 vs. 11.61 ± 0.64, *$p < 0.01$). ■ = rt-PA group ($n = 6$), □ = white emboli group ($n = 6$) Vertical bars represent SEM

chosen. The blood parameters, mainly including platelet and fibrinogen, in the supernatant are at the similar levels. To avoid affecting the antifibrinolytic ability of thrombi, we did not use any anticoagulants in emboli preparation [18]. By operating quickly, we could guarantee that the supernatant did not coagulate before the silicone tube shaping step. From the SEM analysis, it was clear that white emboli with compacted structure mainly consist of a dense mass of fibrin. Secondly, the size, length and number of thrombi can be controlled and the locations of thrombi in coronary artery were similar. Through the guidance of catheter positioning, emboli were sent to anterior descending coronary artery and could be stuck in LAD with similar diameters. This model mimics the clinical situation that the fresh clot was broken off and carried through the flow into distal coronary artery at early stage of myocardial infarction. Thrombolytic therapy in myocardial infarction is a dynamic process due to the progressive embolus dissolution. In our experiment, we found the white embolus moved forward for a limited distance after using rt-PA during early stage, then it formed eccentrically clot in the distal section of coronary artery. The white

embolus could be completely dissolved and LAD became recanalized in a certain time period.

The anti-fibrinolytic ability of the embolus is very important. Looser or more rigid thrombi do not behave like the endogenous thrombi in STEMI and therefore may not provide accurate information concerning the efficacy and safety of different thrombolytic drugs. There are no universal criteria to evaluate autologous emboli, and the different methods resulted in different experimental outcomes [18]. In current experiments, we used the autologous white embolism model to examine the thrombolytic actions of rt-PA. This drug is commonly used in clinical practice because of its rapid clearance and ability to be co-administered with heparin. The average time to reperfusion was 43.2 ± 7.4 min and the patency rate in this model was 5/6(83 %) in 90 min, which was similar to those in clinical study (73–84 %) [8, 19, 20]. The size ratio of myocardial infarct in rt-PA group reduced significantly compared to control group, which confirmed that use of thrombolytic drugs timely could improve the prognosis of patients with STEMI.

As determined by microscopic examination, there was no obvious bleeding-induced damage to skin, mucosa, heart, brain, lungs, liver, spleen, kidneys or other important organs. It may be related to the safer dose adopted in healthy animals. There is no perfect system to predict bleeding risk associated with thrombolysis in clinical treatment, so the animal experiments to evaluate bleeding risk is needed for further studies. Because the time window of thrombolytic treatment is relatively short [19, 21, 22], fast thrombolysis is very important for developing new thrombolytic agents. In conclusion, our model can be used to compare the rates and time of recanalization among different thrombolytic drugs in their safe dose ranges.

Catheter-based delivery of the autologous emboli was shown to be effective in our study. We selected the axillary artery branch instead of carotid artery or femoral artery as the puncture path for the first time, which could shorten the length of interventional devices in the body, reduce the risk of postoperative infection and decrease hemorrhage at the puncture point. In terms of detection, coronary angiography was effective at instantaneously ascertaining the degree of coronary artery stenosis, allowing the progress of thrombolysis to be carefully monitored. Because of its gentle temperament and homogenous genetic background, the beagle is widely used in preclinical drug evaluation. However, the diameter of coronary arteries in beagle is small and no specialized coronary artery catheters are currently available for these animals. Our protocol resolved this bottleneck problem.

At present, the methods for evaluating thrombolytic therapy in large animal models mainly include electrical injury [23], open chest thrombosis injection [24], balloon occlusion and thrombin injection [25] and copper coil-induced coronary thrombosis [26]. The first two methods require open chest operation, with complex operations and a larger trauma. The thrombus in the last two models may have different compositions from those seen in STEMI patients. Although the thrombus induced by electrical injury have similar composition to human coronary artery thrombi, this method takes a long time (3.2 ± 0.4 h) to complete coronary occlusion and the size of thrombus cannot be controlled [23]. The present model was a simple, efficient and inexpensive method with a smaller trauma. Furthermore, the artificially produced fibrin-rich white thrombus has uniform size and clinical features of coronary thrombi in time window of intravenous thrombolysis of STEMI.

Conclusions

We established, for the first time to our knowledge, the coronary artery embolism model with white thrombus which had better stability, uniformity and a higher success rate. Importantly, the model produced thrombi with characteristics similar to those in STEMI patients in time window of thrombolytic therapy and was amenable to evaluation of thrombolytic therapies. This model can be used to evaluate new thrombolytic drugs for the treatment of STEMI.

Abbreviations

ECG: Electrocardiogram; E/I: Expiration/inspiration; FMC: First medical contact; LAD: Left anterior descending artery; PCI: Percutaneous coronary intervention; rt-PA: Recombinant tissue plasminogen activator; SEM: Scanning electron microscope; SIMV: Synchronized intermittent mandatory ventilation; STEMI: ST-segment elevation; TIMI: thrombolysis in myocardial infarction; TTC: 2,3,5-triphenyltetrazolium chloride.

Competing interests

The authors declare that they have no competing interests.

Authors' contributions

HZ and YCC participated in the design of the study and drafted the manuscript. YT, WMY, JZY and PP participated in the operation. KL performed the data collection. XPL and DZ performed the statistical analysis. ALW participated in its coordination. ZZ and YT helped to draft the manuscript. All authors read and approved the final manuscript.

Acknowledgments

This work was supported by Beijing Municipal Science & Technology Commission (Project No: Z101107052210004).

References

1. O'Gara PT, Kushner FG, Ascheim DD, Casey Jr DE, Chung MK, de Lemos JA, et al. 2013 ACCF/AHA guideline for the management of ST-elevation myocardial infarction: a report of the American College of Cardiology Foundation/American Heart Association Task Force on Practice Guidelines. Circulation. 2013;127(4):e362–425.
2. Task Force on the management of STseamiotESoC, Steg PG, James SK, Atar D, Badano LP, Blomstrom-Lundqvist C, et al. ESC Guidelines for the management of acute myocardial infarction in patients presenting with ST-segment elevation. Eur Heart J. 2012;33(20):2569–619.
3. Armstrong PW, Gershlick AH, Goldstein P, Wilcox R, Danays T, Lambert Y, et al. Fibrinolysis or primary PCI in ST-segment elevation myocardial infarction. N Engl J Med. 2013;368(15):1379–87.
4. Meunier JM, Holland CK, Pancioli AM, Lindsell CJ, Shaw GJ. Effect of low frequency ultrasound on combined rt-PA and eptifibatide thrombolysis in human clots. Thromb Res. 2009;123(3):528–36.
5. Mehta RH, Parsons L, Rao SV, Peterson ED, National Registry of Myocardial Infarction I. Association of bleeding and in-hospital mortality in black and white patients with st-segment-elevation myocardial infarction receiving reperfusion. Circulation. 2012;125(14):1727–34.
6. Silvain J, Collet JP, Nagaswami C, Beygui F, Edmondson KE, Bellemain-Appaix A, et al. Composition of coronary thrombus in acute myocardial infarction. J Am Coll Cardiol. 2011;57(12):1359–67.
7. Kirchhof K, Welzel T, Zoubaa S, Lichy C, Sikinger M, de Ruiz HL, et al. New Method of Embolus Preparation for Standardized Embolic Stroke in Rabbits. Stroke. 2002;33(9):2329–33.
8. The GUSTO Angiographic Investigators. The effects of tissue plasminogen activator, streptokinase, or both on coronary-artery patency, ventricular function, and survival after acute myocardial infarction. N Engl J Med. 1993;329(22):1615–22.
9. Kido H, Hayashi K, Uchida T, Watanabe M. Low incidence of hemorrhagic infarction following coronary reperfusion with nasaruplase in a canine model of acute myocardial infarction. Comparison with recombinant t-PA. Jpn Heart J. 1995;36(1):61–79.
10. Ugander M, Bagi PS, Oki AJ, Chen B, Hsu LY, Aletras AH, et al. Myocardial edema as detected by pre-contrast T1 and T2 CMR delineates area at risk associated with acute myocardial infarction. JACC Cardiovascular imaging. 2012;5(6):596–603.
11. Siegel RJ, Atar S, Fishbein MC, Brasch AV, Peterson TM, Nagai T, et al. Noninvasive, Transthoracic, Low-Frequency Ultrasound Augments Thrombolysis in a Canine Model of Acute Myocardial Infarction. Circulation. 2000;101(17):2026–9.
12. Farb A, Burke AP, Tang AL, Liang TY, Mannan P, Smialek J, et al. Coronary plaque erosion without rupture into a lipid core. A frequent cause of coronary thrombosis in sudden coronary death. Circulation. 1996;93(7):1354–63.
13. Maseri A, Chierchia S, Davies G. Pathophysiology of coronary occlusion in acute infarction. Circulation. 1986;73(2):233–9.
14. Schwartz SM, Galis ZS, Rosenfeld ME, Falk E. Plaque rupture in humans and mice. Arteriosclerosis, thrombosis, and vascular biology. 2007;27(4):705–13.
15. Vlaar PJ, Svilaas T, Vogelzang M, Diercks GF, de Smet BJ, van den Heuvel AF, et al. A comparison of 2 thrombus aspiration devices with histopathological analysis of retrieved material in patients presenting with ST-segment elevation myocardial infarction. JACC Cardiovascular interventions. 2008;1(3):258–64.
16. Yunoki K, Naruko T, Sugioka K, Inaba M, Iwasa Y, Komatsu R, et al. Erythrocyte-rich thrombus aspirated from patients with ST-elevation myocardial infarction: association with oxidative stress and its impact on myocardial reperfusion. European heart journal. 2012;33(12):1480–90.
17. Bolotin G, Raman J, Williams U, Bacha E, Kocherginsky M, Jeevanandam V. Glutamine improves myocardial function following ischemia-reperfusion injury. Asian cardiovascular & thoracic annals. 2007;15(6):463–7.
18. Krueger K, Deissler P, Coburger S, Fries JW, Lackner K. How thrombus model impacts the in vitro study of interventional thrombectomy procedures. Investigative radiology. 2004;39(10):641–8.
19. Bode C, Smalling RW, Berg G, Burnett C, Lorch G, Kalbfleisch JM, et al. Randomized comparison of coronary thrombolysis achieved with double-bolus reteplase (recombinant plasminogen activator) and front-loaded, accelerated alteplase (recombinant tissue plasminogen activator) in patients with acute myocardial infarction The RAPID II Investigators. Circulation. 1996;94(5):891–8.
20. Neuhaus KL, von Essen R, Tebbe U, Vogt A, Roth M, Riess M, et al. Improved thrombolysis in acute myocardial infarction with front-loaded administration of alteplase: results of the rt-PA-APSAC patency study (TAPS). Journal of the American College of Cardiology. 1992;19(5):885–91.
21. Indications for fibrinolytic therapy in suspected acute myocardial infarction. collaborative overview of early mortality and major morbidity results from all randomised trials of more than 1000 patients. Fibrinolytic Therapy Trialists' (FTT) Collaborative Group. Lancet. 1994;343(8893):311–22.
22. Wilcox RG, von der Lippe G, Olsson CG, Jensen G, Skene AM, Hampton JR. Trial of tissue plasminogen activator for mortality reduction in acute

myocardial infarction. Anglo-Scandinavian Study of Early Thrombolysis
(ASSET). Lancet. 1988;2(8610):525–30.

23. Romson JL, Haack DW, Abrams GD, Lucchesi BR. Prevention of occlusive
coronary artery thrombosis by prostacyclin infusion in the dog. Circulation.
1981;64(5):906–14.

24. Lee G, Giddens J, Krieg P, Dajee A, Suzuki M, Kozina JA, et al.
Experimental reversal of acute coronary thrombotic occlusion and
myocardial injury in animals utilizing streptokinase. American heart
journal. 1981;102(6 Pt 2):1139–44.

25. Suzuki M, Asano H, Tanaka H, Usuda S. Development and evaluation of a
new canine myocardial infarction model using a closed-chest injection of
thrombogenic material. Japanese circulation journal. 1999;63(11):900–5.

26. Kordenat RK, Kezdi P, Stanley EL. A new catheter technique for producing
experimental coronary thrombosis and selective coronary visualization.
American heart journal. 1972;83(3):360–4.

9

Multimarker approach for the prediction of microvascular obstruction after acute ST-segment elevation myocardial infarction

Hans-Josef Feistritzer[1], Sebastian Johannes Reinstadler[1], Gert Klug[1], Martin Reindl[1], Sebastian Wöhrer[1], Christoph Brenner[1], Agnes Mayr[2], Johannes Mair[1] and Bernhard Metzler[1*]

Abstract

Background: Presence of microvascular obstruction (MVO) derived from cardiac magnetic resonance (CMR) imaging is among the strongest outcome predictors after ST-segment elevation myocardial infarction (STEMI). We aimed to investigate the comparative predictive values of different biomarkers for the occurrence of MVO in a large cohort of reperfused STEMI patients.

Methods: This study included 128 STEMI patients. CMR imaging was performed within the first week after infarction to assess infarct characteristics, including MVO. Admission and peak concentrations of high-sensitivity cardiac troponin T (hs-cTnT), creatine kinase (CK), N-terminal pro-B-type natriuretic peptide (NT-proBNP), high-sensitivity C-reactive protein (hs-CRP), lactate dehydrogenase (LDH), aspartate transaminase (AST) and alanine transaminase (ALT) were measured.

Results: MVO was detected in 69 patients (54%). hs-cTnT, CK, hs-CRP, LDH, AST and ALT peak concentrations showed similar prognostic value for the prediction of MVO (area under the curve (AUC) = 0.77, 0.77, 0.68, 0.79, 0.78 and 0.73, all $p > 0.05$), whereas the prognostic utility of NT-proBNP was weakly lower (AUC = 0.64, $p < 0.05$). Combination of these biomarkers did not increase predictive utility compared to hs-cTnT alone ($p = 0.349$).

Conclusions: hs-cTnT, CK, hs-CRP, LDH, AST and ALT peak concentrations provided similar prognostic value for the prediction of MVO. The prognostic utility of NT-proBNP was lower. Combining these biomarkers could not further improve predictive utility compared to hs-cTnT alone.

Keywords: Myocardial infarction, Biomarker, Cardiovascular magnetic resonance imaging

Background

The broad implementation of early primary percutaneous coronary intervention (PPCI) for acute ST-segment elevation myocardial infarction (STEMI) resulted in a significant improvement of clinical outcomes [1, 2]. Nevertheless, despite restoration of epicardial blood flow, adequate myocardial reperfusion cannot be achieved in a significant portion of patients-a phenomenon called 'no reflow' [3]. Three distinct pathophysiological processes are critical in the development of 'no reflow' after PPCI for STEMI: distal embolization, ischemia-reperfusion injury, and individual susceptibility [4].

Today cardiac magnetic resonance (CMR) imaging allows a comprehensive infarct characterization including the assessment of microvascular injury [5]. Microvascular injury detected by the use of CMR imaging is generally called 'microvascular obstruction' (MVO) [6]. In the so far largest prospective, multicenter study comprising more than 700 STEMI patients MVO provided independent and incremental prognostic value for the occurrence of major adverse cardiac events within 1 year after infarction [7]. In the study by Cochet et al. MVO provided 84% sensitivity and 65% specificity for the prediction of major adverse cardiac events 1 year after

* Correspondence: Bernhard.Metzler@tirol-kliniken.at
[1]University Clinic of Internal Medicine III, Cardiology and Angiology, Medical University of Innsbruck, Anichstraße 35, A-6020 Innsbruck, Austria
Full list of author information is available at the end of the article

reperfused AMI [8]. Another study in STEMI patients proved MVO as an independent outcome predictor during a median long-term follow-up of 52 months [9]. Importantly, presence of MVO provides incremental information over traditional outcome parameters like left ventricular (LV) ejection fraction and infarct size (IS) [3, 10]. Identification of MVO, therefore, could allow for ideal risk stratification in the early stage after acute STEMI, but is still hampered due to the limited availability of CMR in clinical routine [11]. A biomarker model for prediction of MVO, which could easily be applied in a broad range of STEMI patients, might provide a practicable and cost effective alternative to CMR.

An association between serially measured cardiac troponin concentrations and CMR derived MVO has previously been reported for this patient cohort [12, 13]. However, these studies were hampered either due to a small sample size or the use of non-high-sensitivity troponin assays. Furthermore, N-terminal pro-B-type natriuretic peptide (NT-proBNP) levels obtained upon hospital admission for acute STEMI might be predictive for the presence of MVO [14]. However, limited data are available regarding the relation of CMR derived MVO and other clinically available biomarkers apart from cardiac troponin and NT-proBNP [12–14]. Therefore, the aims of the present study were 1) to investigate the association of CMR-determined MVO with admission and peak concentrations of routinely measured laboratory markers (high-sensitivity cardiac troponin T (hs-cTnT), creatine kinase (CK), NT-proBNP, high-sensitivity C-reactive protein (hs-CRP), lactate dehydrogenase (LDH), aspartate transaminase (AST) and alanine transaminase (ALT)), 2) to assess the prognostic value of these biomarkers for the prediction of MVO and 3) to analyze the prognostic utility of a combined biomarker panel.

Methods

Study population

One hundred and twenty-eight patients with first STEMI admitted to our coronary care unit were recruited to this single-center, prospective, observational study. Diagnosis of STEMI was based on the redefined ESC/ACC committee criteria [15]. Inclusion criteria were reperfusion by PPCI and no contraindication for CMR examination. Exclusion criteria were age below 18 years, an estimated glomerular filtration rate < 30 ml/min/1.73 m^2 and Killip class ≥ 3 at admission. Data on patient characteristics were acquired with the help of a standardized questionnaire during hospitalization. Ischemia time was defined as the delay from symptom onset to the time-point of first balloon-inflation. The study complies with the ethical guidelines of the 1975 Declaration of Helsinki and was approved by the local ethics committee of Medical

University of Innsbruck. Written informed consent was obtained from all patients before inclusion into the study.

Biochemical analysis

Blood samples were taken from a peripheral vein and immediately analyzed at our central laboratory. High-sensitivity cardiac troponin T (hs-cTnT) concentrations were measured using a fifth-generation high-sensitivity assay (Roche Diagnostics, Mannheim, Germany) [16, 17]. The analytical limit of detection was 5 ng/l and the 99th percentile upper reference limit was 14 ng/l. The 10% coefficient of variation was 13 ng/l. Plasma NT-proBNP concentrations were measured as described in detail previously [18, 19]. The analytical limit of detection of NT-proBNP was 5 ng/l. Creatine kinase (CK), high-sensitivity C-reactive protein (hs-CRP), lactate dehydrogenase (LDH), aspartate transaminase (AST), and alanine transaminase (ALT) activities were measured by routine assays as described previously [16, 18].

hs-cTnT concentrations were determined on admission, subsequently three times during the first 24 h and then daily until day 4 or discharge. All other biomarkers were measured on admission and subsequently once daily up to day 4 after PPCI or discharge. Biomarker peak concentrations are regarded as the highest values in the concentration time-course.

Cardiac magnetic resonance imaging

All CMR scans were performed on a 1.5 Tesla Magnetom Avanto scanner (Siemens, Erlangen, Germany). The imaging protocol has been described in detail previously [12]. In brief, true fast imaging steady-state precession (true-FISP) bright-blood sequences in the LV short axis were acquired to assess LV function and morphology. Image post-processing was performed using standard software (ARGUS, Siemens). IS and presence of MVO were derived from late gadolinium-enhanced images as previously described [9]. A threshold of + 5 standard deviations was defined as 'hyperenhancement' [20]. MVO was defined as a persisting area of hypoenhancement within hyperenhanced myocardium [9].

Statistical analysis

Statistical analysis was performed using SPSS Statistics 22.0.0 (IBM, Armonk, NY, USA) and MedCalc 15.8 (Ostend, Belgium). To test for normal distribution (ND), Shapiro-Wilk test was used. Continuous data are expressed as mean ± standard deviation (SD) or as median with interquartile range (IQR) as appropriate. Categorical data are expressed as numbers with corresponding percentages. Pearson's (if ND) or Spearman's rank (if not ND) correlation coefficients were calculated. Differences in continuous variables between groups were calculated by Student's t-test, if ND. Otherwise, Mann-Whitney U test was used. To test for group-differences of categorical variables χ^2-test was applied.

Receiver operator characteristics (ROC) analysis was used to determine the predictive value (area under the curve (AUC)) of biomarkers. Biomarkers which significantly differed between patients with and without MVO were included into ROC analyses. Binary logistic regression analysis was used as a statistical tool to combine biomarkers as previously described [17]. The potentially incremental information of a combined biomarker model for the prediction of MVO was assessed by c-statistics. C-statistic results were compared using the method previously described by DeLong et al [21]. Two-tailed p-values < 0.05 were considered statistically significant.

Results

Patients and infarct-related characteristics

Mean age of the study cohort was 58 ± 10 years; 12 patients (9%) were female. Baseline characteristics of the study cohort are shown in Table 1. The median delay to reperfusion was 220 min (IQR 155–417 min). Sixty-one patients (48%) presented with anterior infarct location. Seventy (56%), 34 (27%) and 21 (17%) patients showed 1-, 2- and 3-vessel disease according to coronary angiography, respectively. Culprit only PPCI was performed in all 128 patients. The culprit vessel was the right coronary artery in 55 (43%), the left anterior descending artery in 60 (47%), the left circumflex artery in 12 (9%) and the ramus intermedius in 1 (1%) cases.

CMR scans were performed at a median of 3 days after infarction (IQR 2–4 days). Median IS was 13% (IQR 8–25%). Mean LVEF was $54 \pm 10\%$. MVO was present in 69 patients (54%).

Predictors of MVO

The delay from symptom onset to mechanical reperfusion did not significantly differ between patients with and without MVO (median = 213 min, IQR 149–399 min vs median = 240 min, IQR 154–424 min; $p = 0.469$). Patients showing MVO were more likely to have anterior infarcts compared to patients without MVO ($n = 39$, 57% vs $n = 22$, 37%; $p = 0.030$). No association was detected between the presence of MVO and the number of diseased epicardial coronary arteries ($p = 0.480$).

Patients with presence of MVO showed significantly higher IS (median = 21%, IQR 14–30% vs median = 9%, IQR 3–13%; $p < 0.001$), EDV (153 ± 30 ml vs 140 ± 26 ml; $p = 0.010$), ESV (median = 73 ml, IQR 60–90 ml vs median = 56 ml, IQR 44–72 ml; $p < 0.001$) and lower LVEF ($50 \pm 9\%$ vs $59 \pm 10\%$; $p < 0.001$). The occurrence of MVO did not significantly differ between patients with one- and multivessel disease ($p = 0.286$).

Differences in biomarker levels between patients with and without MVO are shown in Table 1.

hs-cTnT concentrations at admission provided an AUC value of 0.61 (95% CI 0.52–0.69) for the prediction of MVO (Fig. 1a). AUCs did not significantly differ between admission hs-cTnT, CK, NT-proBNP, hs-CRP, LDH, AST and ALT (range 0.54, 95% CI 0.45–0.62 to 0.66, 95% CI 0.57–0.74; all $p > 0.080$).

Biomarker peak concentrations provided significantly higher prognostic value for the prediction of MVO than corresponding admission values (all $p < 0.050$) (Fig. 1).

Peak hs-cTnT concentrations provided an AUC of 0.77 (95% CI 0.68–0.85) for the prediction of MVO. Peak CK (AUC = 0.77, 95% CI 0.69–0.84; $p = 0.882$), hs-CRP (AUC = 0.68, 95% CI 0.60–0.76; $p = 0.108$), LDH (AUC = 0.79, 95% CI 0.71–0.86; $p = 0.336$), AST (AUC = 0.78, 95% CI 0.70–0.85; $p = 0.517$) and ALT (AUC = 0.73, 95% CI 0.64–0.80; $p = 0.312$) showed similar AUCs for the prediction of MVO compared to hs-cTnT. NT-proBNP peak concentrations (AUC = 0.64, 95% CI 0.55–0.73) exhibited significantly lower predictive utility compared to peak hs-cTnT ($p = 0.027$), CK ($p = 0.031$), LDH ($p = 0.007$) and AST ($p = 0.016$) concentrations. Optimal biomarker cut-off values with corresponding sensitivity, specificity as well as positive and negative predictive values for the prediction of MVO are summarized in Table 2.

Including peak CK, NT-proBNP, hs-CRP, LDH, AST and ALT concentrations additionally to peak hs-cTnT levels did not result in a significantly higher accuracy for the prediction of MVO (AUC = 0.79, 95% CI 0.71–0.87 vs AUC = 0.77, 95% CI 0.68–0.85; $p = 0.349$) (Fig. 2).

Discussion

This study for the first time comprehensively assessed the incremental value of routine biomarkers for the prediction of MVO after reperfused STEMI. The major findings were that 1) presence of MVO was associated with higher plasma concentrations of hs-cTnT, CK, hs-CRP, LDH, AST and ALT; 2) biomarker peak concentrations provided significantly higher prognostic value compared to admission values; 3) peak concentrations of hs-cTnT, CK, hs-CRP, LDH, AST and ALT showed similar prognostic value for the prediction of MVO, whereas the prognostic utility of peak NT-proBNP was lower; and 4) a model including peak CK, NT-proBNP, hs-CRP, LDH, AST and ALT concentrations additionally to hs-cTnT did not result in a significantly higher accuracy for the prediction of MVO.

Inadequate myocardial reperfusion despite restoration of epicardial coronary artery patency is attributed to microvascular injury [22]. As previously shown, application of modern antiplatelet therapy partly improves microvascular perfusion [23]. Interestingly, removal of thrombotic material by thrombus aspiration is ineffective in improvement of myocardial reperfusion [24]. In the

Table 1 Patient characteristic of the overall cohort (*n* = 128) and after stratification for presence of MVO

Patient characteristics	Overall cohort	Presence of MVO		
	(*n* = 128)	no (*n* = 59, 46%)	yes (*n* = 69, 54%)	*p*
Age, years	58 ± 10	57 ± 10	58 ± 10	0.925
Female, n (%)	12 (9)	8 (14)	4 (6)	0.223
Body mass index, kg/m^2	26 (25–30)	27 (26–29)	26 (24–30)	0.522
Family history for AMI, n (%)	34 (27)	19 (32)	15 (22)	0.229
Current smokers, n (%)	63 (49)	28 (48)	35 (51)	0.727
RR$_{sys}$, mmHg	125 ± 24	126 ± 23	123 ± 24	0.491
RR$_{dia}$, mmHg	77 ± 15	78 ± 14	76 ± 15	0.309
Leucocyte count admission, G/l	11.7 (8.8–14.5)	11.5 (8.5–14.5)	12.0 (9.0–14.6)	0.649
Leucocyte count max, G/l	12.7 (10.8–15.8)	11.9 (10.3–15.2)	13.1 (11.7–16.4)	0.061
Total cholesterol, mg/dl	192 ± 44	185 ± 41	198 ± 47	0.108
Low-density lipoprotein, mg/dl	128 ± 42	123 ± 39	132 ± 44	0.230
High-density lipoprotein, mg/dl	42 (36–49)	40 (33–53)	43 (38–49)	0.320
Triglycerides, mg/dl	102 (78–151)	108 (80–163)	96 (77–142)	0.276
Plasma glucose admission, mg/dl	135 (115–161)	134 (116–163)	137 (112–160)	0.728
HbA1c, %	5.6 (5.4–6.0)	5.6 (5.4–6.1)	5.6 (5.3–5.9)	0.792
Creatinine admission, mg/dl	0.93 (0.82–1.05)	0.92 (0.76–1.07)	0.93 (0.83–1.04)	0.877
Creatinine max, mg/dl	1.04 (0.92–1.15)	1.03 (0.91–1.13)	1.06 (0.96–1.20)	0.261
hs-cTnT admission, ng/l	226 (29–2168)	201 (18–1388)	523 (34–4001)	**0.036**
hs-cTnT max, ng/l	5254 (2169–8735)	2866 (1026–5524)	6985 (4193–13639)	**<0.001**
CK admission, U/l	353 (174–1182)	301 (148–862)	435 (207–2433)	**0.048**
CK max, U/l	2111 (1168–3674)	1228 (625–2323)	2776 (1749–4686)	**<0.001**
NT-proBNP admission, ng/l	139 (66–511)	128 (66–360)	159 (71–687)	0.487
NT-proBNP max, ng/l	717 (184–1700)	360 (131–924)	1084 (312–2649)	**0.003**
hs-CRP admission, mg/dl	0.23 (0.11–0.61)	0.34 (0.15–0.66)	0.19 (0.09–0.56)	0.119
hs-CRP max, mg/dl	2.20 (0.96–4.56)	1.53 (0.64 3.02)	2.84 (1.68–7.44)	**<0.001**
LDH admission, U/l	238 (196–364)	222 (182–301)	257 (207–493)	**0.009**
LDH max, U/l	593 (354–882)	358 (271–624)	742 (534–1182)	**<0.001**
AST admission, U/l	82 (34–210)	57 (31–113)	126 (40–306)	**0.008**
AST max, U/l	239 (128–423)	151 (75–256)	340 (213–547)	**<0.001**
ALT admission, U/l	37 (27–58)	31 (25–46)	45 (32–75)	**0.003**
ALT max, U/l	60 (42–87)	47 (32–69)	71 (52–111)	**<0.001**
γGT admission, U/l	37 (25–52)	36 (26–50)	39 (23–59)	0.857
γGT max, U/l	40 (26–63)	37 (26–51)	41 (26–71)	0.482
AP admission, U/l	64 (53–79)	64 (52–80)	63 (54–76)	0.918
AP max, U/l	64 (53–81)	64 (52–83)	64 (54–81)	0.951
Total bilirubin admission, mg/dl	0.49 (0.38–0.69)	0.44 (0.37–0.65)	0.52 (0.40–0.73)	0.160
Total bilirubin max, mg/dl	0.62 (0.43–0.84)	0.60 (0.42–0.84)	0.62 (0.45–0.85)	0.668

MVO Microvascular Obstruction, *AMI* Acute Myocardial Infarction, *RR$_{sys}$* Systolic Blood Pressure, *RR$_{dia}$* Diastolic Blood Pressure, *hs-cTnT* High-Sensitivity Cardiac Troponin T, *CK* Creatine Kinase, *NT-proBNP* N-terminal pro-B-type natriuretic peptide, *hs-CRP* High-Sensitivity C-Reactive Protein, *LDH* Lactate Dehydrogenase, *AST* Aspartate Transaminase, *ALT* Alanine Transaminase, *γGT* Gamma-Glutamyltransferase, *AP* Alkaline Phosphatase
Bold data indicate statistical significance

present study microvascular injury, defined as the presence or absence of CMR derived MVO, was detected in 54% of patients. This is in line with data from literature, reporting an up to 60% rate of MVO in patients receiving primary PCI for acute STEMI [3]. In the present study culprit only revascularization was performed during PPCI.

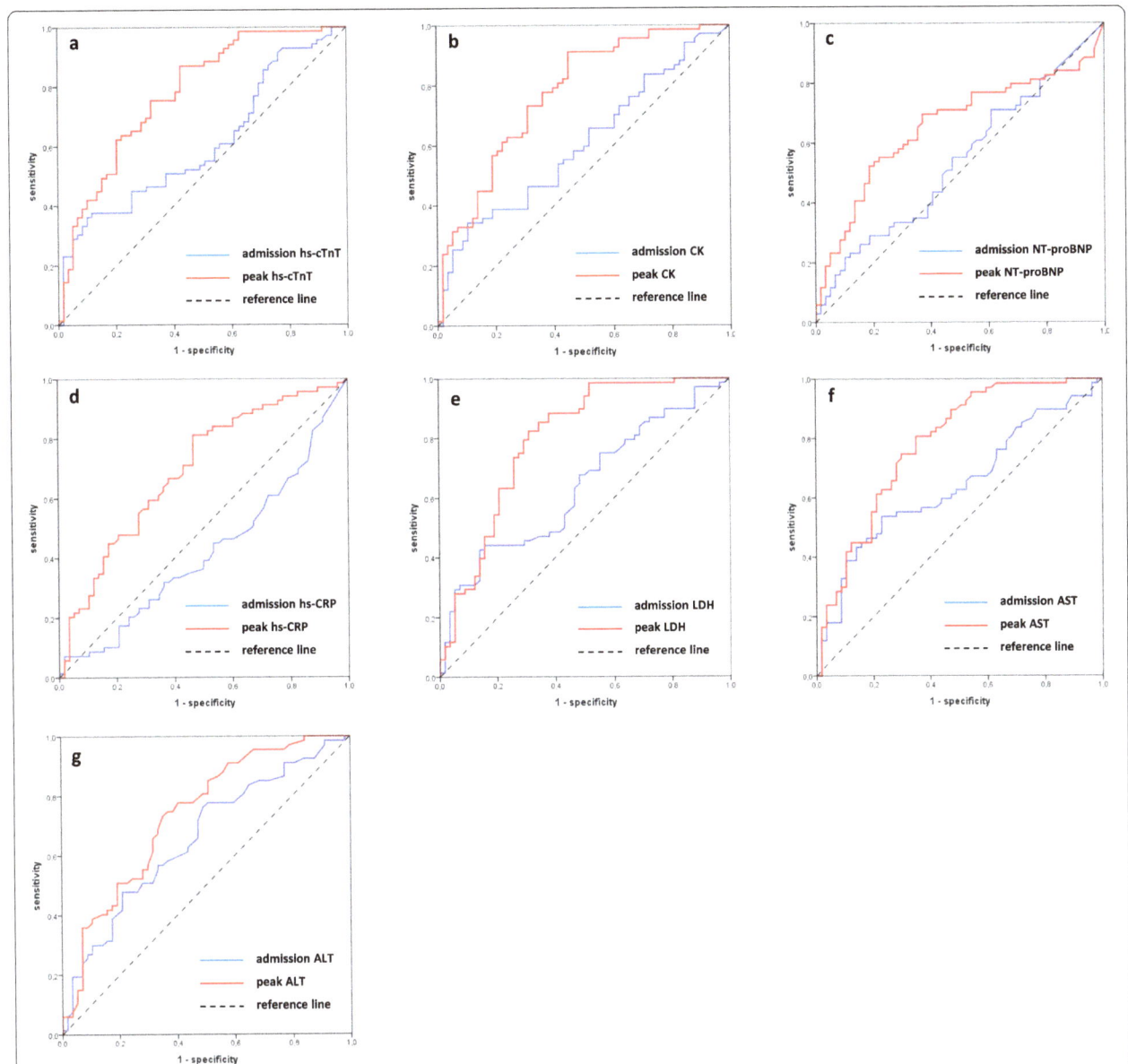

Fig. 1 Receiver operator characteristics (ROC) analyses comparing the predictive utility of admission and peak concentrations of **a**) hs-cTnT (AUC = 0.61, 95% CI 0.52–0.69 vs AUC = 0.77, 95% CI 0.68–0.85; p < 0.001), **b**) CK (AUC = 0.60, 95% CI 0.51–0.69 vs AUC = 0.77, 95% CI 0.69–0.84; p = 0.001), **c**) NT-proBNP (AUC = 0.54, 95% CI 0.45–0.62 vs AUC = 0.64, 95% CI 0.55–0.73; p = 0.011) **d**) hs-CRP (AUC = 0.58, 95% CI 0.49–0.67 vs AUC = 0.68, 95% CI 0.60–0.76; p = NA), **e**) LDH (AUC = 0.64, 95% CI 0.54–0.72 vs AUC = 0.79, 95% CI 0.71–0.86; p = 0.003), **f**) AST (AUC = 0.64, 95% CI 0.55–0.72 vs AUC = 0.78, 95% CI 0.70–0.85, p = 0.005) and **g**) ALT (AUC = 0.66, 95% CI 0.57–0.74 vs AUC = 0.73, 95% CI 0.64–0.80; p = 0.049). hs-cTnT = High-Sensitivity Cardiac Troponin T; CK = Creatine Kinase; NT-proBNP = N-terminal pro-B-type natriuretic peptide; hs-CRP = High-Sensitivity C-Reactive Protein; LDH = Lactate Dehydrogenase; AST = Aspartate Transaminase; ALT = Alanine Transaminase

Thus, the impact of culprit only versus complete PPCI on MVO could not be analysed in the present study. This important topic was recently investigated in a well-conducted meta-analysis [25].

Besides its ability for accurate quantification of ventricular function, morphology and infarct size, CMR imaging has emerged as the most reliable imaging modality to detect microvascular injury and is therefore more and more used to define surrogate endpoints in clinical trials [5, 26, 27]. There is strong evidence that presence of MVO derived from late gadolinium-enhanced images is the best CMR prognosticator regarding clinical outcome after acute reperfused STEMI [3, 7]. Nevertheless, its determination is hampered since CMR is still a rarely available, expensive tool with restricted application in clinical routine. Thus, implementation of a biomarker model, which reliably allows for the prediction of MVO, is of clinical and prognostic importance [28].

Table 2 Biomarker cut-off values providing optimal sensitivity, specificity as well as positive and negative predictive values

	optimal cut-off	sensitivity	specificity	PPV	NPV
hs-cTnT max, ng/l	4387	75	68	73	70
CK max, U/l	1959	73	69	73	69
NT-proBNP max, ng/l	551	70	63	69	64
hs-CRP max, mg/dl	2,11	67	63	68	62
LDH max, U/l	496	82	70	76	77
AST max, U/l	224	75	71	75	71
ALT max, U/l	57	73	64	70	67

hs-cTnT High-Sensitivity Cardiac Troponin T, *CK* Creatine Kinase, *NT-proBNP* N-terminal pro-B-type natriuretic peptide, *hs-CRP* High-Sensitivity C-Reactive Protein, *LDH* Lactate Dehydrogenase, *AST* Aspartate Transaminase, *ALT* Alanine Transaminase

In the present study, time to reperfusion did not differ between patients with and without MVO. Presumably, this is due to the fact that microvascular dysfunction might persist even after restoration of epicardial blood flow [3, 29].

In line with data from literature, we detected a relation between the presence of MVO and infarct size, LV systolic function and morphology [30–32].

An association between cardiac troponin concentrations and CMR derived MVO has already been reported by several studies [13, 33, 34]. Notably, the significance of these studies is limited due to an either small sample size and poorly defined patient selection (STEMI and non-STEMI patients included) or inconsistent reperfusion strategies. These limitations were obviated in the study by Mayr et al, since the relation between MVO and cardiac troponin levels was confirmed in a large, well-defined cohort of STEMI patients [12]. However, in this study a non-high-sensitivity cardiac troponin T assay was used. These assays provide lower prognostic value and are associated with a longer troponin-blind period compared to new-generation high-sensitivity assays [35]. This fact might particularly impact on the prognostic utility of admission troponin levels.

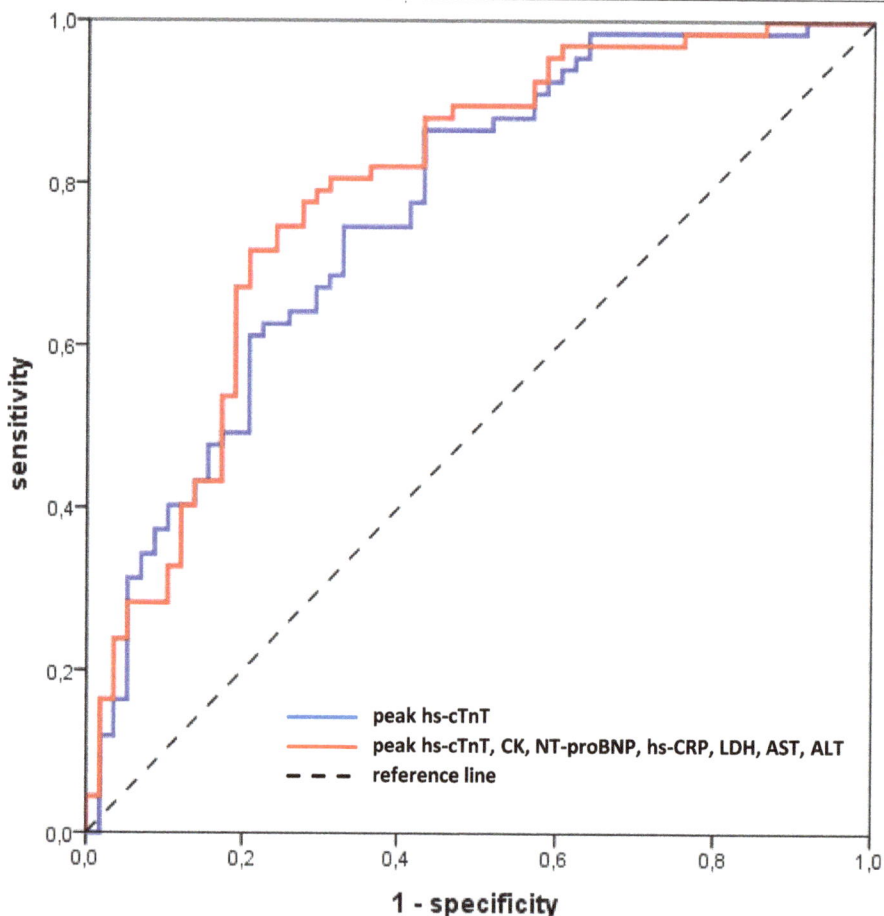

Fig. 2 Receiver operator characteristics (ROC) curves of peak hs-cTnT concentrations and a combined biomarker model. Combination of biomarkers did not result in significantly higher prognostic value for the prediction of MVO compared to hs-cTnT alone (AUC = 0.79, 95% CI 0.71–0.87 vs AUC = 0.77, 95% CI 0.68–0.85; p = 0.349). hs-cTnT = High-Sensitivity Cardiac Troponin T; CK = Creatine Kinase; NT-proBNP = N-terminal pro-B-type natriuretic peptide; hs-CRP = High-Sensitivity C-Reactive Protein; LDH = Lactate Dehydrogenase; AST = Aspartate Transaminase; ALT = Alanine Transaminase

The present study extends previous findings, as we investigated the predictive value of a broad range of routinely used laboratory markers including high-sensitivity cardiac troponin T. All patients were exclusively reperfused by primary PCI, which is of importance since reperfusion strategy might influence the occurrence of MVO. Furthermore, high patient selection, as performed in the present study, reduced the presence of co-morbidities and consequently allowed to investigate predictors of MVO independently of concomitant cardiovascular disease.

Interestingly, peak concentrations of hs-cTnT, CK, hs-CRP, LDH, AST and ALT provided similar prognostic values for the prediction of MVO. This might be of practical significance, in particular if high-sensitivity troponin assays are not available in clinical routine. On the other hand, combining hs-cTnT with other biomarkers did not further improve the prognostic value compared to a model solely including hs-cTnT.

To a certain extent, biomarkers investigated in the present study have already been linked to clinical outcome following AMI [36]. Moreover, in AMI patients prognostic utility was even proved for novel, upcoming biomarkers like galectin-3 [37]. Although an association between biomarkers and hard clinical endpoints was shown in previous studies, the present study adds some causal relation, particularly since MVO is among the strongest predictors of poor outcome after STEMI [7].

Besides its prognostic value, the therapeutic relevance of MVO has been demonstrated in several studies. For instance, modern antiplatelet therapy might improve microvascular perfusion [23]. Moreover, in patients with successfully reperfused AMI treatment with statins before infarction was associated with a reduction of microvascular injury [38].

Limitations

This is the largest CMR study investigating a comprehensive biomarker model for the prediction of MVO. Nevertheless, further confirmation in larger cohorts is necessary. Remarkably, sensitivity and specificity is less than 80% for almost all biomarkers observed in the present study. These biomarkers reflect myocardial injury, haemodynamic alterations and inflammation. However, the occurrence of MVO is a rather complex pathophysiological process and, to a certain extent, a still unresolved topic [39]. Possibly, the analysis of other, upcoming chemical markers might further improve the predictive value for the occurrence of MVO and should be investigated in future studies [36, 40].

In the present study the proportion of female patients was very low. Out of twelve female patients totally included only four patients developed MVO. Therefore, gender-specific, valid statistical analysis could not be performed.

However, the impact of gender on outcome in STEMI patients has already been shown [41]. Thus, further studies are needed investigating gender-specific differences in the prediction of MVO.

The present study focused on the prediction of MVO derived from CMR. Therefore, angiographic assessment of myocardial blush grade and the relatively novel wire-based technique to measure the index of microcirculatory resistance were not performed in this study [42].

Conclusions

hs-cTnT, CK, hs-CRP, LDH, AST and ALT peak concentrations provided similar prognostic value for the prediction of CMR derived MVO in acute STEMI patients reperfused by PPCI. In comparison, the prognostic utility of peak NT-proBNP was lower. Combination of these biomarkers did not add any additional prognostic value. Since presence of MVO is among the strongest surrogate end-points for adverse clinical outcome after acute STEMI, our findings could contribute to optimize risk stratification early after the acute event.

Abbreviations

ALT: Alanine transaminase; AST: Aspartate transaminase; AUC: Area under the curve; CK: Creatine kinase; CMR: Cardiac magnetic resonance; EDV: End-diastolic volume; ESV: End-systolic volume; hs-CRP: High-sensitivity C-reactive protein; hs-cTnT: High-sensitivity cardiac troponin T; IQR: Interquartile range; IS: Infarct size; LDH: Lactate dehydrogenase; LV: Left ventricular; LVEF: Left ventricular ejection fraction; MVO: Microvascular obstruction; ND: Normal distribution; NT-proBNP: N-terminal pro-B-type natriuretic peptide; PPCI: Primary percutaneous coronary intervention; ROC: Receiver operator characteristics; SD: Standard deviation; STEMI: ST-segment elevation myocardial infarction; True-FISP: True fast imaging steady-state precession

Acknowledgements

The abstract of the present manuscript was previously published and selected for poster presentation at an international congress.

Funding

This study was supported by grants from the *Austrian Society of Cardiology* as well as from the intramural funding programme of Medical University of Innsbruck – *MUI-START* (2015-06-013) to HJF, GK and SJR and by a grant from the 'Hans and Blanca-Moser Stiftung' to SJR.

Authors' contribution

HJF, SJR, GK, MR, SW, CB, AM, JM and BM substantially contributed in the design of the study, or acquisition, or analysis and interpretation of the data. HJF, SJR, GK, MR, SW, CB, AM, JM and BM were involved in drafting of the manuscript and revised it critically for important intellectual content. Each author participated sufficiently in the work and gave final approval for publication. All authors agreed to be accountable for all aspects of the work in ensuring that questions related to the accuracy or integrity of any part of the work are appropriately investigated and resolved.

Competing interests

The authors declare that they have no competing interests.

Author details

[1]University Clinic of Internal Medicine III, Cardiology and Angiology, Medical University of Innsbruck, Anichstraße 35, A-6020 Innsbruck, Austria.
[2]Department of Radiology, Medical University of Innsbruck, Anichstraße 35, A-6020 Innsbruck, Austria.

References

1. Jernberg T, Johanson P, Held C, Svennblad B, Lindback J, Wallentin L. Association between adoption of evidence-based treatment and survival for patients with ST-elevation myocardial infarction. JAMA. 2011;305:1677–84.

2. Gjesing A, Gislason GH, Kober L, Gustav Smith J, Christensen SB, Gustafsson F, Olsen AM, Torp-Pedersen C, Andersson C. Nationwide trends in development of heart failure and mortality after first-time myocardial infarction 1997–2010: A Danish cohort study. Eur J Intern Med. 2014;25:731–8.

3. van Kranenburg M, Magro M, Thiele H, de Waha S, Eitel I, Cochet A, Cottin Y, Atar D, Buser P, Wu E, Lee D, Bodi V, Klug G, Metzler B, Delewi R, Bernhardt P, Rottbauer W, Boersma E, Zijlstra F, van Geuns RJ. Prognostic value of microvascular obstruction and infarct size, as measured by CMR in STEMI patients. JACC Cardiovasc Imaging. 2014;7:930–9.

4. Niccoli G, Scalone G, Lerman A, Crea F. Coronary microvascular obstruction in acute myocardial infarction. Eur Heart J. 2016;37:1024–33.

5. Klug G, Metzler B. Assessing myocardial recovery following ST-segment elevation myocardial infarction: short- and long-term perspectives using cardiovascular magnetic resonance. Expert Rev Cardiovasc Ther. 2013;11:203–19.

6. Schaaf MJ, Mewton N, Rioufol G, Angoulvant D, Cayla G, Delarche N, Jouve B, Guerin P, Vanzetto G, Coste P, Morel O, Roubille F, Elbaz M, Roth O, Prunier F, Cung TT, Piot C, Sanchez I, Bonnefoy-Cudraz E, Revel D, Giraud C, Croisille P, Ovize M. Pre-PCI angiographic TIMI flow in the culprit coronary artery influences infarct size and microvascular obstruction in STEMI patients. J Cardiol. 2016;67:248–53.

7. Eitel I, de Waha S, Wohrle J, Fuernau G, Lurz P, Pauschinger M, Desch S, Schuler G, Thiele H. Comprehensive prognosis assessment by CMR imaging after ST-segment elevation myocardial infarction. J Am Coll Cardiol. 2014;64: 1217–26.

8. Cochet AA, Lorgis L, Lalande A, Zeller M, Beer JC, Walker PM, Touzery C, Wolf JE, Brunotte F, Cottin Y. Major prognostic impact of persistent microvascular obstruction as assessed by contrast-enhanced cardiac magnetic resonance in reperfused acute myocardial infarction. Eur Radiol. 2009;19:2117–26.

9. Klug G, Mayr A, Schenk S, Esterhammer R, Schocke M, Nocker M, Jaschke W, Pachinger O, Metzler B. Prognostic value at 5 years of microvascular obstruction after acute myocardial infarction assessed by cardiovascular magnetic resonance. J Cardiovasc Magn Reson. 2012;14:46.

10. de Waha S, Eitel I, Desch S, Fuernau G, Lurz P, Stiermaier T, Blazek S, Schuler G, Thiele H. Prognosis after ST-elevation myocardial infarction: a study on cardiac magnetic resonance imaging versus clinical routine. Trials. 2014;15:249.

11. Watanabe N, Isobe S, Okumura T, Mori H, Yamada T, Nishimura K, Miura M, Sakai S, Murohara T. Relationship between QRS score and microvascular obstruction after acute anterior myocardial infarction. J Cardiol. 2016;67:321–6.

12. Mayr A, Klug G, Schocke M, Trieb T, Mair J, Pedarnig K, Pachinger O, Jaschke W, Metzler B. Late microvascular obstruction after acute myocardial infarction: relation with cardiac and inflammatory markers. Int J Cardiol. 2012;157:391–6.

13. Pernet K, Ecarnot F, Chopard R, Seronde MF, Plastaras P, Schiele F, Meneveau N. Microvascular obstruction assessed by 3-tesla magnetic resonance imaging in acute myocardial infarction is correlated with plasma troponin I levels. BMC Cardiovasc Disord. 2014;14:57.

14. Kim MK, Chung WY, Cho YS, Choi SI, Chae IH, Choi DJ, Park YB. Serum N-terminal pro-B-type natriuretic peptide levels at the time of hospital admission predict of microvascular obstructions after primary percutaneous coronary intervention for acute ST-segment elevation myocardial infarction. J Interv Cardiol. 2011;24:34–41.

15. Thygesen K, Alpert JS, Jaffe AS, Simoons ML, Chaitman BR, White HD, Katus HA, Apple FS, Lindahl B, Morrow DA, Chaitman BA, Clemmensen PM, Johanson P, Hod H, Underwood R, Bax JJ, Bonow RO, Pinto F, Gibbons RJ, Fox KA, Atar D, Newby LK, Galvani M, Hamm CW, Uretsky BF, Steg PG, Wijns W, Bassand JP, Menasche P, Ravkilde J, Ohman EM, Antman EM, Wallentin LC, Armstrong PW, Januzzi JL, Nieminen MS, Gheorghiade M, Filippatos G, Luepker RV, Fortmann SP, Rosamond WD, Levy D, Wood D, Smith SC, Hu D, Lopez-Sendon JL, Robertson RM, Weaver D, Tendera M, Bove AA, Parkhomenko AN, Vasilieva EJ, Mendis S.

Third universal definition of myocardial infarction. Eur Heart J. 2012;33: 2551–67.

16. Feistritzer HJ, Klug G, Reinstadler SJ, Mair J, Seidner B, Mayr A, Franz WM, Metzler B. Aortic stiffness is associated with elevated high-sensitivity cardiac troponin T concentrations at a chronic stage after ST-segment elevation myocardial infarction. J Hypertens. 2015;33:1970–6.

17. Reinstadler SJ, Feistritzer HJ, Klug G, Mair J, Tu AM, Kofler M, Henninger B, Franz WM, Metzler B. High-sensitivity troponin T for prediction of left ventricular function and infarct size one year following ST-elevation myocardial infarction. Int J Cardiol. 2016;202:188–93.

18. Feistritzer HJ, Reinstadler SJ, Klug G, Kremser C, Rederlechner A, Mair J, Mueller S, Franz WM, Metzler B. N-terminal pro-B-type natriuretic peptide is associated with aortic stiffness in patients presenting with acute myocardial infarction. Eur Heart J Acute Cardiovasc Care 2015;Epub ahead of print.

19. Mayr A, Mair J, Schocke M, Klug G, Pedarnig K, Haubner BJ, Nowosielski M, Grubinger T, Pachinger O, Metzler B. Predictive value of NT-pro BNP after acute myocardial infarction: relation with acute and chronic infarct size and myocardial function. Int J Cardiol. 2011;147:118–23.

20. Bondarenko O, Beek AM, Hofman MB, Kuhl HP, Twisk JW, van Dockum WG, Visser CA, van Rossum AC. Standardizing the definition of hyperenhancement in the quantitative assessment of infarct size and myocardial viability using delayed contrast-enhanced CMR. J Cardiovasc Magn Reson. 2005;7:481–5.

21. DeLong ER, DeLong DM, Clarke-Pearson DL. Comparing the areas under two or more correlated receiver operating characteristic curves: a nonparametric approach. Biometrics. 1988;44:837–45.

22. Bekkers SC, Yazdani SK, Virmani R, Waltenberger J. Microvascular obstruction: underlying pathophysiology and clinical diagnosis. J Am Coll Cardiol. 2010;55:1649–60.

23. Montalescot G, Barragan P, Wittenberg O, Ecollan P, Elhadad S, Villain P, Boulenc JM, Morice MC, Maillard L, Pansieri M, Choussat R, Pinton P. Platelet glycoprotein IIb/IIIa inhibition with coronary stenting for acute myocardial infarction. N Engl J Med. 2001;344:1895–903.

24. Carrick D, Oldroyd KG, McEntegart M, Haig C, Petrie MC, Eteiba H, Hood S, Owens C, Watkins S, Layland J, Lindsay M, Peat E, Rae A, Behan M, Sood A, Hillis WS, Mordi I, Mahrous A, Ahmed N, Wilson R, Lasalle L, Genereux P, Ford I, Berry C. A randomized trial of deferred stenting versus immediate stenting to prevent no- or slow-reflow in acute ST-segment elevation myocardial infarction (DEFER-STEMI). J Am Coll Cardiol. 2014;63:2088–98.

25. Moretti C, D'Ascenzo F, Quadri G, Omede P, Montefusco A, Taha S, Cerrato E, Colaci C, Chen SL, Biondi-Zoccai G, Gaita F. Management of multivessel coronary disease in STEMI patients: a systematic review and meta-analysis. Int J Cardiol. 2015;179:552–7.

26. Bajwa HZ, Do L, Suhail M, Hetts SW, Wilson MW, Saeed M. MRI demonstrates a decrease in myocardial infarct healing and increase in compensatory ventricular hypertrophy following mechanical microvascular obstruction. J Magn Reson Imaging. 2014;40:906–14.

27. Khan JN, Greenwood JP, Nazir SA, Lai FY, Dalby M, Curzen N, Hetherington S, Kelly DJ, Blackman D, Peebles C, Wong J, Flather M, Swanton H, Gershlick AH, McCann GP. Infarct Size Following Treatment With Second- Versus Third-Generation P2Y12 Antagonists in Patients With Multivessel Coronary Disease at ST-Segment Elevation Myocardial Infarction in the CvLPRIT Study. J Am Heart Assoc. 2016;5:e003403.

28. O'Donoghue ML, Morrow DA, Cannon CP, Jarolim P, Desai NR, Sherwood MW, Murphy SA, Gerszten RE, Sabatine MS. Multimarker Risk Stratification in Patients With Acute Myocardial Infarction. J Am Heart Assoc. 2016;5:002586.

29. De Luca G, Van't Hof AW, de Boer MJ, Ottervanger JP, Hoorntje JC, Gosselink AT, Dambrink JH, Zijlstra F, Suryapranata H. Time-to-treatment significantly affects the extent of ST-segment resolution and myocardial blush in patients with acute myocardial infarction treated by primary angioplasty. Eur Heart J. 2004;25:1009–13.

30. de Waha S, Desch S, Eitel I, Fuernau G, Lurz P, Leuschner A, Grothoff M, Gutberlet M, Schuler G, Thiele H. Relationship and prognostic value of microvascular obstruction and infarct size in ST-elevation myocardial infarction as visualized by magnetic resonance imaging. Clin Res Cardiol. 2012;101:487–95.

31. Hamirani YS, Wong A, Kramer CM, Salerno M. Effect of microvascular obstruction and intramyocardial hemorrhage by CMR on LV remodeling and outcomes after myocardial infarction: a systematic review and meta-analysis. JACC Cardiovasc Imaging. 2014;7:940–52.

32. Lombardo A, Niccoli G, Natale L, Bernardini A, Cosentino N, Bonomo L, Crea F. Impact of microvascular obstruction and infarct size on left ventricular remodeling in reperfused myocardial infarction: a contrast-enhanced cardiac magnetic resonance imaging study. Int J Cardiovasc Imaging. 2012; 28:835–42.

33. Neizel M, Futterer S, Steen H, Giannitsis E, Reinhardt L, Lossnitzer D, Lehrke S, Jaffe AS, Katus HA. Predicting microvascular obstruction with cardiac troponin T after acute myocardial infarction: a correlative study with contrast-enhanced magnetic resonance imaging. Clin Res Cardiol. 2009;98:555–62.

34. Younger JF, Plein S, Barth J, Ridgway JP, Ball SG, Greenwood JP. Troponin-I concentration 72 h after myocardial infarction correlates with infarct size and presence of microvascular obstruction. Heart. 2007;93:1547–51.

35. Reichlin T, Hochholzer W, Bassetti S, Steuer S, Stelzig C, Hartwiger S, Biedert S, Schaub N, Buerge C, Potocki M, Noveanu M, Breidthardt T, Twerenbold R, Winkler K, Bingisser R, Mueller C. Early diagnosis of myocardial infarction with sensitive cardiac troponin assays. N Engl J Med. 2009;361:858–67.

36. Feistritzer HJ, Klug G, Reinstadler SJ, Reindl M, Mayr A, Mair J, Metzler B. Novel biomarkers predicting cardiac function after acute myocardial infarction. Br Med Bull. 2016;119:63–74.

37. George M, Shanmugam E, Srivatsan V, Vasanth K, Ramraj B, Rajaram M, Jena A, Sridhar A, Chaudhury M, Kaliappan I. Value of pentraxin-3 and galectin-3 in acute coronary syndrome: a short-term prospective cohort study. Ther Adv Cardiovasc Dis. 2015;9:275–84.

38. Iwakura K, Ito H, Kawano S, Okamura A, Kurotobi T, Date M, Inoue K, Fujii K. Chronic pre-treatment of statins is associated with the reduction of the no-reflow phenomenon in the patients with reperfused acute myocardial infarction. Eur Heart J. 2006;27:534–9.

39. Reinstadler SJ, Stiermaier T, Fuernau G, de Waha S, Desch S, Metzler B, Thiele H, Eitel I. The challenges and impact of microvascular injury in ST-elevation myocardial infarction. Expert Rev Cardiovasc Ther. 2016;14:431–43.

40. George M, Ganesh MR, Sridhar A, Jena A, Rajaram M, Shanmugam E, Dhandapani VE. Evaluation of Endothelial and Platelet Derived Microparticles in Patients with Acute Coronary Syndrome. J Clin Diagn Res. 2015;9:OC09–13.

41. Karim MA, Majumder AA, Islam KQ, Alam MB, Paul ML, Islam MS, Chowdhury KN, Islam SM. Risk factors and in-hospital outcome of acute ST segment elevation myocardial infarction in young Bangladeshi adults. BMC Cardiovasc Disord. 2015;15:73.

42. Payne AR, Berry C, Doolin O, McEntegart M, Petrie MC, Lindsay MM, Hood S, Carrick D, Tzemos N, Weale P, McComb C, Foster J, Ford I, Oldroyd KG. Microvascular Resistance Predicts Myocardial Salvage and Infarct Characteristics in ST-Elevation Myocardial Infarction. J Am Heart Assoc. 2012;1:e002246.

10

Independent prognostic value of left atrial function by two-dimensional speckle tracking imaging in patients with non -ST-segment-elevation acute myocardial infarction

Chunlai Shao[†], Jing Zhu[†], Jianchang Chen and Weiting Xu[*]

Abstract

Background: The objective of this study is to evaluate left atrial(LA) function and its prognostic value by two-dimensional speckle tracking echocardiography (STE) in patients with non-ST-segment-elevation acute myocardial infarction (NSTEAMI).

Methods: Global longitudinal LA S/SR data obtained by 2D speckle imaging with automated software (Echo PAC, GE Medical).

Results: Clinical variables and angiographic, echocardiographic, and STE parameters were studied in 65 patients with NSTEAMI (51 males and 14 females; mean age of 60.7 ± 9.8 years) who underwent elective PCI. The final study population consisted of 51 individuals (43 males and 8 females; mean age of 62.9 ± 11.1 years) and a 12 ± 3 months follow-up was performed. A total of 22 combined cardiovascular events(20 patients) occurred. With the use of Univariable Cox regression, all parameters were evaluated in the prediction of cardiac events, ischemic events, and/or cardiac death. According to ROC analysis, baseline mean global left atrial SRs (ROC area 0.82, $p = 0.001$) and baseline mean global left atrial SRe (ROC area 0.68, $p = 0.036$) were the only predictive variables.

Conclusions: In patients with NSTEAMI, we found that the novel global strain parameter of left atrial function is a valuable predictor of combined cardiovascular events over conventional echocardiography and may therefore be an important clinical tool for risk stratification in the acute phase of NSTEAMI.

Keywords: Two-dimensional speckle tracking imaging, Strain, Strain rate, Left atrial function, Non-ST-segment-elevation acute myocardial infarction

Background

Coronary artery diseases (CAD) are the most common cardiac disease, which affect more than twenty million adults in China. Acute myocardial infarction (AMI), acting as a canonical component of CAD, contributes to approximately one million identified cardiac events every year. When ST elevation of AMI patient is present, treatment is aimed at reperfusion by opening the occluded coronary artery, either by thrombolysis or by percutaneous coronary intervention (PCI). Due to presence of more sensitive biochemical markers of myocardial necrosis, an increasing number of patients with non-ST-segment-elevation acute myocardial infarction(NSTEAMI) are diagnosed [1]. These patients may develop substantial myocardial infarction (MI), but criteria for acute reperfusion therapy is rarely fulfilled [2] and clinical outcome is doubted, when compared with patients with ST-segment-elevation acute myocardial infarction.

According to previous studies, LA function index is a powerful predictor of mortality in AMI patients and

* Correspondence: xuwt1968@aliyun.com
[†]Equal contributors
Department of Cardiology, The Second Affiliated Hospital of Soochow University, Sanxiang Street 1055, Suzhou, China

provides prognostic information incremental to clinical data as well as reduced left ventricular ejection fraction (LVEF) [3]. Recently, two-dimensional speckle tracking echocardiography (STE) has been introduced as an accurate technique for quantifying regional LA function, with more comprehensive and reliable echocardiographic resolution compared with traditional methods [4]. In contrast to tissue Doppler imaging, STE shows the advantage of angle-independence, as well as being less affected by reverberations, side lobes and drop out artifacts [5]. Recently, strain echocardiography had been validated as a prognostic indicator of cardiovascular diseases [6, 7].We hypothesized that patients with NSTEAMI have impaired function of LA as well as left ventricular (LV). The aim of our study is to explore the utility of strain echocardiography in the assessment of LA function and prognostic value in patients with NSTEAMI undergoing elective PCI.

Methods
Patient selection
A total of 65 patients (51 males and 14 females; mean age of 60.7 ± 9.8 years) with a diagnosis of NSTEAMI confirmed at the referring hospital by elevated troponin I above the 99 % percentile and positive ECG (Evidence of ischemia was defined as any ST-deviation >0.5 mm or symmetrical T-wave inversion >3 mm in two or more contiguous leads) were enrolled from March 2012 to March 2013. All patients were considered clinically and hemodynamically stable during index admission, and none were referred for urgent coronary intervention. Time from hospital admission to elective PCI was 5.2 ± 0.8 days (range, 2 to 7 days). Patients with atrial fibrillation or flutter, valvular heart disease (of mild or greater severity), or a history of previous myocardial infarction were excluded.

All the patients had received optimized anti-ischemic (beta-blockers, nitrates), dual antiplatelet and antithrombotic therapy (aspirin, clopidogrel, enoxaparin and GP IIb/IIIa antagonists if indicated according to recent international guidelines). The study protocol was approved by the Ethics Committee of The Second Affiliated Hospital of Soochow University (Suzhou, China). Each participant provided written informed consent to be included in the study.

Coronary angiographic procedure
Coronary angiography was performed on clinical indication by standard (Judkins) technique using digital imaging acquisition and storage. Direct stenting was allowed and various kinds of pre-dilatation devices and manual aspiration devices were allowed in case of acute myocardial infarction with severe thrombus in target artery.

Standard echocardiography
The patients were investigated by transthoracic echocardiography immediately prior to coronary angiography and after 6 months of follow-up on a Vivid7 ultrasound system (GE, USA) equipped with a phased array transducer (frequency range of 1.7–3.4 MHz). M-mode echocardiography was used to measure LA diameter and LV end-diastolic and end-systolic diameters. LV ejection fraction (LVEF) was calculated from 4-chamber and 2-chamber view, using the modified Simpson rule. Three separate LA volumes were computed following American Society of Echocardiography guidelines using biplane modified Simpson's method [5]. Left atrial maximum volume (LAVmax) at the end of LV systole, just before the opening of mitral valve and LA minimum volume (LAVmin) at the end of LV diastole, right after the closure of the mitral valve, were measured and LA pre-atrial volume (LAVp) was obtained from the diastolic frame before initial mitral valve reopening elicited by atrial contraction. Left atrial volume index (LAI) = left atrial maximum volume/body surface area; LA reservoir function was assessed using the following equation: LA total EF = (LAVmax-LAVmin)/LAVmax; Passive left atrial ejection fraction (LAPEF) = (LAVmax-LAVp)/LAVmax; Left atrial active ejection fraction (LAAEF) = (LAVp - LAVmin) / LAVp.

Tissue doppler imaging echocardiography
LV diastolic function was explored by pulsed Tissue Doppler imaging, placing the sample volume at the level of mitral lateral and septal annulus from the apical four chamber view. Mean peak systolic (S), early diastolic (E'), and late diastolic (A') annular velocities were obtained by averaging respective values measured at the septal and lateral sides of the mitral annulus. Mean Em and the derived mean E'/A' ratio were used as load-independent markers of ventricular diastolic relaxation. Mean E/E' ratio was also calculated.

Two-dimensional speckle tracking echocardiography(STE)
In the setting of 2D-STE analysis, three consecutive heart cycles were recorded and averaged. The frame rate was set between 60 and 90 frames per second. Echocardiograms were digitally stored and later analyzed off-line using acoustic-tracking software (Echo-Pac version 7.0, GE Vingmed). LA endocardial surface was manually traced in each view with a point-and-click approach. An epicardial surface tracing was then automatically generated by the software, creating a region of interest (ROI). Afterwards, The ROI was divided into three segments: annular, mid and roof, whereas the resultant tracking quality for each segment is automatically scored for evaluation as either acceptable or non-acceptable. Finally, the software generated strain and strain rate curves for each atrial segment

[8]. We acquired global longitudinal LA peak negative strain during atrial systole (GLSs), peak positive strain during ventricle systole (GLSr), peak positive strain rate during ventricle systole (GLSRs), peak negative strain rate during early ventricular diastole (GLSRe) and peak negative strain rate during late ventricular diastole (GLSRa) (Figs. 1 and 2), respectively [9]. Mean global longitudinal LA S/SR of three views was calculated as following: (LA S/SR in apical long axis view + LA S/SR in 4-chamber + LA S/SR in 2-chamber view)/3. We identified 65 subjects in our database. Of these patients, 14 subjects were excluded from analysis for inadequate electrocardiograms or inadequate imaging quality due to acquisition with low frame rates ($n = 8$), LA foreshortening or inadequate acoustic windows ($n = 6$). The final study population consisted of 51 individuals (43 males and 8 females; mean age of 62.9 ± 11.1 years).

Follow-up and study endpoints

Fifty one NSTEAMI patients were followed from March 2011 to March 2013 with follow-up telephone conversations or review of medical records. Patients were monitored regularly for the occurrence of cardiac mortality and adverse cardiac events. The primary end point of this study was combined cardiac events, which were defined as combined cardiac-cause mortality and re-hospitalization due to adverse cardiac events such as exacerbation of heart failure or acute myocardial ischemia. Cardiac death was defined by clinical data of acute myocardial infarction and/or fatal cardiac arrhythmias and/or refractory congestive heart failure. The date of the last interview or review was used to calculate the follow-up duration.

Statistical analysis

Data was analyzed using the statistical software package (SPSS, Rel 13.0, Chicago: SPSS Inc.). Continuous data were presented as mean ± SD. Differences between the baseline and 6 months groups were compared using the independent t-test. Categorical parameters are presented as numbers (%), and were analyzed by χ^2 test. Univariable Cox proportional-hazards regression models were used to identify independent predictors of late cardiac events. The risk of a given variable was expressed by a hazard ratio (HR) with corresponding 95 % confidence intervals. Receiver-operating characteristic (ROC) curves were constructed, and areas under curves were measured to determine cutoff values with maximum sensitivity and

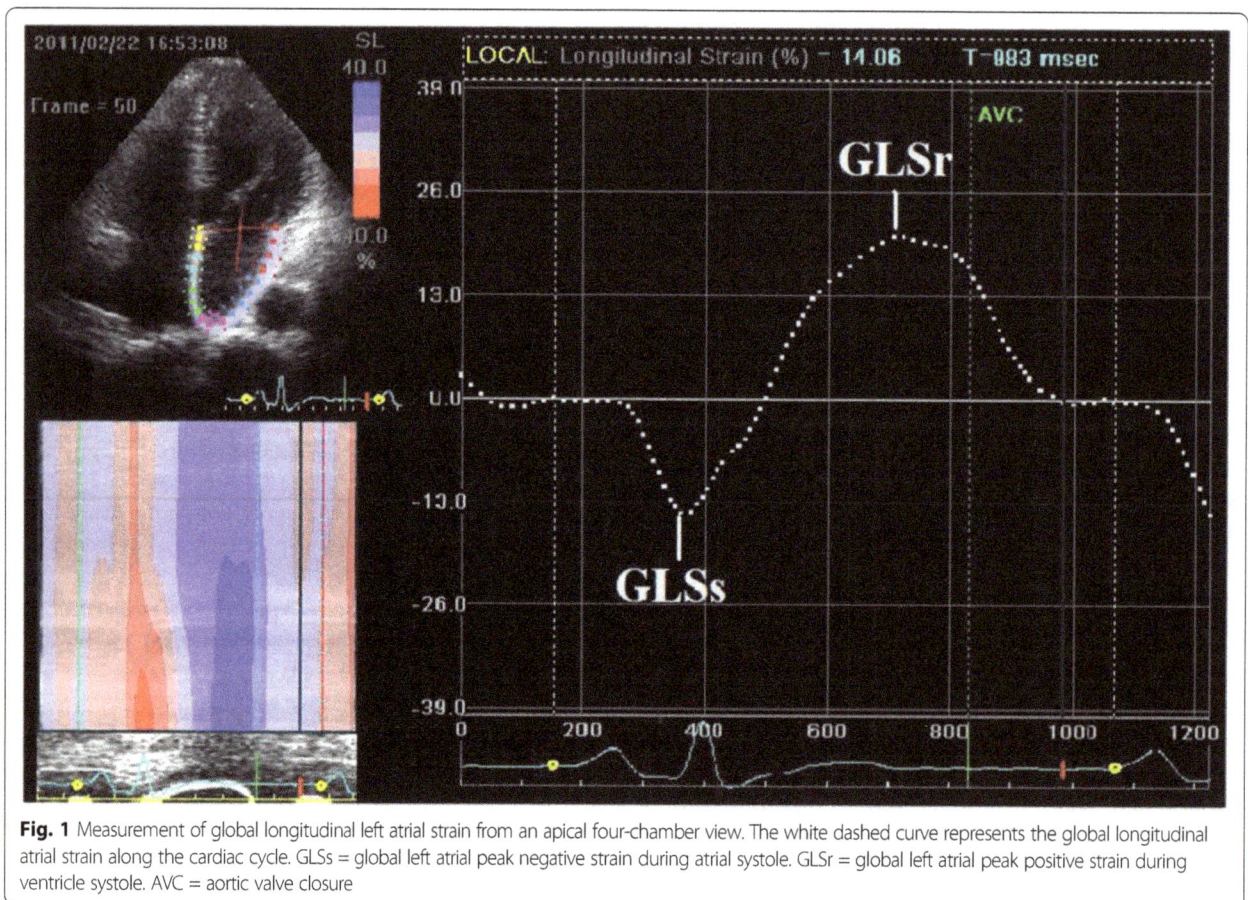

Fig. 1 Measurement of global longitudinal left atrial strain from an apical four-chamber view. The white dashed curve represents the global longitudinal atrial strain along the cardiac cycle. GLSs = global left atrial peak negative strain during atrial systole. GLSr = global left atrial peak positive strain during ventricle systole. AVC = aortic valve closure

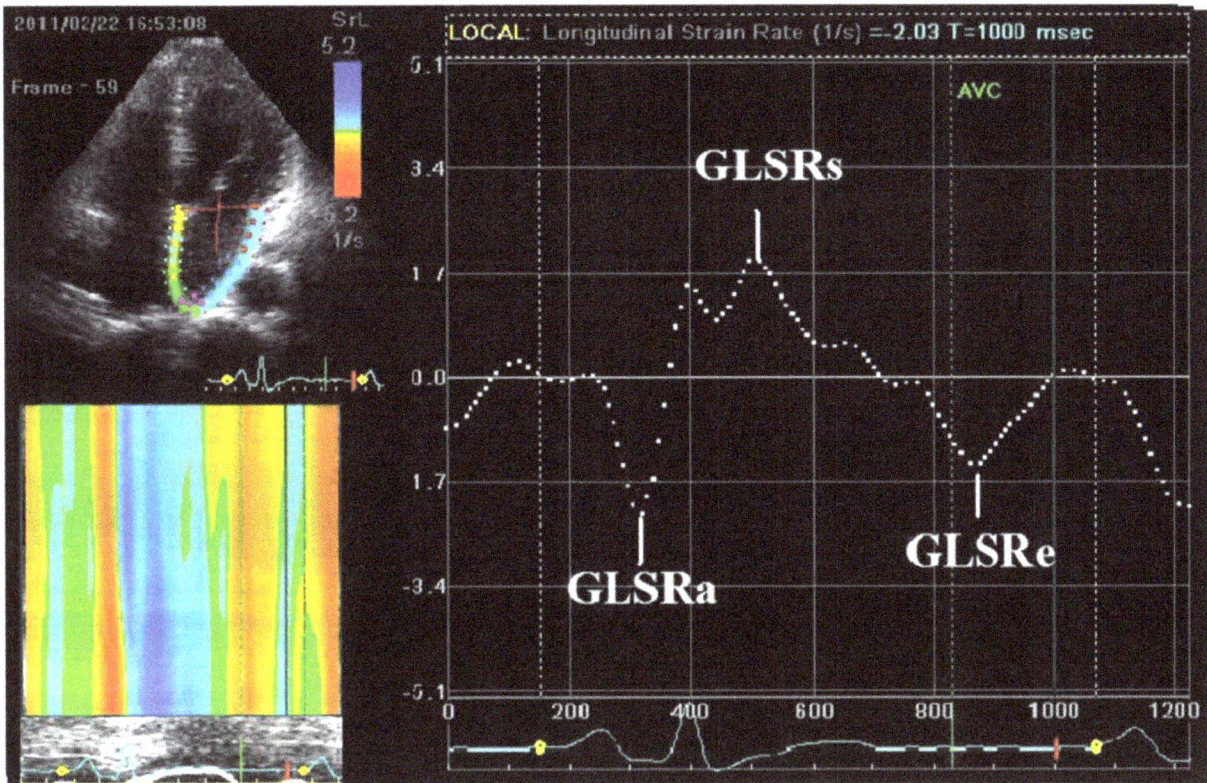

Fig. 2 Measurement of global longitudinal left atrial strain rate from an apical four-chamber view. The white dashed curve represents the global longitudinal strain rate during the cardiac cycle. GLSRa = global left atrial peak negative strain rate during late ventricular diastole. GLSRs = global left atrial peak positive strain rate during ventricle systole. GLSRe = global left atrial peak negative strain rate during early ventricular diastole . AVC = aortic valve closure

specificity. A 2-tailed p-value < 0.05 was considered significant for statistical inference.

Results

Over an average of 12 months (range 6 to 17 months, 12 ± 3 months) follow-up, a sum of 22 cardiovascular events(20 patients) have been recorded, including 2 patients death (9.1 %) due to a cardiac cause, 11 progressive heart failure (50.0 %), and 9 recurrent acute coronary syndrome(ACS) (40.9 %) (Table 1). According to clinical follow-up results, the overall population was divided into two groups: patients with ($n = 20$) and without ($n = 31$) cardiac events.

Clinical and angiographic characteristics

Baseline clinical and angiographic characteristics of two groups are shown in Table 2. No significant differences were evidenced between the two groups, except for a higher prevalence of Hyperlipidemia and less final TIMI 3 flow in had events patients.

Echocardiography characteristics

Conventional and TDI echocardiography parameters of LA and LV function are shown in Table 3. Table 4 displays baseline STE data on three views and baseline mean electrocardiographic data, as well as 6 months mean echocardiography data for the entire study patients. Patients with cardiac events had significantly decreased LAPEF(25.16 ± 12.26 vs 29.02 ± 10.22, $p = 0.028$), baseline mean GLASRs(1.39 ± 0.48 vs 1.62 ± 0.55, $p = 0.003$), mean Glaser(-1.07 ± 0.42 vs-1.25 ± 0.48, $p = 0.013$) and 6 months mean GLASRs(1.73 ± 0.48 vs 1.98 ± 0.61, $p = 0.017$),but increased E/E' ratio(6.9 ± 2.7 vs 5.8 ± 1.8, $p = 0.037$).

Table 1 Follow-up combined cardiovascular events

Cardiovascular Events	$n = 22$(20 patients)
Cardiovascular death	2 (9.10 %)
Re-hospitalization	20 (90.90 %)
Progressive heart failure	11 (50 %)
Recurrent ACS	9 (40.90 %)

ACS acute coronary syndrome

Table 2 Clinical and catheterization data of the study population of NSTEAMI patients Stratified by Event Status ($n = 51$)

Characteristics	Had events ($n = 20$)	No events ($n = 31$)	p
Clinical data			
Age (years)(means)	63.2 ± 9.46	60.9 ± 12.17	0.274
Male (%)	18(90.0 %)	25(80.6 %)	0.138
Female (%)	2 (10.0 %)	6 (19.4 %)	0.068
Body mass index (kg/m^2)	1.81 ± 0.17	1.78 ± 0.21	0.454
Heart rate (beats/min)	78 ± 8.11	74 ± 10.23	0.228
Systolic blood pressure (mmHg)	144 ± 18	138 ± 12	0.152
Diastolic blood pressure (mmHg)	68 ± 19	65 ± 17	0.098
Diabetesmellitus (%)	6(30.0 %)	11(35.5 %)	0.148
Hyperlipidemia (%)	12(60.0 %)	14(45.2 %)	0.048*
Catheterization data			
Native diseased vessel (%)			
One vessel	7(35.0 %)	11(35.5 %)	0.216
Two vessels	3(15.0 %)	7(22.6 %)	0.192
Three vessels	10(50.0 %)	13(41.9 %)	0.323
Treated vessel, n (%)			
LAD	5(25.0 %)	6(19.4 %)	0.277
LCX	3(15.0 %)	5(16.1 %)	0.284
RCA	1(5.0 %)	2(6.5 %)	0.408
Final TIMI flow (%)			
3	19(95 %)	29(93.5 %)	0.054
<3	3	0	<0.001**

LCX left circumflex coronary artery, LAD left anterior descending, RCA right coronary artery, TIMI thrombolysis in myocardial infarction
*$P < 0.05$, **$P < 0.01$, between Had events group and No events group

Prediction of clinical and echocardiography characteristics
Correlations of cardiac events were assessed using multivariable Cox proportional hazards models (Table 5), containing four echocardiography variables, which were significant predictors of combined cardiovascular events: LAPEF (HR = 1.05, 95 % CI 1.02 to 1.08, $p =$ 0.003), LA total EF (HR = 1.02, 95%CI 0.99 to 1.05, $p =$ 0.048), baseline mean GLSRs (HR = 1.27, 95 % CI 1.01 to 1.59, $p =$ 0.044) and baseline mean GLSRe (HR = 6.95, 95 % CI 2.00 to 24.94, $p =$ 0.002). Other clinical variables (age, sex, BMI, hypertension, diabetes mellitus, and hyperlipidemia), angiographic variables (native diseased vessel, natively occluded coronary artery, final TIMI flow, and ACC/AHA lesion type after PTCA), conventional electrocardiographic characteristics (LAVmax, LAVmin, LAVp, LAAEF, LAVI and LVEF) and STE variables (baseline mean GLSs, GLSr, GLSRa, 6-month mean GLSs, GLSr, GLSRa, GLSRs and GLSRe) tested were not significant predictors of diagnostic accuracy of cardiac events.

In accordance to the ROC analysis, baseline mean GLSRs (ROC area 0.82, $p =$ 0.001) and baseline mean GLSRe (ROC area 0.68, $p =$ 0.036) displayed a better prognostic value in predicting cardiac events than LAPEF (ROC area 0.64, $p =$ 0.094) and LA total EF (ROC area 0.39, $p =$ 0.174). The "optimal" cut off values of baseline mean GLSRs and baseline mean Glare for cardiac events were 1.62 (s^{-1}) and –1.16 (s^{-1}), respectively (Table 6 and Fig. 3).

Discussion
The left atrium serves as a blood reservoir during ventricular systole and a conduit for the passage of blood from the pulmonary veins into the left ventricle during early and middle ventricular diastole, as well as a booster pump increasing LV filling during late diastole [10]. Using conventional echocardiography to perform LA function analysis, three different parameters (LA total EF, LAPEF, and LAAEF) can be obtained which may latterly be used to evaluate the reservoir, conduit, and booster pump components of LA function. Chinali et al. [11] have reported that the LA ejection force has been proposed as an independent predictor of LV diastolic properties and subsequent cardiovascular events. In the present investigation, similar findings were observed. In concert with their studies, our data showed that LAPEF and LA total EF were significant predictors of cardiac

Table 3 Conventional and TDI electrocardiographic characteristics of patients

Characteristic	Had events (n = 20)	No events (n = 31)	p
LAVmax (ml)	62.18 ± 17.64	59.32 ± 11.77	0.104
LAVmin (ml)	26.56 ± 12.59	25.17 ± 9.58	0.262
LAVp (ml)	43.81 ± 15.59	43.06 ± 16.17	0.303
LAI (ml/m^2)	35.78 ± 10.15	34.88 ± 11.51	0.089
LAPEF (%)	25.16 ± 12.26	29.02 ± 10.22	0.028*
LAAEF (%)	43.19 ± 9.67	45.33 ± 12.71	0.078
LA total EF (%)	58.06 ± 11.04	60.12 ± 10.52	0.054
LVEF (%)	56.18 ± 10.01	62.44 ± 11.92	0.089
E (cm/s)	77 ± 22	74 ± 16	0.434
A (cm/s)	82 ± 17	88 ± 11	0.118
E/A ratio	0.8 ± 0.2	0.8 ± 0.3	0.787
DT, ms	258 ± 44	230 ± 56	0.668
E' (cm/s)	11.2 ± 2.5	12.5 ± 1.9	0.184
A' (cm/s)	12.8 ± 2.2	11.6 ± 1.4	0.098
E/E' ratio	6.9 ± 2.7	5.8 ± 1.8	0.037*

TDI Tissue Doppler Imaging, *LAVmax* Left atrial maximum volume, *LAVmin* LA minimum volume, *LAVp* LA pre-atrial volume, *LAI* Left atrial volume index, *LAPEF* left atrial passive ejection fraction, *LAAEF* Left atrial active ejection fraction, *LA total EF* left atrial total ejection fraction, *LVEF* left ventricular ejection fraction, *E:*mitral early diastolic peak velocity, *A* mitral late diastolic peak velocity, *E/A* ratio of early to late diastolic transmitral flow velocity, *DT* deceleration time, *E'* myocardial early diastolic peak velocity, *A'* myocardial late diastolic peak velocity, *E/E' ratio* ratio of mitral to myocardial early diastolic peak velocity
*$P < 0.05$, between Had events group and No events group

Table 4 Left atrial STE characteristics of NSTEAMI patients

Characteristic	Had events (n = 20)	No events (n = 31)	p
Apical long axis			
GLSs (%)	−13.46 ± 7.70	−14.59 ± 7.62	0.607
GLSr (%)	13.02 ± 9.64	16.86 ± 9.31	0.163
GLSRs (s^{-1})	1.57 ± 0.58	2.04 ± 0.82	0.027*
GLSRe (s^{-1})	−1.31 ± 0.77	−1.51 ± 0.77	0.366
GLSRa (s^{-1})	−1.87 ± 1.10	−2.08 ± 0.95	0.489
Four-chamber			
GLSs (%)	−12.32 ± 5.65	−15.42 ± 7.31	0.095
GLSr (%)	11.33 ± 7.37	14.74 ± 7.62	0.116
GLSRs (s^{-1})	1.38 ± 0.79	1.56 ± 0.84	0.441
GLSRe (s^{-1})	−1.04 ± 0.47	−1.30 ± 0.59	0.084
GLSRa(s^{-1})	−1.52 ± 0.85	−1.99 ± 1.08	0.092
Two-chamber			
GLSs (%)	−11.85 ± 3.77	−13.67 ± 2.92	0.071
GLSr (%)	9.78 ± 5.63	11.30 ± 4.98	0.314
GLSRs (s^{-1})	1.21 ± 0.45	1.25 ± 0.36	0.739
GLSRe (s^{-1})	−0.87 ± 0.51	−1.03 ± 0.47	0.271
GLSRa(s^{-1})	−1.51 ± 0.62	−1.81 ± 0.48	0.057
Baseline Mean			
GLSs (%)	−12.54 ± 4.61	−14.56 ± 4.76	0.136
GLSr (%)	11.38 ± 5.10	14.30 ± 5.58	0.059
GLSRs (s^{-1})	1.39 ± 0.48	1.62 ± 0.55	0.003**
GLSRe (s^{-1})	−1.07 ± 0.42	−1.25 ± 0.48	0.013*
GLSRa(s^{-1})	−1.64 ± 0.67	−1.86 ± 0.71	0.138
6 months Mean			
GLSs (%)	−12.76 ± 4.78	−13.88 ± 5.21	0.094
GLSr (%)	13.22 ± 5.42	14.74 ± 6.89	0.228
GLSRs (s^{-1})	1.73 ± 0.48	1.98 ± 0.61	0.017*
GLSRe (s^{-1})	−1.69 ± 0.46	−1.75 ± 0.52	0.064
GLSRa(s^{-1})	−1.84 ± 0.49	−1.98 ± 0.37	0.445

GLSs global longitudinal left atrial peak negative strain during atrial systole, *GLSr* global longitudinal left atrial peak positive strain during ventricle systole, *GLSRs* global longitudinal left atrial peak positive strain rate during ventricle systole, *GLSRe* global longitudinal left atrial peak negative strain rate during early ventricular diastole, *GLSRa* global longitudinal left atrial peak negative strain rate during late ventricular diastole
*$P < 0.05$, **$P < 0.01$, between Had events group and No events group

events (HR = 1.05, $p = 0.003$ and HR = 1.02, $p = 0.048$, respectively) in patients with NSTEAMI after PCI.

Strain rate imaging on the basis of speckle-tracking technique represents the velocity gradient between two spatial points in relation to each other and overcomes noise artifacts associated with Doppler velocity imaging [12]. Quantification method of LA myocardial function using speckle tracking has been recently proposed [13]. In concert with conventional echocardiography, Inaba Y et al. [14] found that SRs corresponds to reservoir function and SRe corresponds to conduit function while SRa corresponds to booster pump function. Compared with S, SR seems to be less load-dependent, might be a better measure of contractility, and is theoretically more sensitive than S to myocardial pathology [15, 16].

The prognostic value of longitudinal LV strain in patients with NSTEAMI was consistent with previous reports. Park et al. [17], who studied 50 patients with acute anterior MI and primary reperfusion (PCI in 44 patients and thrombolysis in six patients) and assessed longitudinal strain by both tissue Doppler imaging (TDI) and STE in seven LV segments related to the vascular territory of the LAD artery territory. A total of 22 patients showed LV remodeling (LV dilatation with an increase in LVEDV >15 % during follow-up). Both strain assessed by TDI and assessed by speckle-tracking imaging were independent predictors of LV remodeling (odds ratio 1.430 and 1.307, respectively) and death as well as development of congestive heart failure during follow-up (odds ratio1.436 and 1.455, respectively). Recently, in a group of more than 600 patients from the Valsartan In Acute Myocardial Infarction (VALIANT) trial, Hung et al. demonstrated that both strain and strain rate (by speckle-tracking imaging) were independent

Table 5 Multivariable Predictors of Combined Cardiovascular Events by Cox Proportional Hazards Analysis

Variables	Hazard Ratio	95 % CI	Wald χ^2	P Value
Age	0.8	0.5–1.44	2.85	0.095
LAPEF (%)	1.05	1.02–1.08	8.88	0.003**
LA total EF (%)	1.02	0.99–1.05	3.89	0.048*
E/E' ratio	0.96	0.93–0.98	12.64	0.001**
Baseline mean GLSRs (s^{-1})	1.27	1.01–1.59	4.05	0.044*
Baseline mean GLSRe (s^{-1})	6.95	2.00–24.95	9.58	0.002**

LAPEF left atrial passive ejection fraction, *LA total EF* left atrial total ejection fraction, *E/E' ratio* ratio of mitral to myocardial early diastolic peak velocity, *GLSRs* global longitudinal left atrial peak positive strain rate during ventricle systole, *GLSRe* global longitudinal left atrial peak negative strain rate during early ventricular diastole
*$P < 0.05$, **$P < 0.01$

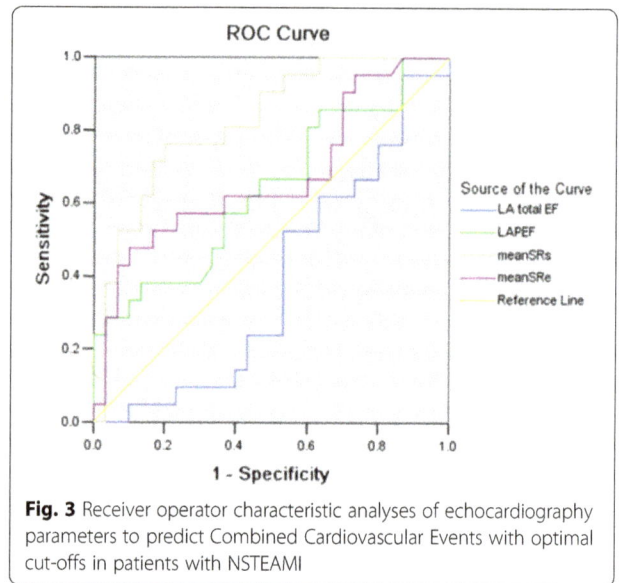

Fig. 3 Receiver operator characteristic analyses of echocardiography parameters to predict Combined Cardiovascular Events with optimal cut-offs in patients with NSTEAMI

predictors for death. In particular, strain rate imaging provided incremental prognostic information beyond LVEF after AMI [18]. However, there were few previous studies on the prognostic value of LA strain and strain rate in patients with NSTEAMI. In the current study, we observed the independent prognostic value of both left atrial traditional echocardiography parameters and longitudinal S and SR imaging and clinical variables in patients with NSTEAMI.As a result, multivariable Cox regression analysis showed that baseline LA Strain Rate (mean GLSRs, mean GLSRe), LAPEF and LA total EF were the independent predictor of combined cardiovascular events. Furthermore ROC analysis demonstrated that the diagnostic content of conventional echocardiography on predictor of cardiac events was less in LAPEF (ROC area 0.64, $p = 0.094$) and LA total EF (ROC area 0.39, $p = 0.174$) than STE in baseline mean GLSRs (ROC area 0.82, $p = 0.001$) and mean GLSRe (ROC area 0.68, $p = 0.036$). A cutoff value of baseline mean GLSRs 1.62 s^{-1} and mean GLSRe –1.16 s^{-1} predicted cardiac events with a sensitivity of 71.4 and 61.9 %, specificity of 83.3 and 63.3 %, respectively. Nevertheless, LAPEF and LA total EF identified cardiac events with a sensitivity of 52.4 %, 66.7 % and a specificity of 46.7 %, 53.3 %, respectively, which were lower than that

of baseline mean GLSRs and mean GLSRe (Table 6 and Fig. 3). Accordingly, LA longitudinal SRs and SRe further added incremental value beyond LA ejection force in the prediction of all cause cardiovascular events. As generally accepted, LV diastolic dysfunction is a hallmark of the severity of cardiac disease, whereas the degree of diastolic impairment correlates with symptoms and prognosis more closely than LV contractive dysfunction in patients with AMI [19]. LA dysfunction represents a strong predictive marker since the atrial chamber is a window allowing comprehensive evaluation of LV diastolic dysfunction which is often difficult to analyze directly. Our study reconfirmed these findings and extended them further.

On the basis of the superiority of global SR to S and other traditional echocardiography in predicting infarct size and assessment of myocardial viability from these previous studies, we hypothesized that the average SR from all three views(long apical axis, 4-chamber and 2-chamber view) reflecting the total extent of the whole LA function damage—might provide a better prediction of clinical outcomes after MI. Our study demonstrated

Table 6 Receiver operating characteristics analysis of echocardiographic parameters to predict cardiovascular events

Variables	Cut off Value	ROC Area (95 % CI)	Univariate P Value	Se %	Sp %
LAPEF (%)	31.69	0.52(0.36–0.69)	0.781	52.4	46.7
LA total EF (%)	61.54	0.41(0.25–0.57)	0.267	46.7	43.3
E/E' ratio	5.94	0.46(0.29–0.63)	0.605	47.6	46.7
Baseline mean GLSRs (s^{-1})	1.68	0.78(0.64–0.91)	0.001**	76.4	67.7
Baseline mean GLSRe (s^{-1})	−1.24	0.82(0.70–0.94)	0.001**	85.7	76.7

ROC Receiver operator characteristic, *Se* sensitivity, *Sp* specificity, *LAPEF* left atrial passive ejection fraction, *LA total EF* left atrial total ejection fraction, *GLSRs* global longitudinal left atrial peak positive strain rate during ventricle systole, *GLSRe* global longitudinal left atrial peak negative strain rate during early ventricular diastole
*$P < 0.05$, **$P < 0.01$

that both mean GLSRs and mean GLSRe improved significantly from baseline to 6-month, suggesting that LA reservoir and conduit function were restored to a certain extent in patients with NSTEAMI after PCI.

To our perspective, this study provides evidence that noninvasive provides prognostic information about the success of PCI procedure is highly desirable. With the use of this definition, mean GLSRs and mean GLSRe of left atrium, represents an optimal method with high specificity and sensitivity for the prediction of patients with NSTEAMI. In this regard, the value of 2D STE arises from its ability to directly measure atrial myocardium deformation that can be used at the bedside and provide additional information about atrial function of NSTEAMI to what can be obtained from a conventional echocardiographic analysis.

Conclusions

2D-STE provides important insights into the mechanism and temporal sequence of left atrial dysfunction after NSTEAMI. As confirmed in our study, mean GLSRs and mean GLSRe, the new LA function parameters, which are measured by 2D-STE, exert better prognostic value in predicting cardiac events over conventional echocardiography and should be the preferred method in patients with NSTEAMI.

Abbreviations
NSTEAMI: Non-ST-segment-elevation acute myocardial infarction; STE: Speckle tracking echocardiography.

Competing interests
The authors declare that they have no competing interests.

Authors' contributions
CS has designed, written, reviewed the article and has given final approval of the version to be published. JZ cowrited the article designed the tables, collected the data and revised the final manuscript and helped with the organization of references. JC also provided the figures from his own collection. WX were involved in the neurological revising of data. All authors read and approved the manuscript.

Acknowledgments
This study was approved by the International Review Board (IRB) of the 2nd affiliated hospital of Soochow University.

Work limitations
A number of several obvious limitations of our study are to be outlined. Firstly, the 2D-STE analysis software that was originally designed for the left ventricle was applied to the left atrium in our study. Secondly, strain and SR can be measured in all dimensions (longitudinal, radial, and circumferential), but we only quantified the longitudinal strain and SR assuming that the contraction of the left atrium is predominantly longitudinal. Thirdly, a relatively large number of studies with low-quality LA images could not be analyzed. It suggested that patients may not have been consecutive and that there was a bias in patient selection. Fourthly, the relatively small number of patients eligible for analysis in the present study may render it difficult to generalize the results and apply them to other patient populations. Further larger prospective studies are warranted to determine the predictive value of this new tool to evaluate LA function in patients with NSTEAMI.

References

1. Roger VL, Killian JM, Weston SA, Jaffe AS, Kors J, Santrach PJ, et al. Redefinition of myocardial infarction: prospective evaluation in the community. Circulation. 2006;114:790–7.
2. Bassand JP, Hamm CW, Ardissino D, Boersma E, Budaj A, Fernandez-Aviles F, et al. Guidelines for the diagnosis and treatment of non-ST-segment elevation acute coronary syndromes. Eur Heart J. 2007;28:1598–660.
3. Moller JE, Hillis GS, Oh JK, Seward JB, Reeder GS, Wright RS, et al. Left atrial volume: a powerful predictor of survival after acute myocardial infarction. Circulation. 2003;107:2207–12.
4. Wang Z, Tan H, Zhong M, Jiang G, Zhang Y, Zhang W, et al. Strain rate imaging for noninvasive functional quantification of the left atrium in hypertensive patients with paroxysmal atrial fibrillation. Cardiology. 2008;109:15–24.
5. Lang RM, Bierig M, Devereux RB, Flachskampf FA, Foster E, Pellikka PA, et al. Recommendations for chamber quantification: a report from the american society of Echocardiography's guidelines and standards committee and the chamber quantification writing group, developed in conjunction with the european association of echocardiography, a branch of the european society of cardiology. J Am Soc Echocardiogr. 2005;18:1440–63.
6. Cho GY, Marwick TH, Kim HS, Kim MK, Hong KS, Oh DJ. Global 2-dimensional strain as a new prognosticator in patients with heart failure. J Am Coll Cardiol. 2009;54:618–24.
7. Stanton T, Leano R, Marwick TH. Prediction of all-cause mortality from global longitudinal speckle strain: comparison with ejection fraction and wall motion scoring. Circ Cardiovasc Imaging. 2009;2:356–64.
8. Serri K, Reant P, Lafitte M, Berhouet M, Le Bouffos V, Roudaut R, et al. Global and regional myocardial function quantification by two-dimensional strain: application in hypertrophic cardiomyopathy. J Am Coll Cardiol. 2006;47:1175–81.
9. Kim DG, Lee KJ, Lee S, Jeong SY, Lee YS, Choi YJ, et al. Feasibility of two-dimensional global longitudinal strain and strain rate imaging for the assessment of left atrial function: a study in subjects with a low probability of cardiovascular disease and normal exercise capacity. Echocardiography. 2009;26:1179–87.
10. Abhayaratna WP, Seward JB, Appleton CP, Douglas PS, Oh JK, Tajik AJ, et al. Left atrial size: physiologic determinants and clinical applications. J Am Coll Cardiol. 2006;47:2357–63.
11. Chinali M, de Simone G, Roman MJ, Bella JN, Liu JE, Lee ET, et al. Left atrial systolic force and cardiovascular outcome. The Strong Heart Study. Am J Hypertens. 2005;18:1570–6. 1577.
12. Hashimoto I, Li X, Hejmadi BA, Jones M, Zetts AD, Sahn DJ, et al. Myocardial strain rate is a superior method for evaluation of left ventricular subendocardial function compared with tissue doppler imaging. J Am Coll Cardiol. 2003;42:1574–83.
13. D'Andrea A, Caso P, Romano S, Scarafile R, Cuomo S, Salerno G, et al. Association between left atrial myocardial function and exercise capacity in patients with either idiopathic or ischemic dilated cardiomyopathy: a two-dimensional speckle strain study. Int J Cardiol. 2009;132:354–63.
14. Inaba Y, Yuda S, Kobayashi N, Hashimoto A, Uno K, Nakata T, et al. Strain rate imaging for noninvasive functional quantification of the left atrium: comparative studies in controls and patients with atrial fibrillation. J Am Soc Echocardiogr. 2005;18:729–36.
15. Greenberg NL, Firstenberg MS, Castro PL, Main M, Travaglini A, Odabashian JA, et al. Doppler-derived myocardial systolic strain rate is a strong index of left ventricular contractility. Circulation. 2002;105:99–105.
16. Thomas JD, Popovic ZB. Assessment of left ventricular function by cardiac ultrasound. J Am Coll Cardiol. 2006;48:2012–25.
17. Park YH, Kang SJ, Song JK, Lee EY, Song JM, Kang DH, et al. Prognostic value of longitudinal strain after primary reperfusion therapy in patients with anterior-wall acute myocardial infarction. J Am Soc Echocardiogr. 2008;21:262–7.
18. Hung CH, Shin SH, Hassanein A. Strain and strain rate imaging are independent predictors of mortality after high-risk myocardial infarction[abstract]. J Am Coll Cardiol. 2008;10:A142.
19. Poulsen SH, Jensen SE, Moller JE, Egstrup K. Prognostic value of left ventricular diastolic function and association with heart rate variability after a first acute myocardial infarction. Heart. 2001;86:376–80.

11

Analysis of risk factors of ST-segment elevation myocardial infarction in young patients

Wang Yunyun[1], Li Tong[1*], Liu Yingwu[1], Liu Bojiang[1], Wang Yu[1], Hu Xiaomin[1], Li Xin[1], Peng Wenjin[1] and JinFang Li[2]

Abstract

Background: Acute myocardial infarction (AMI) is often present in old populations and rare in young people. Its incidence significantly increased recent years. The mechanism and disease course of AMI in young people are probably different from that in old population. The aim of this study was to analyze clinical risk factors of STEMI in young patients.

Methods: Data was collected from consecutive patients ≤ 44 years of age (young; $n = 86$) and 60–74 years of age (old; $n = 65$) diagnosed with STEMI, and 79 young age-matched patients without coronary artery disease (CAD), hospitalized between January 2009 and June 2013.

Results: The young STEMI group had a significantly higher proportion of males (88.37 vs. 53.16%; $P < 0.01$), smokers (82.56 vs. 49.37%; $P < 0.01$) and patients with a family history of early CAD (54.65 vs. 32.91%; $P < 0.05$) than age-matched controls. Young STEMI patients also had significantly higher levels of fasting blood sugar (6.39 vs. 5.25 mmol/L; $P < 0.001$), glycated hemoglobin (HbA1c) (6.26 vs. 5.45%; $P < 0.05$), total cholesterol (5.14 vs. 4.65 mmol/L, $P < 0.05$), and fibrinogen (Fib) (3.39 vs. 2.87; $P < 0.01$). Compared with the old STEMI group, young STEMI patients had significantly higher proportions of males (88.37 vs. 63.08%; $P < 0.01$) smokers (82.56 vs. 41.54%; $P < 0.01$), and those with a family history of early CAD (54.65 vs. 18.46%; $P < 0.01$). Young STEMI patients also lower Fib (3.39 vs. 3.88 g/L; $P < 0.01$), less frequent occurrence of angina pectoris before STEMI (13.95 vs. 29.23%; $P < 0.05$) compared with the old STEMI group. Logistic regression analysis indicated that male sex (OR = 5.891), smoking (OR = 3.500), family history of early CAD (OR = 3.194), Fib (OR = 2.414) and HbA1c (OR = 1.515) are associated with STEMI in young patients.

Conclusion: In addition to previously recognized risk factors (male sex, smoking and family history of early CAD), Fib and HbA1c are associated with STEMI in individuals ≤ 44 years of age without antecedent angina pectoris.

Keywords: Antecedent angina pectoris, Fibrinogen, Glycated hemoglobin, Risk factors, ST-segment elevation myocardial infarction, Young patients

Background

Acute myocardial infarction (AMI) is a major cause of death worldwide. AMI is less frequent in adults younger than 45 years of age than in elderly adults [1,2], but is of increasing clinical interest in young adults because of the potential of premature death and long-term disability [3]. The incidence of AMI in young people was as low as 2–6% [1,2], but has recently begun to rise. The protection offered by young age is countered by increased prevalence of risk factors for coronary artery disease (CAD), such as impaired glucose tolerance and obesity, in adolescence [4]. Ignorance of CAD combined with a false sense of security likely prevents younger individuals from seeking medical advice. Early recognition and risk factor modification in this population is of key importance [5].

The mechanism and disease course of AMI in young patients are likely different from those in an older population, and knowing of theses differences may help to prevent the disease and improve the prognosis [6]. However, there are few studies investigating risk factor profiles and patterns of coronary artery involvement in ST-segment elevation myocardial infarction (STEMI) in younger individuals. This

* Correspondence: litong3zx@sina.com
[1]Cardiac Center, Third Central Hospital of Tian Jin, Tian Jin 300170, China
Full list of author information is available at the end of the article

paper retrospectively analyzed risk factors and clinical features in young patients with STEMI to characterize this medical condition.

Methods

Ethics statement

This study was approved by ethics committee of The Third Central Hospital of Tian Jin. The study protocols comply with the ethical guidelines of the Declaration of Helsinki. All subjects provided informed consent.

Subjects

This was a retrospective study of 86 consecutive young patients (18–44 years of age) with STEMI selected from a total of 2460 AMI patients enrolled between January 2009 and June 2013 at The Third Central hospital of Tianjin. A group of 79 young adults of the same age range who made consecutive visits to the hospital during the same period, were enrolled as controls. Coronary heart disease was excluded in this group by coronary angiography. An additional group of 65 consecutive old patients (60–74 years of age) with STEMI were included for comparison.

Inclusion criteria

Patients included in the study were diagnosed with STEMI, defined by the typical rise and fall of cardiac markers of myocardial necrosis with at least one of the following [7]: i) symptoms of ischemia; ii) echocardiogram changes indicative of new ischemia (≥ 0.1 mV in two or more standard leads, ≥ 0.2 mV in two or more contiguous pre-cordial leads, or a new left bundle branch block); iii) 12 h after symptoms, levels of creating kinase and its isoform (CKMB) were twice the normal upper limit or a troponin level was increased to the standard of MI (according to the normal local laboratory value). All patients had complete medical records and had undergone coronary angiography.

Exclusion criteria

Patients with the following conditions were excluded: congenital heart disease, cardiomyopathy, myocarditis, Takayasu's arteritis or vascular dysplasia; coronary artery embolism; AMI secondary to aortic dissection, severe aorta valve stenosis, myocardial hypertrophy, and history of AMI without evidence from angiography showing narrowing of the coronary arteries.

Data collection

Demographic and baseline data were collected by questionnaire at patient interviews and by review of medical records. Medical records were analyzed for the patients' CAD risk factor profiles. Baseline data included gender, age, body mass index, history of smoking or drinking, family history of CAD, medical history of hypertension, type II diabetes mellitus, cranial vascular accidents, systolic and diastolic pressure, and the presence of other diseases. A TBA-120FR auto-biochemical analyzer (Toshiba, Japan) and Sysmex kx-21 hematology analyzer (Sysmex, Japan) were used to measure fasting blood sugar, glycated hemoglobin (HbA1c), creatine kinase and CKMB, troponin I (normal range 0.05–0.40 ng/mL), triglycerides (TG), total cholesterol (TC), non-high-density lipoprotein cholesterol (NHDL-C), HDL-C, and fibrinogen (Fib) in the morning after hospital admission, following an overnight fast.

Criteria for other conditions

Hypertension was defined as a systolic pressure ≥ 140 mmHg and/or a diastolic pressure ≥ 90 mmHg [8]; a history of hypertension was noted in patients using anti-hypertension medications. Type II diabetes was noted in patients who met the 1999 WHO diagnosis criteria [9]. Unstable angina pectoris (AP) before AMI included initial AP on effort, exacerbation of effort AP, spontaneous AP, mixed AP, variant angina, and angina that occurred within one month of AMI, each episode lasting 2–20 min [10]. Smoking was defined as smoking for six months or longer, and a smoking index was calculated as the number of daily cigarettes × years of smoking [11]. A family history of early CAD was recorded in patients where it was first diagnosed in the father at ≤ 55 or the mother at ≤ 65 years of age.

Coronary angiography

Due to delays for hospital admittance in some patients, coronary angiography was performed within one month after STEMI via the radial artery using a multifunction catheter or via the femoral artery using the Judkins method. The results were interpreted by two experienced physicians.

Statistical analysis

SPSS 17.0 software (SPSS Inc., Chicago, IL, USA) was used for all data analysis. Normally distributed numeric data are presented as means ± standard deviation and intergroup comparisons were conducted with a Student's t-test. Non-normally distributed numeric data are presented as medians and quartiles (M [Q1, Q3]) and intergroup comparisons were conducted with the Mann–Whitney U test. Categorical data were tested with the χ^2 test. A logistic regression model was used to identify risk factors of STEMI in young patients. All tests were two sided and $P < 0.05$ was regarded as significant.

Results

Comparison between young STEMI and control patients

Baseline clinical and laboratory test data in the young STEMI and young control groups are summarized in

Table 1. The proportions of smokers and patients with a family history of early CAD, and the smoking index values in the STEMI group were significantly higher than those in the control group (Ps < 0.05). STEMI patients had significantly higher fasting blood sugar, HbA1c, TC, NHDL-C and Fib levels than controls (Ps < 0.05). There were no differences between the two groups in age, blood pressure, TG, HDL-C, hypertension, type II diabetes, cerebrovascular diseases, or drinking.

Comparison between young and old STEMI patients

Baseline clinical and laboratory test data in the young and old STEMI groups are summarized in Table 2. The gender, diastolic pressure, pulse pressure, smoking, smoking index values, and family history of early CAD were significantly different between the two groups (Ps < 0.05). Patients in the

Table 1 Clinical data from the young groups

Variable	STEMI (n = 86)	Control (n = 79)	P
Age, y	40.00 (23, 44)	39.94 (27, 44)	0.317
Male, n (%)	76 (88.37)	42 (53.16)	<0.001
BMI (kg/m^2)	27.96 ± 2.80	25.16 ± 3.15	0.127
Systolic pressure (mmHg)	133.59 (90, 200)	134.82 (100, 190)	0.629
Diastolic pressure (mmHg)	81.03 (50, 124)	83.37 (60, 140)	0.957
Pulse pressure (mmHg)	52.67 (25, 90)	51.71 (30, 90)	0.608
Fasting blood sugar (mmol/L)	6.39 (3.76, 18.00)	5.25 (3.25, 12.35)	<0.001
HbA1C (%)	6.26 ± 1.69	5.45 ± 1.12	0.018
CK (U/L)	1950.28 ± 1639.52	81.15 ± 44.60	<0.001
CKMB (U/L)	163.99 ± 127.38	14.77 ± 13.35	<0.001
TNI (ng/mL)	3.08 (0.11, 30)	0.07 (0.05, 0.3)	<0.001
TG (mmol/L)	2.37 ± 2.48	2.25 ± 1.26	0.201
TC (mmol/L)	5.14 ± 1.39	4.65 ± 0.87	0.002
NHDL-C (mmol/L)	4.06 ± 1.35	3.53 ± 0.87	0.002
HDL-C (mmol/L)	1.07 ± 0.27	1.12 ± 0.26	0.856
Fib (g/L)	3.39 (1.90, 7.52)	2.87 (1.78, 5.30)	<0.001
Hypertension, n (%)	41 (47.67)	35 (44.30)	0.755
Type II diabetes, n (%)	18 (20.93)	17 (21.52)	1.000
Cerebrovascular diseases, n (%)	6 (6.98)	2 (2.53)	0.281
Alcohol drinking, n (%)	25 (29.07)	19 (24.05)	0.486
Smoking, n (%)	71 (82.56)	39 (49.37)	<0.001
Smoking index	329.53 (0, 1200)	179.49 (0, 900)	<0.001
Family history of early CAD, n (%)	47 (54.65)	26 (32.91)	0.007

Abbreviations: *BMI* body mass index, *CAD* coronary artery disease, *CK* creatine kinase, *CKMB* isoform of CK, *Fib* fibrinogen, *HbA1c* glycated hemoglobin, *HDL-C* high-density lipoprotein cholesterol, *MI* myocardial infarction, *NHDL-C* non-HDL-C, *TC* total cholesterol, *TG* triglyceride, *TNI* troponin I, *STEMI* ST-segment elevation myocardial infarction.
Note: Data are expressed as mean ± standard deviation or medians (Q1, Q3).

Table 2 Comparison of young and old STEMI groups

Variable	Young (n = 86)	Old (n = 65)	P
Age, y	40.00 (23, 44)	69.15 (63,74)	< 0.001
Male, n (%)	76 (88.37)	41 (63.08)	0.001
BMI, kg/m^2	27.96 ± 2.80	26.18 ± 2.30	0.346
Systolic pressure, mmHg	133.59 (90, 200)	131.09 (96,180)	0.885
Diastolic pressure, mmHg	81.03 (50, 124)	73.20 (46, 120)	0.005
Pulse pressure, mmHg	52.67 (25, 90)	57.89 (30, 100)	0.030
Fasting blood sugar (mmol/L)	6.39 (3.76, 18.00)	6.02 (3.61, 12.00)	0.682
HbA1C (%)	6.26 ± 1.69	6.29 ± 1.47	0.458
CK (U/L)	1950.28 ± 1639.52	1691.35 ± 1411.02	0.533
CKMB (U/L)	163.99 ± 127.38	189.14 ± 173.26	0.066
TNI (ng/mL)	3.08 (0.11, 30)	3.40 (0.17, 30)	0.664
TG (mmol/L)	2.37 ± 2.48	1.29 ± 0.48	0.001
TC (mmol/L)	5.14 ± 1.39	4.74 ± 0.85	0.005
NHDL-C (mmol/L)	4.06 ± 1.35	3.60 ± 0.76	0.003
HDL-C (mmol/L)	1.07 ± 0.27	1.14 ± 0.24	0.760
Fib (g/L)	3.39 (1.90, 7.52)	3.88 (2.06, 10.94)	< 0.001
Hypertension, n (%)	41 (47.67)	35 (53.85)	0.512
Type II diabetes, n (%)	18 (20.93)	21 (32.30)	0.135
Cerebrovascular diseases, n (%)	6 (6.98)	18 (27.69)	< 0.001
Alcohol drinking, n (%)	25 (29.07)	7 (10.77)	0.008
Smoking, n (%)	71 (82.56%)	27 (41.54)	< 0.001
Smoking index	329.53 (0, 1200)	263.54 (0, 2400)	< 0.001
Family history of early CAD, n (%)	47 (54.65)	12 (18.46)	< 0.001
Angina pectoris before MI, n (%)	12 (13.95)	19 (29.23)	0.026

Abbreviations: *BMI* body mass index, *CAD* coronary artery disease, *CK* creatine kinase, *CKMB* isoform of CK, *Fib* fibrinogen, *HbA1c* glycated hemoglobin, *HDL-C* high-density lipoprotein cholesterol, *MI* myocardial infarction, *NHDL-C* non-HDL-C, *STEMI* ST-segment elevation myocardial infarction, *TC* total cholesterol, *TG* triglyceride, *TNI* troponin I.
Note: Data are expressed as mean ± standard deviation or medians (Q1, Q3).

young group were less likely to have cerebrovascular diseases or experience AP before STEMI than the older patients. TG, TC, and NHDL-C levels were higher, and serum Fib was lower, in young compared with old STEMI patients (Ps < 0.05). Smoking and imbalance of lipid metabolism were more common in young STEMI patients than in old patients (Ps < 0.05).

Risk factors of STEMI

Using STEMI as a dependent variable, independent risk factors among young patients were determined as those with a $P < 0.25$ in Student's t-tests, including gender, smoking history, smoking index, family history of early CAD, and levels of blood sugar, HbA1c, TC, NHDL-C, and Fib, and assessed by a logistic regression analysis. The analysis revealed that gender, smoking, family history of CAD, Fib, and HbA1c levels were independent risk factors for STEMI in young individuals ($Ps < 0.05$) (Table 3).

Discussion

The lifestyles of young people, characterized by high work stress, fast pace, overwork, smoking, drinking alcohol, and overeating, likely cause disturbances in the internal environment, such as coronary atherosclerosis, that increase the incidence of AMI [12]. Atherosclerosis, which is affected by many factors, may cause coronary spasms or broken plaque in coronary arteries resulting in acute blockage [13]. In this study, we found that STEMI tended to occur suddenly in young patients and in those without a history of AP.

Conventional risk factors for STEMI include male sex, smoking, and a family history of early CAD [14]. In accordance with this and another study [15], we found that male sex was an important risk factor for STEMI in young patients. Androgen was shown to negatively correlate with the incidence of STEMI, and physiologic levels can prevent atherosclerosis [16]. Androgen levels, which peak at age 20–24 and then decline gradually, are significantly reduced in atherosclerosis patients, and low androgen levels can induce heart diseases and predict AMI [17]. The unhealthy habits such as smoking, drinking, and eating high-fat or high-purine diets may also increase the risk of AMI in young men compared with older male and young female populations. This may explain why the group of young STEMI patients included a significantly higher proportion of males than the old group.

A recent study published by Cases and Rate [18] found that among 6892 STEMI who received percutaneous coronary intervention, 46.4% were smokers, compared with 20.5% in the general population. Studies in China and other countries demonstrated that young AMI patients have smoking rates as high as 70–90% [5,19]. As our data show, young STEMI patients are more likely

than older patients to be smokers. The risk of AMI decreases after smokers quit, and the benefit of quitting is correlated with amount smoked [11]. Moreover, smoking cessation can help prevent cardiovascular events, especially in young people [18].

The results of our study show that 58.33% of young patients have a family history of early CAD, which is higher than the 30–40% of young AMI patients reported by Colkesen et al. [20]. Patients with a family history of CAD have more severe disease progression than those without a history [21], more lipid metabolism disorders, and more likely to have insulin resistance and be obese, possibly resulting from hereditary factors [22].

An important finding from our study is that levels of HbA1c and Fib were independent risk factors for STEMI in young patients. Fib is associated with vascular endothelial injury, and enhances the coagulation of platelets and increase in blood viscosity to induce thrombosis. Fib level is significantly associated with coronary artery calcification and sclerosis [23], and levels are significantly higher in patients who die from coronary diseases than in those who survive [24]. A study by Tatli et al. [25] showed that Fib can predict the extent of coronary artery narrowing in young AMI patients. In this study, the Fib levels were significantly higher in young STEMI patients compared with controls, and logistic regression analysis indicated it was an independent risk factor of STEMI, further confirming the role of coagulation disorders in STEMI in the young population. Old STEMI patients also had higher Fib levels, suggesting that its effect in this population is even more important.

Although diabetes is an important risk factor for coronary disease, its incidence was not significantly higher in the young versus the old STEMI patients. However, many studies report that non-diabetic AMI patients have increased blood sugar, compromised glucose tolerance, and insulin resistance [26,27]. There is a significant correlation between HbA1c level, an indicator of long-term glycemic control, and the development and prognosis of coronary diseases; this correlation is less frequently reported in young patients [28]. In our study, STEMI patients were younger than the peak age of diabetes incidence, though baseline fasting blood sugar and HbA1c were significantly higher, suggesting that a higher proportion of patients had undetected diabetics or prediabetes. As pre-diabetic conditions can influence the course of STEMI, medical intervention in young people may help prevent STEMI. The findings of this study show that whereas fasting blood sugar level is a dependent risk factor, HbA1c is an independent risk factor, indicating that HbA1c is more strongly correlated with STEMI in young people.

Unstable AP before AMI is a clinical manifestation of ischemic preconditioning; repeated AP prepares the

Table 3 Logistic regression analysis of STEMI risk factors in young patients

Factors	B value	SE	Wald	OR	95% CI	P
Male	1.7731	0.508	12.177	5.891	2.176–15.950	<0.001
Smoking history	1.253	0.473	7.016	3.500	1.385–8.842	0.008
Family history of early CAD	1.161	0.409	8.059	3.194	1.433–7.122	0.005
Fib	0.881	0.288	9.366	2.414	1.373–4.245	0.002
HbA1c	0.415	0.165	6.370	1.515	1.097–2.091	0.012

Abbreviations: CAD coronary artery disease, CI confidence interval, Fib fibrinogen, HbA1c glycated hemoglobin, OR odds ratio, SE standard error, STEMI ST-segment elevation myocardial infarction.

myocardium, reducing myocardial injury, cardiac dysfunction and severe cardiac arrhythmia following AMI [29]. Klein *et al.* [30] found that young patients seldom experience AP before MI, but that AP quickly progresses to AMI. Consistent with their findings, only 12% of the young STEMI patients in our study experienced AP before STEMI, a significantly smaller percentage than in old STEMI patients. STEMI in young patients generally has no ischemic preconditioning, and occurs and progresses faster than it does in older patients. However, troponin I values were similar between the young and old STEMI groups, and there were no differences in the degree of myocardial necrosis.

Study limitations

This study is subject to the usual limitations associated with a retrospective design. Because of the low incidence of STEMI in young people, the sample size of this study was small. Despite adjusting for multiple risk factors, it is possible that there may have been residual confounding conditions and medications. In addition, no data were collected about coronary artery disease extension. Therefore, the influence of some confounders and biases cannot be completely excluded. Multicenter studies with large sample sizes will further elucidate the mechanism of STEMI in the young population. Nevertheless, this study provides a clinical reference for healthcare professionals to more fully understand risk factors in young STEMI patients and to develop early preventative interventions.

Conclusion

In conclusion, STEMI in young people has some clinical features that are different from those in older patients. In addition to the conventional risk factors, Fib and HbA1c are associated with the initiation of STEMI, and can provide inexpensive and powerful prognostic factors for STEMI in young patients. STEMI in young patients is often accompanied by disorders of glucose metabolism and abnormal coagulation, though AP before STEMI is rare.

Competing interests
The authors declare that they have no competing interests.

Authors' contributions
WY carried out the studies of coronary heart disease. WY and LT designed the study and drafted the manuscript. LY and LT conceived of the study. LB, WY, HX, LX and PW participated in the collection of data. LJF helped to draft the manuscript. All authors read and approved the final manuscript.

Acknowledgements
I would like to express my gratitude to all those who helped me during the writing of this paper.
My deepest gratitude goes first and foremost to Professor Li Tong for his constant encouragement and guidance. He has walked me through all the stages of the writing of this paper. Without his consistent and illuminating instruction, this paper could not have reached its present form.
Second, I would like to express my heartfelt gratitude to Professor Liu Yingwu, who conceived of the study and helped to draft the manuscript. I am also greatly indebted to the professors and teachers at the Department of Cardiac Center: Liu Bojiang, Wang Yu, Hu Xiaomin, Li Xin and Peng Wenjin, who have instructed and helped me a lot in the past two years. I am also deeply indebted to Professor JinFang Li,whose profound knowledge of English triggers my love for this beautiful language and whose earnest attitude tells me how to learn English.
Last my thanks would go to my beloved family for their loving considerations and great confidence in me all through these years.

Author details
[1]Cardiac Center, Third Central Hospital of Tian Jin, Tian Jin 300170, China.
[2]Essen Medical Associates, P.C.2015 Grand concourse, Bronx, NY 10453, USA.

References
1. Fournier J, Sanchez A, Quero J, Fernandez-Cortacero J, González-Barrero A: **Myocardial infarction in men aged 40 years or less: a prospective clinical-angiographic study.** *Clin Cardiol* 1996, **19**(8):631–636.
2. Garoufalis S, Kouvaras G, Vitsias G, Perdikouris K, Markatou P, Hatzisavas J, Kassinos N, Karidis K, Foussas S: **Comparison of angiographic findings, risk factors, and long term follow-up between young and old patients with a history of myocardial infarction.** *Int J Cardiol* 1998, **67**(1):75–80.
3. Weinberger I, Rotenberg Z, Fuchs J, Sagy A, Friedmann J, Agmon J: **Myocardial infarction in young adults under 30 years: risk factors and clinical course.** *Clin Cardiol* 1987, **10**(1):9–15.
4. Sinha R, Fisch G, Teague B, Tamborlane WV, Banyas B, Allen K, Savoye M, Rieger V, Taksali S, Barbetta G, Sherwin RS, Caprio S: **Prevalence of impaired glucose tolerance among children and adolescents with marked obesity.** *N Engl J Med* 2002, **346**:802–810.
5. Jamil G, Jamil M, Alkhazraji H, Haque A, Chedid F, Balasubramanian M, Khairallah B, Qureshi A: **Risk factor assessment of young patients with ST-segment elevation myocardial infarction.** *Am J Cardiovasc Dis* 2013, **3**(3):170–174.
6. Egred M, Viswanathan G, Davis G: **Myocardial infarction in young adults.** *Postgrad Med* 2005, **81**(962):741–745.
7. Chinese Society of Cardiology of Chinese Medical Association, Editorial committee of Chinese Journal of Cardiology, Editorial committee of Chinese Circulation Journal: **Acute myocardial infarction diagnosis and treatment guidelines.** *Chin J Cardiol (Chin)* 2001, **29**:710–725.
8. Chinese Hypertension Prevention and Treatment Guide Revision Committee: **Chinese hypertension prevention and treatment guide 2004.** *Chin J Cardiol* 2004, **32**:1060–1064.
9. Ye RG, Lu ZY, Xie Y, Wang C: *Internal Medicine.* 6th edition. China: People's Medical Publishing House; 2006:918.
10. Yang YJ, Hua W, Gao RL: *Fuwai Cardiovascular Medicine Manual.* 1st edition. China: People's Medical Publishing House; 2006:154–173.
11. Zhao J, Hu D-y, Ding R-j, Li XB, Zhang P, Wang L, Yu XJ, Guo JH, Wang XQ, Li L, Zhang FF, Huang ZW: **Coronary characteristics of young smokers with coronary heart disease and the effects of tobacco control on smoking cessation [J].** *Zhonghua Yi Xue Za Zhi* 2010, **38**(12):1077–1080.
12. Wang XY: **Analysis of 56 young patients with acute myocardial infarction.** *J Med Theory Pract* 2012, **25**:917–918.
13. Ma CT, Jiang YX, Du WJ, Liu ZF, Wang J: **The correlation analysis of serum BNP, hypersentive C-creative protein and left ventricular ejection fraction of acute myocardial infarction patients.** *Chin Crit Care* 2012, **24**(4):247–248.
14. Schoenenberger AW, Radovanovic D, Stauffer JC, Windecker S, Urban P, Niedermaier G, Keller PF, Gutzwiller F, Erne P: **Acute coronary syndromes in young patients: presentation, treatment and outcome.** *Int J Cardiol* 2011, **148**(3):300–304.
15. Egiziano G, Akhtari S, Pilote L, Daskalopoulou S: **Sex differences in young patients with acute myocardial infarction.** *Diabet Med* 2013, **30**(3):e108–e114.
16. Provotorov V: **Age-related androgen deficiency in men with ischemic heart disease.** *Adv Gerontol* 2007, **21**(2):311–313.
17. Zhang X, Li X, Cao T, Ye L: **Correlation of endogenous androgen and androgen receptor level with coronary artery diseases in elderly males].** *Zhonghua Yi Xue Za Zhi* 2011, **91**(14):984.
18. Cases N, Rate ES: **The ongoing importance of smoking as a powerful risk factor for ST-segment elevation myocardial infarction in young patients.** *JAMA* 2013, **173**(13):1261.

19. Barbash G, White H, Modan M, Diaz R, Hampton J, Heikkila J, Kristinsson A, Moulopoulos S, Paolasso E, Werf TV: Acute myocardial infarction in the young-the role of smoking. *Eur Heart* 1995, **16**(3):313–316.

20. Colkesen AY, Acil T, Demircan S, Sezgin AT, Muderrisoglu H: Coronary lesion type, location, and characteristics of acute ST elevation myocardial infarction in young adults under 35 years of age. *Coron Artery Dis* 2008, **19**(5):345–347.

21. Gaeta G, De Michele M, Cuomo S, Guarini P, Foglia MC, Bond MG, Trevisan M: Arterial abnormalities in the offspring of patients with premature myocardial infarction. *N Engl J Med* 2000, **343**(12):840–846.

22. Berenson GS, Srinivasan SR, Bao W, Newman WP, Tracy RE, Wattigney WA: Association between multiple cardiovascular risk factors and atherosclerosis in children and young adults. *N Engl J Med* 1998, **338**(23):1650–1656.

23. Bielak LF, Klee GG, Sheedy PF, Turner ST, Schwartz RS, Peyser PA: Association of fibrinogen with quantity of coronary artery calcification measured by electron beam computed tomography. *Arterioscler Thromb Vasc Biol* 2000, **20**(9):2167–2171.

24. Meade T, Chakrabarti R, Haines A, North W, Stirling Y, Thompson S, Brozović M: Haemostatic function and cardiovascular death: early results of a prospective study. *Lancet* 1980, **315**(8177):1050–1054.

25. Tatli E, Ozcelik F, Aktoz M: Plasma fibrinogen level may predict critical coronary artery stenosis in young adults with myocardial infarction. *Cardiol J* 2009, **16**(4):317–320.

26. Tandjung K, van Houwelingen KG, Jansen H, Basalus MW, Sen H, Löwik MM, Stoel MG, Louwerenburg JHW, de Man FH, Linssen G: Comparison of frequency of periprocedural myocardial infarction in patients with and without diabetes mellitus to those with previously unknown but elevated glycated hemoglobin levels (from the TWENTE trial). *Am J Cardiol* 2012, **110**(11):1561–1567.

27. Lazzeri C, Valente S, Chiostri M, Picariello C, Attanà P, Gensini GF: Glycated hemoglobin in ST-elevation myocardial infarction without previously known diabetes: Its short and long term prognostic role. *Diabetes Res Clin Pract* 2012, **95**(1):e14–e16.

28. Timmer JR, Hoekstra M, Nijsten MW, van der Horst IC, Ottervanger JP, Slingerland RJ, Dambrink J-HE, Bilo HJ, Zijlstra F, van't Hof AW: Prognostic value of admission glycosylated hemoglobin and glucose in nondiabetic patients with ST-segment–elevation myocardial infarction treated with percutaneous coronary intervention. *Circulation* 2011, **124**(6):704–711.

29. Przyklenk K, Whittaker P: Brief antecedent ischemia enhances recombinant tissue plasminogen activator–induced coronary thrombolysis by adenosine-mediated mechanism. *Circulation* 2000, **102**(1):88–95.

30. Klein LW, Agarwal JB, Herlich MB, Leary TM, Helfant RH: Prognosis of symptomatic coronary artery disease in young adults aged 40 years or less. *Am J Cardiol* 1987, **60**(16):1269–1272.

12

N-terminal pro-brain natriuretic peptide improves the C-ACS risk score prediction of clinical outcomes in patients with ST-elevation myocardial infarction

Peng-cheng He[1†], Chong-yang Duan[2,3†], Yuan-hui Liu[1], Xue-biao Wei[1] and Shu-guang Lin[1*]

Abstract

Background: It remained unclear whether the combination of the Canada Acute Coronary Syndrome Risk Score (CACS-RS) and N-terminal pro-brain natriuretic peptide (NT-pro-BNP) could have a better performance in predicting clinical outcomes in acute ST-elevation myocardial infarction (STEMI) patients with primary percutaneous coronary intervention.

Methods: A total of 589 consecutive STEMI patients were enrolled. The potential additional predictive value of NT-pro-BNP with the CACS-RS was estimated. Primary endpoint was in-hospital mortality and long-term poor outcomes.

Results: The incidence of in-hospital death was 3.1%. Patients with higher NT-pro-BNP and CACS-RS had a greater incidence of in hospital death. After adjustment for the CACS-RS, elevated NT-pro-BNP (defined as the best cutoff point based on the Youden's index) was significantly associated with in hospital death (odd ratio = 4.55, 95%CI = 1.52–13.65, $p = 0.007$). Elevated NT-pro-BNP added to CACS-RS significantly improved the C-statistics for in-hospital death, as compared with the original score (0.762 vs. 0.683, $p = 0.032$). Furthermore, the addition of NT-pro-BNP to CACS-RS enhanced net reclassification improvement (0.901, $p < 0.001$) and integrated discrimination improvement (0.021, $p = 0.033$), suggesting effective discrimination and reclassification. In addition, the similar result was also demonstrated for in-hospital major adverse clinical events (C-statistics: 0.736 vs. 0.695, $p = 0.017$) or 3-year mortality (0.699 vs. 0.604, $p = 0.004$).

Conclusions: Both NT-pro-BNP and CACS-RS are risk predictors for in hospital poor outcomes in patients with STEMI. A combination of them could derive a more accurate prediction for clinical outcome s in these patients.

Keywords: N-terminal pro-brain natriuretic peptide, Canada Acute Coronary Syndrome Risk Score, Acute ST-elevation myocardial infarction

Background

Despite significant advances in treatment and prevention, patients with ST-elevation myocardial infarction (STEMI) still remained important population with high risk of adverse clinical outcomes [1], especially in developed countries [2]. Accurate and comprehensive simple risk evaluation plays an important role for these patients in appropriate therapeutic decision making. Therefore, several prognostic risk scores have been established to identify high-risk patients and provide important prognostic information, such as the Global Registry of Acute Coronary Events (GRACE) risk score [3, 4]. Recently, Fabrizio D'Ascenzo et al demonstrated that Thrombolysis in Myocardial Infarction (TIMI) and GRACE are the risk scores that up until now have been most extensively investigated, and GRACE was better

---

* Correspondence: gdlinshuguang@126.com

†Equal contributors

[1]Department of Cardiology, Guangdong Cardiovascular Institute, Guangdong Provincial Key Laboratory of Coronary Heart Disease Prevention, Guangdong General Hospital, Guangdong Academy of Medical Sciences, Guangzhou 510080, Guangdong, China

Full list of author information is available at the end of the article

than others [5]. However, these risk scores are not widely used in clinical practice because they contain many variables that may not be easily applicable before hospital admission or in the emergency department, and they require computerized calculation methods. Recently, the Canada Acute Coronary Syndrome Risk Score (CACS-RS), has been shown to permit rapid stratification of patients with acute coronary syndrome (ACS) [6]. Because this risk score is simple and easy to memorize and calculate, it can be comfortably used by health care professionals without advanced medical training. However, the predictive value of CACS-RS in selected STEMI patients remains unknown.

N-terminal-pro-brain natriuretic peptide (NT-pro-BNP) is secreted in response to cardiac hemodynamic stress mediated by volume and pressure overload [7]; NT-pro-BNP is very stable at room temperature and is often measured in clinical practices, especially in the emergency department. NT-pro-BNP has been proposed to provide prognostic information in patients with acute coronary syndrome (ACS) [8]. The current clinical cardiology guidelines also recommended the use of selected newer biomarkers, including NT-pro-BNP, to provide additional prognostic information in patients with non-ST-elevation ACS [9, 10]. However, there has been no simple and effective risk model incorporating NT-pro-BNP for predicting the prognosis of STEMI patients.

Therefore, the present study was conducted to validate the predictive value of CACS-RS for STEMI patients, and to develop a Bio-Clinical CACS-RS (Bio-C-CACS) incorporating NT-pro-BNP to evaluate whether Bio-C-CACS would improve the ability to predict clinical poor outcomes compared with CACS-RS in those patients undergoing primary percutaneous coronary intervention (PPCI).

Methods

Population selection

According to our institute's protocol, we enrolled all consecutive patients who were admitted to Guangdong Cardiovascular Institute of Guangdong General Hospital, Guangdong Academy of Medical Sciences, between March 2008 and October 2012. These patients presented within 12 h of onset of cardiac symptoms with ST-segment elevation undergoing PPCI and admitted to the coronary care unit within at least 48 h of admission. Patients with cardiac shock on admission, patients with chronic peritoneal or hemodialysis treatment were excluded. Patients without pre-procedural NT-pro-BNP levels, or with severe liver or kidney dysfunction, or malignancy were also excluded.

The local ethics committee of our institute approved the study protocol. Written informed consent was obtained from the patients before the procedure,

or from next of kin for patients who could not sign the informed consent themselves.

Study protocol and Risk calculation

The baseline patient demographic data, cardiovascular risk factors, cardiac history, clinical data, and in-hospital medications of all the patients were recorded. NT-pro-BNP was measured using an electro-chemiluminescence immunoassay (Roche Diagnostics, Germany) at hospital admission before the procedure. Other clinical parameters, such as serum creatinine, cardiac troponin I, creatine kinase MB, and levels of electrolytes were measured as a part of standard clinical care. The estimated glomerular filtration rate (eGFR) was calculated using the four-variables of the Modification of Diet in Renal Disease equation for Chinese patients [11].

For each patient, we used the CACS-RS model at admission to estimate the risks for in-hospital and follow-up patient outcomes. The CACS-RS ranged from 0 to 4, with 1 point assigned for the presence of each of these variables: age ≥75 years, Killip > 1, systolic blood pressure <100 mmHg, and heart rate >100 beats/min (Table 1).

PCI procedure and medications

Primary PCI was performed with standard technique according to our institute's protocol and AHA/ACC guidelines for the management of patients with STEMI. The use of anti-platelet agents (aspirin/clopidogrel), β-adrenergic blocking agents, angiotensin-converting enzyme inhibitors, statins, or inotropic drug support was left at the clinician's discretion according to clinical protocols.

Follow-up and Clinical endpoints

All patients were followed up at least 3 years after the PCI procedure. The follow up data were obtained by reviewing medical records or through a telephone interview with patients.

The primary end point was in-hospital mortality. The secondary end point was the incidence of in hospital major adverse clinical events (MACEs: including all causes mortality, nonfatal myocardial infarction, target-vessel revascularization, and cerebrovascular events) and 3-year all cause mortality [12].

Table 1 The variables in the CACS risk score

Variables	Scores
Age ≥75 years	1
Killip > 1	1
Systolic blood pressure < 100 mmHg	1
Heart rate > 100 beats/min	1

Abbreviation: *CACS* Canada Acute Coronary Syndrome

Statistical analysis

Continuous variables were expressed as mean ± standard deviation or median values with interquartile ranges (IQR), where appropriate. Categorical variables were expressed as absolute number (percentage). The Student's t-test and Mann-Whitney U test were applied to compare normally and non-normally distributed continuous variables, respectively. The best cut-off value of NT-pro-BNP for predicting in hospital mortality was determined by the receiver-operating characteristic (ROC) curves analysis. The differences in clinical characteristics between patients with higher or lower than this cut-off value were compared. Multivariable logistic regression was performed by forward stepwise selection to evaluate the independent value of NT-pro-BNP as a categorical variable (based on the cut-off value) for in -hospital mortality, after adjusting the CACS-RS or variables, with p values <0.15 in the univariate analysis. Then, a new score, the Bio-C-CACS was obtained by adding the points based on the association between the CACS-RS regression coefficient and the NT-pro-BNP coefficient, if NT-pro-BNP was higher than its cut-off. The discrimination between NT-pro-BNP, CACS-RS and Bio-C-CACS risk score for in-hospital mortality or MACEs were evaluated with ROC area under the curve (AUC), sensitivity, and specificity.

The AUC was compared using the nonparametric approach of DeLong et al. [13]. Calibration was evaluated using the Hosmere-Lemeshow goodness-of-fit. We also performed net reclassification improvement (NRI) and integrated discrimination improvement (IDI) to analyze the degree to which the addition of NT-pro-BNP to the CACS-RS improved predictive ability [14]. All data analysis was performed using SAS version 9.4 (SAS Institute, Cary, NC). All statistical tests were two-tailed and statistical significance was accepted at $p < 0.05$.

Results

Baseline clinical characteristics and clinical outcomes

A total of 589 patients were included in the study. 16.3% were female. The percentages of patients complicated with diabetes, hypertension, and who were smokers were 21.6%, 54.3% and 48.9%, respectively. The mean age was 63.0 ± 11.9 years, mean eGFR was 77.70 ± 26.5 mL/min/ 1.73m^2. NT-pro-BNP showed a median of 1244 pg/mL (IQR = 515-2704). The CACS-RS showed a median of 1 (IQR = 0-1), with 45.84% being low risk (0-1), 51.61% medium risk (1-3) and 2.55% high risk (≥3).

From the CACS-RS low risk to high risk, there was a positive trend with older age, NT-pro-BNP levels, and the pre-procedural SCr level. There was a negative trend with the pre-procedural renal function and left ventricular ejection fraction (LVEF). However, there were no significant differences in the incidence of hypertension,

diabetes, or previous myocardial infarction among the different risk groups of CACS- RS (Table 2).

Overall, the incidence of in-hospital mortality was 3.1%, and the MACEs were 23.8%. The median follow-up period was 3.54 ± 1.40 years (inter quartile range, 2.61–4.28 years). During patient follow up, 3-year all cause mortality developed in 26 patients (5.9%).

Predictive value of CACS-RS

Patients who developed in-hospital mortality presented with a higher CACS-RS than those without (1.50 vs. 0.71, $p = 0.008$). The similar results were also demonstrated in patients developed in hospital MACEs or 3-year mortality (1.21 vs. 0.59, $p < 0.001$; 1.16 vs. 0.67, $p < 0.001$). The predictive value of CACS-RS for in hospital mortality was 0.683 (95% CI = 0.551-0.816) (Fig. 1). CACS-RS also showed predictive accuracy for in hospital MACEs (Fig. 1) or 3-year all cause mortality, with C-statistics of 0.695 (95% CI = 0.650-0.741), 0.604(95% CI = 0.515- 0.694).

Independent Predictive value of NT-pro-BNP

In addition, the best cut-off value of NT-pro-BNP for predicting in-hospital mortality was 2300 pg/mL with 72.2% sensitivity and 73.0% specificity, based on the Youden index. Furthermore, comparing to patients with low NT-pro-BNP (<2300 pg/mL), patients with NT-pro-BNP ≥2300 pg/mL presented with a significantly higher in-hospital mortality (7.74% vs. 1.19%, $p < 0.001$) or in hospital MACEs (42.86% vs. 16.15%, $p < 0.001$). The Kaplan-Meier curve showed that the incidence of MACEs was higher in those patients with higher NT-pro-BNP levels. Log-rank test on the curves demonstrated significant difference between two groups (Chi square = 15.56, $P < 0.001$).

Univariate logistic regression analysis showed that NT-pro-BNP ≥2300 pg/mL was significantly associated with in-hospital mortality (OR = 6.98, 95% CI = 2.45–19.90, $p < 0.001$). Additional significant variables included CACS-RS (OR = 2.76, 95% CI, 1.64–4.66, $p < 0.001$). The multivariate analysis, together with CACS-RS and NT-pro-BNP (as a categorical variable) demonstrated that CACS-RS and NT-pro- BNP ≥2300 pg/mL remained the significant independent predictor of in hospital mortality (OR = 2.15, 95%CI, 1.24–3.75, $p = 0.007$; OR = 4.55, 95% CI, 1.52–13.65, $p = 0.007$).

Combination of NT-pro-BNP with the CACS-RS

In order to evaluate the additional predictive value of NT-pro-BNP to CACS-RS, the NT-pro-BNP (as a categorical variable, according to the cut-off value) was incorporated into the new score (Bio-C-CACS-RS). Combinations of NT-pro-BNP with CACS-RS might more accurately identify patients at high risk of

Table 2 Baseline characteristics of patients according to C-ACS-RS group

Variables	0 (n = 266)	1 (n = 217)	2 (n = 95)	≥3 (n = 11)	P value
Demographics					
Age, years	58.32 ± 9.84	64.41 ± 11.93	71.08 ± 11.22	77.55 ± 6.31	<0.001
Age ≥ 75 years, n (%)	0 (0.0%)	46 (21.2%)	45 (47.4%)	8 (72.7%)	<0.001
Female, n (%)	34 (12.8%)	41 (18.9%)	20 (21.1%)	1 (9.1%)	0.140
Systolic BP (mmHg)	125.36 ± 16.16	117.79 ± 21.45	113.28 ± 29.40	98.30 ± 27.75	<0.001
Diastolic BP (mmHg)	76.22 ± 40.09	71.02 ± 14.00	67.00 ± 16.34	59.70 ± 14.49	0.028
Heart rate (beat/min)	76.88 ± 11.23	79.77 ± 16.92	85.70 ± 24.54	86.70 ± 18.56	<0.001
Medical history, n (%)					
Diabetes	56 (21.1%)	48 (22.1%)	19 (20.0%)	4 (36.4%)	0.760
Previous myocardial infarction	12 (4.5%)	14 (6.5%)	5 (5.3%)	2 (18.2%)	0.240
Coronary artery bypass graft	11 (4.1%)	6 (2.8%)	10(10.5%)	2(18.2%)	0.005
Hypertension	135 (50.8%)	121 (55.8%)	56 (58.9%)	8 (72.7%)	0.276
Smoking	138 (51.9%)	102 (47.0%)	43 (45.3%)	5 (45.5%)	0.612
Anemia	78 (29.3%)	45 (20.7%)	16 (16.8%)	2 (18.2%)	0.040
Laboratory findings					
NT-pro-BNP, pg/mL(Median)	851.15	1506.00	2414.00	2330.00	<0.001
Lg NT-pro-BNP, pg/mL	6.61 ± 1.27	7.28 ± 1.23	7.81 ± 1.26	7.85 ± 1.46	<0.001
Pre-procedural SCr (μmol/L)	91.24 ± 44.05	101.04 ± 39.58	111.49 ± 52.16	171.92 ± 147.90	<0.001
eGFR, mL/min/1.73 m^2	90.59 ± 94.56	78.16 ± 38.82	66.34 ± 21.50	50.97 ± 26.01	0.008
LVEF, %	55.54 ± 10.42	53.54 ± 10.31	49.04 ± 10.85	51.67 ± 14.62	<0.001
Hemoglobin (g/L)	135.33 ± 16.32	131.13 ± 17.97	127.39 ± 17.10	132.52 ± 18.79	<0.001
Hemoglobin A1c (%)	6.47 ± 1.36	6.62 ± 1.74	6.30 ± 1.39	6.44 ± 0.64	0.554
Serum albumin (g/L)	34.47 ± 5.24	32.71 ± 4.30	31.58 ± 4.47	31.27 ± 4.85	<0.001
Uric acid (μmol/L)	358.13 ± 93.3	377.69 ± 124.2	380.06 ± 117.7	393.11 ± 79.9	0.265
Procedural characteristic					
Contrast volume (mL)	132.80 ± 53.81	132.92 ± 53.00	144.29 ± 43.39	187.50 ± 81.32	0.291
Contrast exposure time (min)	78.89 ± 42.27	82.52 ± 37.72	92.02 ± 42.80	80.00 ± 49.50	0.347
Number of diseased vessels (n)	1.99 ± 1.17	2.08 ± 0.90	2.26 ± 0.94	2.00 ± 0.77	0.197
Number of stents (n)	1.36 ± 0.82	1.40 ± 0.77	1.49 ± 0.84	1.36 ± 0.50	0.587
Total length of stent (mm)	37.04 ± 26.47	35.61 ± 23.55	37.05 ± 24.60	24.00 ± 8.49	0.871

Abbreviation: *C-ACS-RS* Canada Acute Coronary Syndrome risk score, *NT-pro-BNP* N-terminal-pro-brain natriuretic peptide, *SCr* serum creatinine, *eGFR* estimated glomerular filtration rate, *LVEF* left ventricular ejected function

in hospital mortality or MACEs than using CACS-RS only. (Fig. 2)

In addition, ROC analysis demonstrated that the AUC for in hospital mortality increased significantly after the addition of NT-pro-BNP to the CACS-RS (AUC: 0.762 vs. 0.683; $p = 0.032$), as did the Hosmer-Lemeshow goodness of fit ($X^2 = 7.44$, $p = 0.489$). (Fig. 1) More importantly, the inclusion of NT-pro-BNP into the CACS-RS was associated with a NRI of 90.1%, suggesting effective reclassification. The IDI showed that the model diagnostic performance was significantly improved by adding NT-pro-BNP to the CACS-RS (IDI = 0.021, $p = 0.033$).

Meanwhile, applying the same statistic metrics to other clinical endpoints, we found that NT-pro-BNP increased

the AUC, and improved the reclassification and discrimination ability when added to the CACS-RS, with in-hospital MACEs: (AUC: 0.736 vs. 0.695, IDI: 0.032, NRI: 0.601); 3-year all cause mortality: (AUC: 0.699 vs. 0.604, IDI: 0.032, NRI: 0.762).

Discussions

This study demonstrated that CACS-RS is an independent predictor of outcomes in STEMI patients undergoing PPCI, and with good predictive value of poor outcomes. Furthermore, this might be the first study to demonstrate that the measurement of NT-pro-BNP concentrations on patient hospital admission add prognostic information about short- and long-

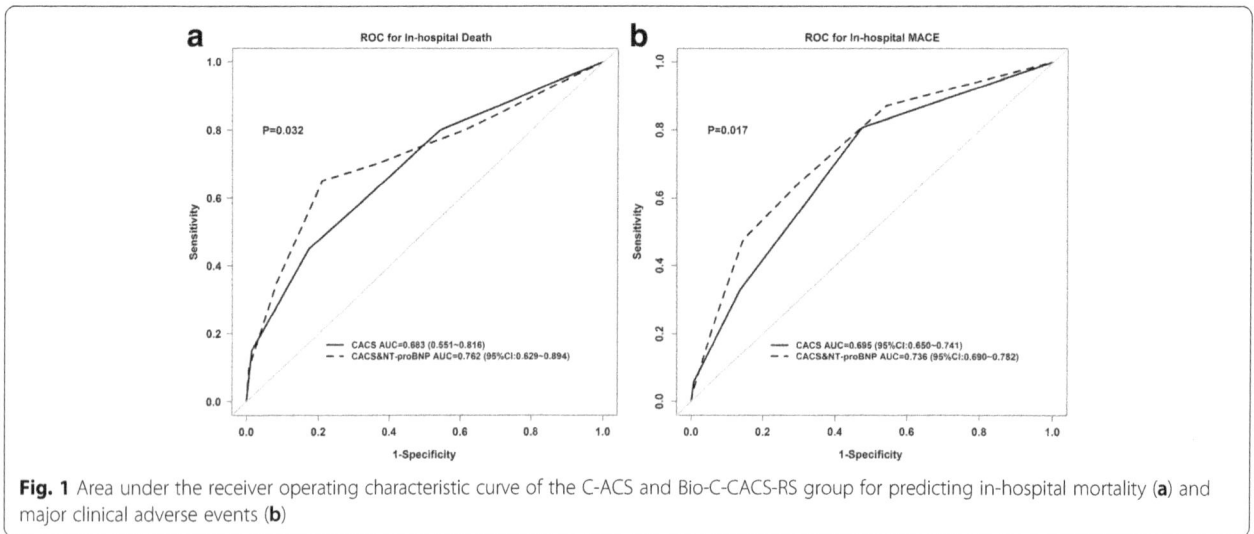

Fig. 1 Area under the receiver operating characteristic curve of the C-ACS and Bio-C-CACS-RS group for predicting in-hospital mortality (**a**) and major clinical adverse events (**b**)

term outcomes to the CACS-RS. This study has described the use of the new Bio-C-CACS.

STEMI patients remain an important clinical population with a risk of adverse clinical outcomes [2]. In the present study, the in hospital mortality of STEMI patients was shown to be 3.1% and the 3-year mortality was 5.9%, which was lower than the incidence of mortality in the study by Campo G et al [15–17]. It might be related to the different percentage of hypertension, previous myocardial

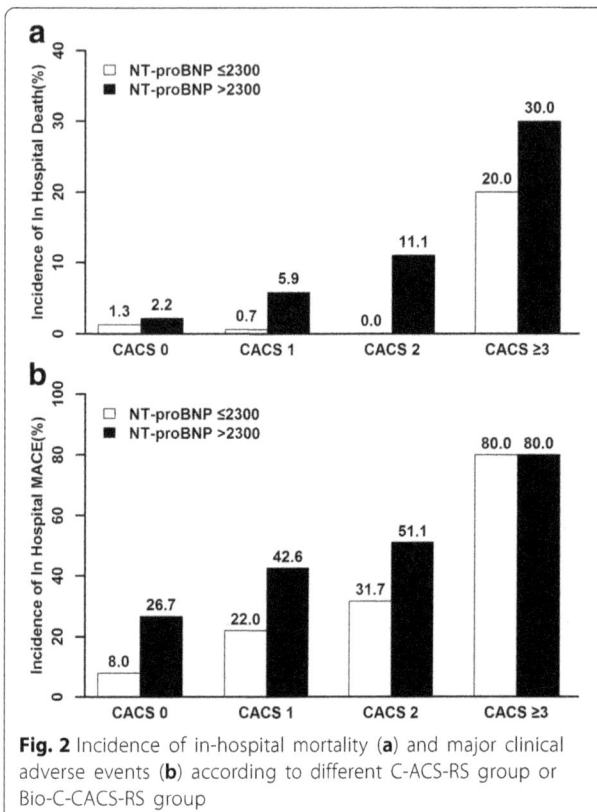

Fig. 2 Incidence of in-hospital mortality (**a**) and major clinical adverse events (**b**) according to different C-ACS-RS group or Bio-C-CACS-RS group

infraction and the type of stent. The findings in present and previous studies support the aim of this study, to develop improved clinical tools to identify STEMI patients at high risk of poor clinical outcome. Accurate and comprehensive simple risk evaluation plays an important role for these patients in appropriate therapeutic decision making. Higher risk scores usually imply that higher-intensity treatments may be appropriate within the context of the patient's health status. However, inappropriate use of aggressive medical management in patients at low-risks may only expose them to experience adverse effects.

Several risk-scoring systems have been proven to evaluate the risk of poor clinical outcomes in STEMI patients. The GRACE risk score is one of the most frequently used models, incorporating clinical investigation (such as an ECG) and cardiac and renal biomarker (such as creatinine kinase MB and serum creatinine levels). However, the GRACE risk score requires computerized calculation methods, and not all clinical information for this assessment may be available at first clinical contact. In addition, the TIMI score for STEMI is an another popular risk-assessment tool, which is simpler to use than the GRACE score, but may also require the availability of an ECG and patient weight on admission [18]. Furthermore, previous research has shown that the Mehran risk score (MRS) for contrast-induced nephropathy can be applied to stratify STEMI patients for poor clinical outcomes both in the short- and long-term follow-up. However, the MRS incorporates eight variables, which include not only the history of previous diseases, but also the procedure-related variables (such as contrast volume), and cannot be used before the procedure [19]. The clinical SYNTAX risk score is used for identifying STEMI patients for poor clinical outcomes, and was based on the anatomy of the coronary diseases following coronary angiography, but this scoring method cannot be used in clinical practice before the PCI.

Although the above risk-scoring systems were demonstrated the good predictive value for the clinical outcomes for STEMI patients, they are limited due to their relative complexity, the requirement of data calculation, and the required the procedure related variables. In contrast, the CACS-RS only requires basic demographic and initial hemodynamic data, which can be acquired in the emergency department, or possibly prior to arrival at the hospital.

Despite its simplicity, the CACS-RS had good predictive value for clinical outcomes. The C statistic of in hospital mortality was 0.683. The CACS-RS was first developed by Huynh et al, who performed their research study to include the ACS patients, most of whom were without ST-segment elevation; the score was demonstrated to have good predictive values for short- and long-term mortality of ACS patients [6]. The C statistic in this previous study was similar to the findings in the present study (0.73 vs. 0.68), which included only STEMI patients. More recently, two published studies have validated the clinical usefulness of CACS-RS in ACS patients. One study reported that CACS-RS performed well in predicting hospital mortality in a contemporary ACS population outside North America [20]. The other study showed that CACS-RS was the strongest predictor of in-hospital mortality in all ACS patients in western Romania [21]. However, we propose that the present study is the first to further validate the predictive value of the C-ACS score in a selected STEMI patient population. The difference in C-statistic analysis among these researches might be related to the differences in patient populations studied, and on the characters of the patients included in the studies. However, the CACS-RS had acceptable predictive value for STEMI patients, and permits rapid stratification of patients with STEMI, and would be welcomed for used by busy clinicians, because it is simple and can be used as an initial risk-assessment tools by health care professionals without advanced medical training.

In addition, although more biomarkers are being added to develop risk clinical scoring systems, many new biomarkers still have not been taken account into the CACS-RS. NT-pro-BNP, which is influenced both by cardiac and renal function, can be quickly measured by the bedside, and is increasingly shown to be predictive of short- and long-term outcomes following STEMI [22]. The current clinical guidelines also recommended that the use of selected newer biomarkers, especially NT-pro-BNP, may provide additional prognostic information in patients with non–ST-elevation ACS. Lee et al found that an improvement in the ability of the clinical SYNTAX score to predict 1-year major adverse cardiovascular events can be achieved by combining the clinical SYNTAX score with

an NT-pro-BNP [23]. Similar results have been found in the study performed by Grabowski et al. Admission of BNP adds significant prognostic information in addition to that of Killip classes and TIMI risk score in STEMI patients [24]. However, another study showed that NT-pro-BNP did not increase the prognostic accuracy of the GRACE risk score in patients with ACS [25]. To date, it has been unclear whether NT-pro-BNP could provide additional predictive value for CACS-RS. The present study found that adding the NT-pro-BNP to the CACS-RS could increase the predictive value for patient clinical outcome. This is unsurprising, because STEMI patients with significant left ventricular dysfunction appear to be at low risk based on the CACS-RS if the blood pressure or heart rate is within the normal range, but the risk increase with increased NT-pro-BNP levels.

It is important to bear in mind that risk scores only based on the clinical characteristic are supplementary tools and are no replacement for clinical judgment or biomarker measurement, but combining them could have a beneficial cumulative effect. According to the guideline's recommendation that risk assessment is a continuous process that should be repeated throughout the hospitalization duration and at time of discharge, after we easily used the CACS-RS to identify patients at risk of poor clinical outcome at the first medical contact, we should re-calculate the CACS-RS, and add the NT-pro-BNP to the CACS-RS to evaluate the risks for patients during in-hospital stay or following hospital discharge.

Clinical implications

The results of the present study may have important clinical implications. The C-ACS-RS permits rapid stratification of STEMI patients. Because it is simple and easy to memorize and calculate, it can be rapidly applied at the first medical contact. In particular, the combined application of the C-ACSRS with the plasma NT-pro-BNP levels on admission serves to identify high-risk patients. The effective risk stratification provided may be of specific value for early therapeutic decision making and patient treatment in the different risk of STEMI patients.

Limitations

The current study had several limitations. Firstly, It was a single-center, observational study, including a relatively small number of STEMI patients. The results of a single study should be interpreted with caution. In addition, we did not measure NT-pro-BNP concentrations at long-term follow up, such as at 3 months or at 1 year. Thirdly, C-ACS-Rs lacks precision, being more of a categorical than a continuous scoring system. The Killip class evaluation is totally dependent on the clinical evaluation and expertise of the examiner. However, this scoring system is simple and easy to apply.

Conclusions

In conclusion, for the fist time, the present study validated the predictive value of C-ACS-RS in STEMI patients. The combination of C-ACS-RS and NT-pro-BNP could result in a more accurate prediction for clinical outcomes in these patients.

Acknowledgements
We are grateful for the efforts of Lei Jiang, MD, of the Department of cardiology, Guangdong General Hospital, Guangzhou, 510100, China.

Funding
This study was supported by a grant from Science and Technology Planning Project of Guangdong Province (grant NO.: 2014A020209053). The funders had no role in the study design, data collection and analysis, the decision to publish, or the preparation of the manuscript. The work was not funded by any industry sponsors.

Authors' contributions
Conception/Design: SGL. Collection and/or assembly of data: HPC, YHL, XBW. Data analysis and interpretation: CYD. Manuscript writing: HPC, LYH. Manuscript revising: SGL. Final approval of the version to be published: All authors. All authors read and approved the final manuscript.

Competing interests
The authors declare that they have no competing interests.

Author details
[1]Department of Cardiology, Guangdong Cardiovascular Institute, Guangdong Provincial Key Laboratory of Coronary Heart Disease Prevention, Guangdong General Hospital, Guangdong Academy of Medical Sciences, Guangzhou 510080, Guangdong, China. [2]State Key Laboratory of Organ Failure Research, National Clinical Research Center for Kidney Disease, Guangzhou, China. [3]Department of Biostatistics, School of Public Health, Southern Medical University, Guangzhou 510515, China.

References
1. Amin ST, Morrow DA, Braunwald E, Sloan S, Contant C, Murphy S, Antman EM. Dynamic TIMI risk score for STEMI. J Am Heart Assoc. 2013;2(1):e003269.
2. Li J, Li X, Wang Q, Hu S, Wang Y, Masoudi FA, Spertus JA, Krumholz HM, Jiang L. ST-segment elevation myocardial infarction in China from 2001 to 2011 (the China PEACE-Retrospective Acute Myocardial Infarction Study): a retrospective analysis of hospital data. Lancet. 2015;385(9966):441–51.
3. American College of Emergency P, Society for Cardiovascular A, Interventions, O'Gara PT, Kushner FG, Ascheim DD, Casey Jr DE, Chung MK, de Lemos JA, Ettinger SM, et al. 2013 ACCF/AHA guideline for the management of ST-elevation myocardial infarction: a report of the American College of Cardiology Foundation/American Heart Association Task Force on Practice Guidelines. J Am Coll Cardiol. 2013;61(4):e78–140.
4. Eagle KA, Goodman SG, Avezum Á, Budaj A, Sullivan CM, López-Sendón J. Practice variation and missed opportunities for reperfusion in ST-segment-elevation myocardial infarction: findings from the Global Registry of Acute Coronary Events (GRACE). Lancet. 2002;359(9304):373–7.
5. D'Ascenzo F, Biondi-Zoccai G, Moretti C, Bollati M, Omede P, Sciuto F, Presutti DG, Modena MG, Gasparini M, Reed MJ, et al. TIMI, GRACE and alternative risk scores in Acute Coronary Syndromes: a meta-analysis of 40 derivation studies on 216,552 patients and of 42 validation studies on 31,625 patients. Contemp Clin Trials. 2012;33(3):507–14.
6. Huynh T, Kouz S, Yan AT, Danchin N, O'Loughlin J, Schampaert E, Yan RT, Rinfret S, Tardif JC, Eisenberg MJ, et al. Canada Acute Coronary Syndrome

7. Risk Score: a new risk score for early prognostication in acute coronary syndromes. Am Heart J. 2013;166(1):58–63.
7. Nadir MA, Witham MD, Szwejkowski BR, Struthers AD. Meta-analysis of B-type natriuretic peptide's ability to identify stress induced myocardial ischemia. Am J Cardiol. 2011;107(5):662–7.
8. Garcia-Alvarez A, Regueiro A, Hernandez J, Kasa G, Sitges M, Bosch X, Heras M. Additional value of B-type natriuretic peptide on discrimination of patients at risk for mortality after a non-ST-segment elevation acute coronary syndrome. Eur Heart J Acute Cardiovasc Care. 2014;3(2):132–40.
9. Weber M, Bazzino O, Navarro Estrada JL, Fuselli JJ, Botto F, Perez de Arenaza D, Mollmann H, Nef HN, Elsasser A, Hamm CW. N-terminal B-type natriuretic peptide assessment provides incremental prognostic information in patients with acute coronary syndromes and normal troponin T values upon admission. J Am Coll Cardiol. 2008;51(12):1188–95.
10. Amsterdam EA, Wenger NK, Brindis RG, Casey Jr DE, Ganiats TG, Holmes Jr DR, Jaffe AS, Jneid H, Kelly RF, Kontos MC, et al. 2014 AHA/ACC Guideline for the Management of Patients with Non-ST-Elevation Acute Coronary Syndromes: a report of the American College of Cardiology/ American Heart Association Task Force on Practice Guidelines. J Am Coll Cardiol. 2014;64(24):e139–228.
11. Ma YC, Zuo L, Chen JH, Luo Q, Yu XQ, Li Y, Xu JS, Huang SM, Wang LN, Huang W, et al. Modified glomerular filtration rate estimating equation for Chinese patients with chronic kidney disease. J Am Soc Nephrol. 2006;17(10):2937–44.
12. Cannon CP, Brindis RG, Chaitman BR, Cohen DJ, Cross JT, Drozda JP, Fesmire FM, Fintel DJ, Fonarow GC, Fox KA, et al. 2013 ACCF/AHA Key Data Elements and Definitions for Measuring the Clinical Management and Outcomes of Patients With Acute Coronary Syndromes and Coronary Artery Disease. J Am Coll Cardiol. 2013;61(9):992–1025.
13. DeLong ERDD, Clarke-Pearson DL. Comparing the areas under two or more correlated receiver operating characteristic curves: a nonparametric approach. Biometrics. 1988;44(3):837–45.
14. Pencina MJDARS, D'Agostino Jr RB, Vasan RS. Evaluating the added predictive ability of a new marker: from area under the ROC curve to reclassification and beyond. Stat Med. 2008;27(2):157–72.
15. Campo G, Guastaroba P, Marzocchi A, Santarelli A, Varani E, Vignali L, Sangiorgio P, Tondi S, Serenelli C, De Palma R, et al. Impact of COPD on Long-term Outcome After ST-Segment Elevation Myocardial Infarction Receiving Primary Percutaneous Coronary Intervention. Chest. 2013;144(3):750–7.
16. Campo G, Saia F, Percoco G, Manari A, Santarelli A, Vignali L, Varani E, Benassi A, Sangiorgio P, Tarantino F, et al. Long-term outcome after drug eluting stenting in patients with ST-segment Elevation Myocardial Infarction. Int J Cardiol. 2010;140(2):154–60.
17. Campo GSF, Guastaroba P, Marchesini J, Varani E, Manari A, Ottani F, Tondi S, De Palma R, Marzocchi A. Prognostic impact of hospital readmissions after primary percutaneous coronary intervention. Arch Intern Med. 2011;171(21):1948–9.
18. DA Morrow AE, Charlesworth A, Cairns R, Murphy SA, de Lemos JA, Giugliano RP, McCabe CH, Braunwald E. TIMI risk score for ST-elevation myocardial infarction: A convenient, bedside, clinical score for risk assessment at presentation: An intravenous nPA for treatment of infarcting myocardium early II trial substudy. Circulation. 2000;102(17):2031–7.
19. Mehran R, Aymong ED, Nikolsky E, Lasic Z, Iakovou I, Fahy M, Mintz GS, Lansky AJ, Moses JW, Stone GW, et al. A simple risk score for prediction of contrast-induced nephropathy after percutaneous coronary intervention: development and initial validation. J Am Coll Cardiol. 2004;44(7):1393–9.
20. AlFaleh HF, Alsheikh-Ali AA, Ullah A, AlHabib KF, Hersi A, Suwaidi JA, Sulaiman K, Saif SA, Almahmeed W, Asaad N, et al. Validation of the Canada Acute Coronary Syndrome Risk Score for Hospital Mortality in the Gulf Registry of Acute Coronary Events-2. Clin Cardiol. 2015;38(9):542–7.
21. Pogorevici A, Citu IM, Bordejevic DA, Caruntu F, Tomescu MC. Canada acute coronary syndrome score was a stronger baseline predictor than age >/=75 years of in-hospital mortality in acute coronary syndrome patients in western Romania. Clin Interv Aging. 2016;11:481–8.
22. Jarai R, Huber K, Bogaerts K, Droogne W, Ezekowitz J, Granger CB, Sinnaeve PR, Ross AM, Zeymer U, Armstrong PW, et al. Plasma N-terminal fragment of the prohormone B-type natriuretic peptide concentrations in relation to time to treatment and Thrombolysis in Myocardial Infarction (TIMI) flow: a substudy of the Assessment of the Safety and Efficacy of a New Treatment Strategy with Percutaneous Coronary Intervention (ASSENT IV-PCI) trial. Am Heart J. 2010;159(1):131–40.

23. Lee JH, Kim JH, Jang SY, Park SH, Bae MH, Yang DH, Park HS, Cho Y, Chae SC. A new tool for the risk stratification of patients undergoing primary percutaneous coronary intervention with ST-segment elevation myocardial infarction: Bio-Clinical SYNTAX score. Int J Cardiol. 2015;187:193–5.

24. Grabowski M, Filipiak KJ, Malek LA, Karpinski G, Huczek Z, Stolarz P, Spiewak M, Kochman J, Rudowski R, Opolski G. Admission B-type natriuretic peptide assessment improves early risk stratification by Killip classes and TIMI risk score in patients with acute ST elevation myocardial infarction treated with primary angioplasty. Int J Cardiol. 2007;115(3):386–90.

25. Valente S, Lazzeri C, Chiostri M, Giglioli C, Sori A, Tigli S, Gensini GF. NT-proBNP on admission for early risk stratification in STEMI patients submitted to PCI. Relation with extension of STEMI and inflammatory markers. Int J Cardiol. 2009;132(1):84–9.

13

Renal insufficiency was correlated with 2-year mortality for rural female patients with ST-segment elevation acute myocardial infarction after reperfusion therapy

Yuan Gao[1*], Daming Jiang[2], Bo Zhang[3], Yujiao Sun[4], Lina Ren[1], Dandan Fan[1] and Guoxian Qi[1]

Abstract

Background: Renal insufficiency (RI) following ST-segment elevation acute myocardial infarction (STEMI) is associated with a worse clinical prognosis. We investigated the impact of RI on long-term mortality in rural female patients with STEMI and evaluated prognostic factors.

Methods: A prospective cohort study of 436 consecutive rural female patients who were successfully treated with reperfusion therapy for STEMI between May 2009 and August 2011 in secondary care hospitals in Liaoning province northeastern China and followed up for 2 years. Patients were divided into three groups by estimated glomerular filtration rate (eGFR): Normal group, eGFR ≥90 mL/min/1.73 m^2 ($n = 233$). Moderate group, eGFR 60–90 mL/min/1.73 m^2 ($n = 108$). RI group, eGFR <60 mL/min/1.73 m^2 ($n = 95$). The primary outcome was 2-year mortality.

Results: During follow-up (mean 741 ± 118 days), the RI group had a significantly higher mortality than the other groups (24.21 % vs. 6.87 % and 10.19 %, $p < 0.001$). The RI group had significantly higher hospital mortality (7.37 % $p = 0.045$ vs. Normal group). RI increased the risk of hospital mortality (hazard ratio (HR) 1.832, 95 % CI 1.017–3.091, $p = 0.033$), and increased the risk of 2-year mortality (HR 3.872, 95 % CI 2.004–6.131, $p < 0.001$). Multivariate analysis showed eGFR <90 ml/min/1.73 m^2 and age ≥75 years as independent predictors of mortality at 2 years. In detail these were eGFR 60–90 ml/min/1.73 m^2 with HR 2.081, 95%CI 1.250–2.842, $p < 0.001$; eGFR <60 ml/min/1.73 m^2 with HR 3.872, 95%CI 2.004–6.131, $p < 0.001$; age ≥75 with HR 1.461, 95%CI 1.011–1.952, $p = 0.024$.

Conclusions: RI had a powerful correlation with long-term mortality for rural female patients with STEMI after reperfusion therapy.

Keywords: ST-segment elevation, Myocardial infarction, Renal insufficiency, Risk factors

Background

At present the incidence of chronic kidney disease is rapidly increasing [1]. Nearly 30 % of patients with ST-segment elevation acute myocardial infarction (STEMI) have combined renal insufficiency (RI) [2]. Widely used early reperfusion therapy, including emergency primary percutaneous coronary intervention (PCI) or thrombolysis therapy has beneficial effects for STEMI [3, 4]. However, RI following STEMI is associated with a worse clinical prognosis [5–7], a 6 to 11-fold increase in hospital risk of death [8], and a 1.76- to 6.18-fold 7-month risk of death [6]. Unfortunately, most STEMI patients with RI are excluded from randomized trials. Renal insufficiency may lead to alteration in lipid metabolism, vascular endothelial injury and dysfunction, trigger the inflammatory response, coagulation and oxidative stress and increase atherosclerosis, by the

* Correspondence: plateau1216@163.com
[1]Department of Cardiology, First Affiliated Hospital of China Medical University, Shenyang, Liaoning 110001, China
Full list of author information is available at the end of the article

sympathetic, neurohormonal pathway and renin angiotensin aldosterone axis activation [9–11].

Most clinical studies into myocardial infarction involve only a minority of female patients. For example women accounted for 29.6 % of the total enrolled patients in the Korea acute myocardial infarction registry study [7]. This is of concern because acute myocardial infarction mortality is higher in females than males and while there have been declines in the risk of death in men; the rate in women remains fairly constant [12]. The risk of in hospital mortality after primary PCI is also significantly higher for females than males [13], and female patients with STEMI show significantly greater death rates than males [14], with younger females at much higher risk than males of the same age [15].

In China the rates of mortality due to cardiac disease are growing, and while they are highest in urban areas, the rate in rural areas is increasing more rapidly [16]. Therefore, female patients with STEMI complicated by RI who reside in rural areas are an often neglected population that may be at high risk of death resulting from their condition. Little is known of the impact of RI on the prognosis in rural female patients with STEMI regardless of reperfusion therapy in Liaoning province in northeastern China.

The objective of this study was to determine the association between RI and the risk of death in STEMI patients successfully treated with PCI or thrombolytic therapy. We hypothesized that RI would be associated with higher 2-year mortality. The results of our prospective cohort study provide convincing evidence of this association in a real world situation.

Methods

Subjects

This was a prospective, multicenter study conducted at 16 hospitals in the Liaoning Province of northeast China from May 2009 to August 2011. The 16 hospitals were: First Affiliated Hospital, China Medical University; First Affiliated Hospital, Dalian Medical University; Changtu xian People's Hospital; Fuxin Mongolian Autonomous County People's Hospital; Yixian People's Hospital; Benxi Steel Company Hospital; Fushun Coal Mining Administration Hospital; Chaoyang Center Hospital; Fuxin Center Hospital; Zhuanghe Center Hospital; Wafangdian Center Hospital; Pulandian Center Hospital; Donggang Center Hospital; Dashiqiao Center Hospital; Zhangwu xian People's Hospital; Kuandian xian Center Hospital.

This study was conducted in accordance with the declaration of Helsinki, and was conducted with approval from the Ethics Committee of China Medical University. Written informed consent was obtained from all participants.

We enrolled 479 consecutive rural female STEMI patients from May 2009 to August 2011 from all of the centers. The inclusion criteria were: (1) STEMI was diagnosed according to European Society of Cardiology (ESC) criteria [3]; (2) it was the first time STEMI was diagnosed; (3) all patients were given primary PCI treatment within 12 h or thrombolytic therapy within 6 h after symptom onset. The exclusion criteria were: (1) acute myocardial infarction patients with acute kidney injury (AKI); (2) patients undergoing dialysis treatment. (3) patients whose non-infarct-related artery was treated during primary PCI; (4) PCI was undertaken after thrombolytic therapy.

Acute renal failure was diagnosed by an increase in serum creatinine levels of 50 % or an absolute increase of $\geq$26.5 µmol/l in 48 h [17].

Demographic and basic clinical data were obtained from all patients, which included age, gender, body mass index and cardiovascular risk factors. Additional clinical data including clinical laboratory tests, coronary imaging data, therapeutic strategies and adverse cardiac events were collected by trained personnel.

eGFR measurement

Kidney function was measured by estimated glomerular filtration rate (eGFR), calculated using the Chronic Kidney Disease Epidemiology Collaboration (CKD-EPI) Modification of Diet in Renal Disease (MDRD) equation [18] [CKD-EPI formula If female and if serum creatinine (Scr) $\leq$0.7 mg/dL:

$$CKD\text{-}EPI = 144 \times Scr(mg/dL)/0.7^{-0.329} \\ \times 0.993^{age(years)}$$

If female and if Scr > 0.7 mg/dL:

$$CKD\text{-}EPI = 144 \times Scr(mg/dL)/0.7^{-1.209} \\ \times 0.993^{age(years)}.$$

Renal insufficiency (RI) was defined as eGFR <60 mL/min/1.73m^2 according to the Kidney Disease: Improving Global Outcomes (KDIGO) guidelines [19] eGFR were calculated by the Scr examination results immediately after admission.

The patients were divided into 3 groups based on their eGFR values; the Normal group (high eGFR group, eGFR $\geq$ 90 mL/min/1.73 m^2, n = 233), the Moderate group (middle eGFR group, 60 mL/min $\cdot$ m^2 < eGFR <89 mL/min/1.73 m^2, n = 108) who had moderate RI, and the RI group (low eGFR group, eGFR <60 mL/min/1.73 m^2, n = 95).

Successful PCI

PCI was considered to be successful if the infarct-related artery residual stenosis was <10 %, and the Thrombolysis in Myocardial Infarction (TIMI) flow level reached 3 [20]. All patients were estimated immediately after PCI.

Successful thrombolytic therapy

1.5 million Units of urokinase were administrated to patients by intravenous infusion within 30 min for thrombolytic therapy.

Thrombolytic therapy was considered successful if more than 2 of 4 criteria were met [9]: ST segment resolved by ≥ 50 % by electrocardiogram (ECG) within 2 h, chest pain disappeared within 2 h; reperfusion arrhythmia occurred; serum myocardial enzyme peaks were detected in advance.

Medication

All patients received the recommended standard management for STEMI, including 300 mg loading dose of aspirin and clopidogrel after admission, aspirin, clopidogrel, low-molecular-weight heparin, beta-blockers, statins and angiotensin-converting enzyme (ACE) inhibitors/angiotensin receptor antagonist (ARB) as appropriate. The details of the medications are included in Appendix 1.

Definition of risk factors

Abnormal body mass index (BMI) was defined as BMI ≥ 25 kg/m [2, 21]. Diabetes was diagnosed by previous medical history or fasting glucose ≥ 7.0 mmol/L and/or 2 h plasma glucose level ≥11.1 mmol/l (measured after 75 g oral glucose load). Hypertension was diagnosed by previous medical history or systolic blood pressure ≥ 140 mmHg and/or diastolic blood pressure ≥ 90 mmHg after admission. Hypercholesterolemia was diagnosed by previous medical history or low-density lipoprotein (LDL) cholesterol ≥ 2.6 mmol/L and/or non high-density lipoprotein (HDL) cholesterol ≥3.3 mmol/L. Definition of contrast-induced nephropathy (CIN) was an increase in serum creatinine ≥ 0.5 mg/dL, occurring 48 h after exposure to contrast media [22]. Current smoker was defined as smoking >300 cigarettes/year.

Outcomes

Major adverse cardiac events (MACE) included: death, recurrent myocardial infarction, target vessel revascularization and stroke.

Key bleeding end points were analyzed on the basis of global use of strategies to open occluded coronary arteries (GUSTO) criteria [23].

CIN, contrast-induced nephropathy was defined as either a greater than 25 % increase of serum creatinine or an absolute increase in serum creatinine of 0.5 mg/dL [24].

Clinical examination and laboratory analysis

Patients underwent physical examination, ECG examination and fasting blood biochemical examination after admission including Scr, serum creatine kinase MB (CKMB), and cardiac troponin I (cTNI). Patients were examined for myocardial necrosis markers and by ECG once every 8 h

in 72 h, then every 24 h they were examined again. Blood leukocyte counts were examined 24 h after admission and echocardiography 48 h after admission.

To ensure the standard of data collection, laboratory procedures, data management and coordination between the multiples centers involved in the study was up to our quality control all the clinicians involved in this study received uniform training before the research began.

Follow up

The patients were followed up by telephone for 2 years; once per year; by the same doctor.

Statistical method

Categorical data were expressed with absolute numbers and percentages and analyzed using the χ^2 test. Continuous data with normal distribution were described with mean and standard deviation (SD) and median and interquartile range (IQR; 25th to 75th). Data among groups were compared using ANOVA. Further Student–Newman–Keuls (SNK) analyses were performed between the three groups. Non-normally distributed data among groups were compared using rank test.

Corresponding Kaplan-Meier curves with the log-rank test were constructed. Univariate analysis of eGFR, Scr, Microalbuminuria, age, gender, diabetes, hypertension, hyperlipidemia, Killip class, heart rate (HR), ejection fraction (EF), white blood cell (WBC) counts, and medication treatment were performed to determine the predictors for mortality. Multiple Cox proportional hazard model was used to estimate associations between significant factors identified in the univariate analysis. Hazard ratios (HR) and 95 % confidence intervals (CI) were calculated and p value <0.05 was considered statistically significant. All analyses were performed using SPSS version 19.0 (SPSS Inc., Chicago, IL, USA).

Results

The flowchart showing inclusion of patients in the study is presented in Fig. 1. In total 479 patients were enrolled in the study, 24 from these were excluded including 8 patients with incomplete data, 4 for whom clinical data were incomplete and 4 whose laboratory data were incomplete. Thus, 455 patients were included and 19 patients were lost to follow up. Finally 436 patients were included in the study 233 in the Normal group, 108 in the Moderate group, and 95 in the RI group (Fig. 1).

Study sample and characteristics

The mean follow-up period was 741 ± 118 days. Among the 436 individuals in the final cohort, the mean age was 67.52 years, and 35.78 % had diabetes (Table 1). Elderly

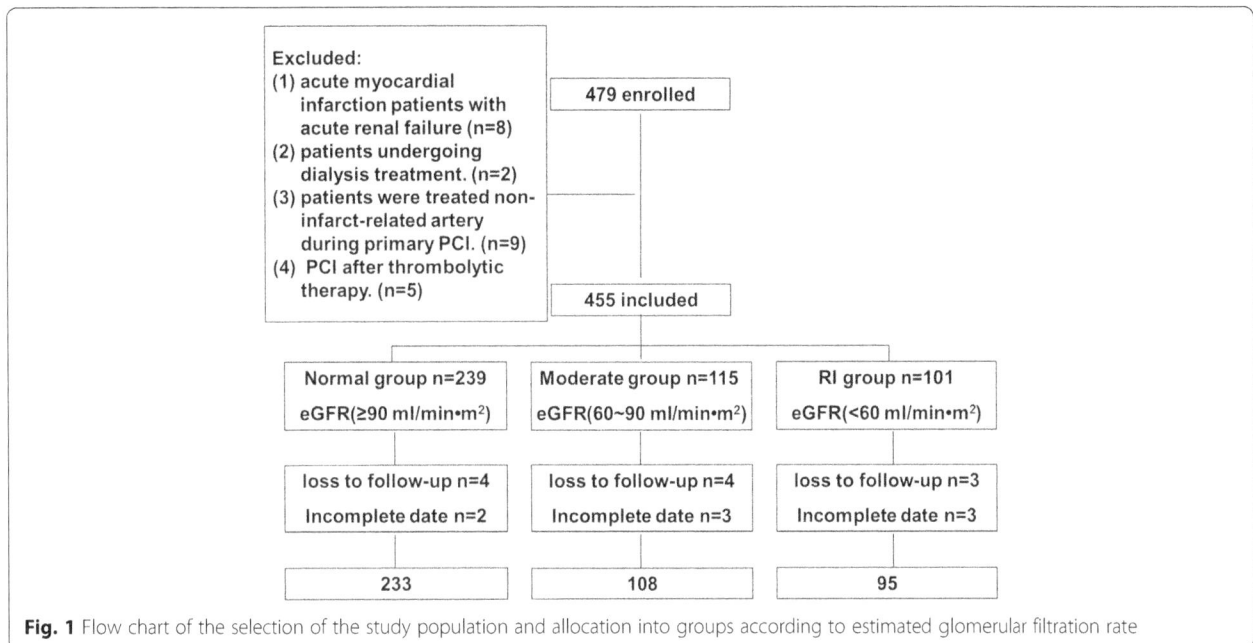

Fig. 1 Flow chart of the selection of the study population and allocation into groups according to estimated glomerular filtration rate

patients and those with hypertension and diabetes accounted for a high proportion of patients in the RI group. Median symptom to door time, door to balloon time and door to needle time were 183, 134 and 56 min, respectively. In the three groups the mean ages were 61.11 ± 8.42 years in the Normal group, 64.08 ± 6.91 years in the Moderate group and 75.57 ± 7.53 years in the RI group with a significant difference between all of the groups ($p < 0.05$). The diabetes rates were 29.61 % in the Normal group, 37.96 % in the Moderate group and 48.42 % in the RI group with a significant difference between the Normal and RI groups ($p < 0.05$). The hypertension rates were 32.19 % in the Normal group 44.44 % in the Moderate group and 52.63 % in the RI group with a significant difference between the Normal and RI group ($p < 0.05$). There were higher proportions in the RI group of Killip ≥ 2 at 21.05 % compared to 9.26 % ($p < 0.05$) in the Moderate group and 9.01 %, ($p < 0.05$) in the Normal group, longer hospital stay at 12.05 ± 5.74 days compared to 8.36 ± 5.11 days ($p < 0.05$) in the Moderate group and 8.53 ± 4.78 days ($p < 0.05$) in the Normal group, low EF values at 44.38 ± 13.05 % compared to 48.92 ± 14.02 % ($p < 0.05$) in the Moderate group and 50.11 ± 13.60 % ($p < 0.05$) in the Normal group, high Scr values at 116.67 ± 59.01 mmol/l compared to 85.47 ± 44.90 mmol/l ($p < 0.05$) in the Moderate group and 78.12 ± 31.13 mmol/l ($p < 0.05$) in the Normal group, and cTnI peak at 45.33 ± 15.26 ng/ml compared to 30.19 ± 18.73 ng/ml ($p < 0.05$) for the Moderate group and 31.06 ± 16.28 ng/ml for the Normal group ($p < 0.05$) (Table 1). There were 298 patients

who underwent primary PCI and 138 thrombolytic therapy.

Clinical outcomes

The mortality rates of the patients in the Normal group, Moderate group and RI group were 1.72 %, 3.7 %, and 7.37 %, respectively, during hospitalization. Patients in the RI group had a significantly higher mortality rate compared with Normal group during hospitalization ($p = 0.045$). There were no significant differences in RMI, TVR, stroke and bleeding between the three groups. In-hospital MACE developed more frequently in the patients in the RI group compared with Normal group ($p = 0.022$). But there was no significant difference in the incidence of CIN (Table 2).

A similar trend was observed during 1 year of follow up after hospital discharge. Patients in the RI group had a significantly higher mortality rate compared with those in the Normal group (16.84 % v.s.4.29 %, $p < 0.001$), and a significantly higher MACE rate compared with the other two groups ($p < 0.001$) (Table 2).

During 2 years of follow up, patients in the RI group had a significantly higher mortality rate compared with the other two groups (24.21 % v.s. 6.87 % and 10.19 %, $p < 0.001$). There were no significant differences in recurrent myocardial infarction (RMI), target vessel revascularization (TVR), stroke and bleeding between the three groups. Compared with the RI group respectively, the Moderate group and the Normal group had higher MACE rates

Table 1 Baseline characteristics

	Normal group (n = 233)	Moderate group (n = 108)	RI group (n = 95)	χ^2 /F	p value
Age (years)	61.11 ± 8.42	64.08 ± 6.91[a]	75.57 ± 7.53[ab]	114.59	<0.001
BMI (kg/m^2)	24.51 ± 4.49	24.03 ± 3.98	23.95 ± 5.08	0.721	0.486
Killip ≥ 2	21 (9.01)	10 (9.26)	20 (21.05)[ab]	10.297	0.006
HR (bpm)	71.58 ± 23.40	73.29 ± 19.17	78.05 ± 25.18	2.823	0.061
Current smoker (%)	96 (41.20)	47 (43.52)	45 (47.37)	1.056	0.59
Diabetes (%)	69 (29.61)	41 (37.96)	46 (48.42)[a]	10.686	0.005
Hypertention (%)	75 (32.19)	48 (44.44)	50 (52.63)[a]	13.145	0.001
Hyperlipidemia (%)	79 (33.91)	36 (33.33)	29 (30.53)	0.799	0.671
Previous MI (%)	15 (6.44)	9 (8.33)	2 (2.11)	3.697	0.157
Previous PCI (%)	11 (4.72)	5 (4.63)	4 (4.21)	0.078	1
Previous stroke	2 (0. 86)	3 (2.78)	4 (4.21)	4.336	0.087
Peripheral vasculardisease (%)	3 (1.29)	1 (0.95)	1 (1.05)	0.261	1
Anterior and/or Lateral wall (%)	113 (57.08)	45 (41.67)	53 (55.79)	4.039	0.133
Inferior and/or Posterior wall	105 (45.06)	60 (55.56)	40 (42.11)	4.437	0.109
Maximum ST segment elevation (mm)	3.16 ± 1.27	2.95 ± 1.08	3.11 ± 1.33	1.072	0.345
Q wave	96 (41.20)	38 (35.19)	41 (42.11)	1.573	0.455
Symptom to door time (min)					
Median (25–75th)	189.46 (130.51–392.26)	170.13 (110.50–337.12)	180.11 (104.39–387.25)	0.978	0.613
Door to balloon time (min)					
Median (25–75th)	123.42 (91.35–210.92)	135.56 (80.49–198.55)	142.6 (98.53–228.11)	3.071	0.215
Door to needle time (min)					
Median (25–75th)	58.21 (28.20–110.83)	50.55 (31.02–126.02)	63.48 (32.01–130.44)	4.335	0.114
Left ventricular ejection fraction (%)	50.11 ± 13.60	48.92 ± 14.02	44.38 ± 13.05[ab]	6.051	0.003
IABP use	3 (1.29)	5 (4.63)	1 (1.05)	3.882	0.143
Successful PCI	166 (71.24)	73 (67.59)	57 (60.00)	3.92	0.141
Successful thrombolysis	40 (17.17)	21 (19.44)	18 (18.95)	0.314	0.855
Serum creatinine (mmol/l)	78.12 ± 31.13	85.47 ± 44.90	116.67 ± 59.01[ab]	28.612	<0.001
Peak troponin (ng/ml)	31.06 ± 16.28	30.19 ± 18.73	45.33 ± 15.26[ab]	28.253	<0.001
Hospitalization days	8.53 ± 4.78	8.36 ± 5.11	12.05 ± 5.74[ab]	18.401	<0.001

BMI body mass index, HR heart rate, MI myocardial infarction, PCI percutaneous coronary intervention, IABP intra-aortic balloon pump
[a] compared to Group A, p < 0.05
[b] compared to Group B, p < 0.05

(36.11 % v.s. 22.32 %, 52.63 % v.s. 22.32 %, p < 0.001) (Table 2).

During 2 years of follow-up, there were 1 case of moderate bleeding and 4 cases of minor bleeding in the RI group. There were 3 cases of minor bleeding in the other two groups, respectively.

Risk factors of 2 year mortality

Variables were analyzed by univariate analysis for significant factors for 2 year mortality and are presented in Table 3, this suggested that eGFR of less than 90 ml/min/1.73 m^2, may be a predictor of 2 year mortality as both 60–90 ml/mim/ m^2 eGFR and

eGFR <60 ml/min/1.73 m^2 were significant (both p > 0.001). Age ≥75 years was another significant factor (p = 0.049) as well as hypertension (p = 0.013), Killip class ≥2 (p = 0.023), and EF <40 (p = 0.025). The Kaplan–Meier survival curves are depicted in Fig. 2. The survival rate of the RI group was significantly lower than in the other two groups (log-rank test, p < 0.001).

Multivariate analysis then identified eGFR <90 ml/min/1.73 m^2 and age ≥75 years as independent predictors of mortality at 2 years. In detail these were eGFR 60–90 ml/min/1.73 m^2 with HR 2.081, 95%CI 1.250–2.842, p < 0.001; eGFR <60 ml/min/1.73 m^2 with HR 3.872, 95%CI

Table 2 Outcomes of patients according to eGFR group

	Normal group (n = 233)	Moderate group (n = 108)	RI group (n = 95)	χ^2	p value
In hospital					
MACE	7 (3.00)	6 (5.56)	10 (10.53)[a]	7.664	0.022
death	4 (1.72)	4 (3.70)	7 (7.37)[a]	6.127	0.045
Recurrent MI	2 (0.86)	1 (0.93)	1 (1.05)	0.472	1
TVR	0	1 (0.93)	1 (1.05)	2.941	0.216
Stroke	0	0	0		NS
Bleeding	1 (0.43)	0	1 (1.05)	1.403	0.45
CIN	0	1 (0.93)	2 (2.11)	4.383	0.06
At 1-year follow-up					
MACE	35 (15.02)	24 (22.22)	36 (37.89)[ab]	20.734	<0.001
death	10 (4.29)	8 (7.41)	16 (16.84)[a]	14.814	<0.001
Recurrent MI	9 (3.86)	4 (3.70)	3 (3.16)	0.117	1
TVR	12 (5.15)	9 (8.33)	12 (12.63)	5.519	0.063
Stroke	1 (0.43)	2 (1.85)	1 (1.05)	2.02	0.424
Bleeding	3 (1.29)	1 (0.93)	4 (4.21)	3.244	0.173
At 2-year follow-up					
MACE	52 (22.32)	39 (36.11)[a]	50 (52.63)[a]	29.275	<0.001
death	16 (6.87)	11 (10.19)	23 (24.21)[ab]	20.227	<0.001
Recurrent MI	13 (5.58)	10 (9.26)	6 (6.32)	1.631	0.442
TVR	17 (7.30)	12 (11.11)	13 (13.68)	3.524	0.172
Stroke	3 (1.29)	3 (2.78)	3 (3.16)	1.919	0.391
Bleeding	3 (1.29)	3 (2.78)	5 (5.26)	4.275	0.109

eGFR estimated glomerular filtration rate, MI myocardial infarction, TVR target vessel revascularization, MACE major adverse cardiac events
[a]compared to Normal group, $p < 0.05$
[b]compared to Moderate group, $p < 0.05$

Table 3 Univariate and multivariate analysis for prediction of 2-year mortality

	Univariate			Multivariate		
	HR	95%CI	p value	HR	95%CI	p value
eGFR ml/min/1.73 m^2						
≥ 90	1			1		
60–90	2.911	1.295–3.731	<0.001*	2.081	1.250–2.842	<0.001*
< 60	5.043	1.585–8.960	<0.001*	3.872	2.004–6.131	<0.001*
Age ≥75	1.368	1.023–1.909	0.049*	1.461	1.011–1.952	0.024*
Diabetes	1.332	0.727–1.936	0.251			
Hypertension	1.241	1.032–1.453	0.013*	1.191	0.904–1.395	0.114
Hyperlipidemia	0.927	0.544–1.147	0.690			
Killip ≥ 2	1.593	1.032–2.301	0.023*	1.131	0.781–1.893	0.586
EF < 40 %	1.227	1.012–1.447	0.025*	0.905	0.451–1.060	0.647

CI confidence interval, eGFR estimated glomerular filtration rate, EF ejection fraction, HR hazard ratio
*$p < 0.05$

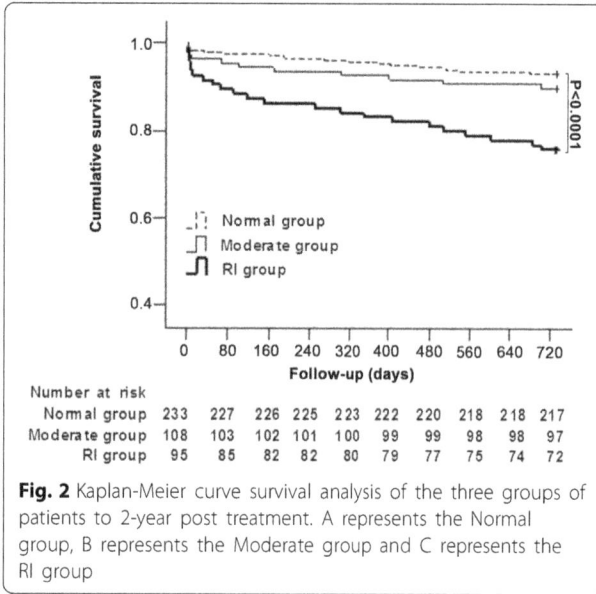

Fig. 2 Kaplan-Meier curve survival analysis of the three groups of patients to 2-year post treatment. A represents the Normal group, B represents the Moderate group and C represents the RI group

2.004–6.131, $p < 0.001$; age ≥ 75 with HR 1.461, 95%CI 1.011–1.952, $p = 0.024$.

Risk factors for in hospital mortality

All variables were also included into univariate analysis to investigate the independent predictors for in hospital mortality. The independent predictors of mortality in hospital were eGFR <60 ml/min/1.73 m^2 and Killip ≥ 2 (Table 4). Further analysis of the significant factors by multiple cox proportional hazard modeling identified independent predictors of mortality. This showed that the independent predictors of hospital mortality were eGFR <60 ml/min/1.73 m^2 [HR 1.832, 95 % CI 1.017–3.091, $p = 0.033$] and Killip ≥ 2 [HR 1.340, 95 % CI 1.012–1.647, $p = 0.018$].

Discussion

The aim of this study was to investigate the effect of RI on the mortality of female rural patients with STEMI. We demonstrated that the in hospitalization and 2-year mortality in the RI group (<60 ml/min/1.73 m^2) were significantly higher than in the other two groups. And RI (eGFR <60 ml/min/1.73 m^2) was an independent predictor of in hospital and 2-year mortality in the female STEMI patients after emergency reperfusion therapy. Compared with the Normal group, there was a 1.8-fold higher risk of death during hospitalization, and 3.9-fold higher risk of 2-year mortality. In the Moderate group (60–89 ml/min/1.73 m^2), there was a 2.1-fold higher risk of 2-year mortality. We found a decreased eGFR was associated with a higher risk of death. Thus, RI was associated with higher rates of death. The most important finding of our study is that the inclusion of RI in the risk model improves the risk in female patients with STEMI in rural areas. We demonstrated hospitalization mortality in the RI group was 7.37 %. Another reported study showed a similar mortality rate of 7.69 % [25]. It has also previously been confirmed that RI is an independent risk factor for poor prognosis in both the short and long term for female STEMI patients [26].

Renal dysfunction is an independent risk factor for death in patients with STEMI [27]. And patients with renal dysfunction have been shown to have a 6 to 11-fold higher in-hospital mortality rate compared to patients with normal renal function [8]. These patients more commonly developed low left ventricular ejection fraction, higher Killip class, cardiogenic shock, hemodynamic instability or malignant arrhythmia during admission [28]. Previous studies have also found that the risk of MACEs and cardiac death at both

Table 4 Univariate and multivariate analysis for prediction of in hospital mortality

	Univariate			Multivariate		
	HR	95%CI	p value	HR	95%CI	p value
eGFR ml/min/1.73 m^2						
≥ 90	1			1		
60–90	0.942	0.653–1.131	0.670	0.865	0.586–1.390	0.220
< 60	2.655	1.147–4.238	0.003*	1.832	1.017–3.091	0.033*
Age ≥75	0.815	0.462–1.536	0.504			
Diabetes	0.893	0.601–1.072	0.443			
Hypertension	0.747	0.352–1.167	0.340			
Hyperlipidemia	0.86	0.317–1.053	0.622			
Killip ≥ 2	1.446	1.009–2.090	0.047*	1.34	1.012–1.647	0.018*
EF < 40 %	0.871	0.592–1.017	0.317			

CI confidence interval, *eGFR* estimated glomerular filtration rate, *EF* ejection fraction, *HR* hazard ratio

*$p < 0.05$

1 month and 1 year increased with lower eGFR [5]. Thus, the results of our study are in agreement with the previous research.

Comparison between the three groups showed that there were higher proportions of Killip class ≥ 2, longer hospital stay, low LVEF values, high serum creatinine levels and cTnI peak in the RI group. The patients had larger myocardial infarction area and worse heart function. These differences may be related to the high mortality in the RI group. The Killip class is a useful prognostic tool for predicting in hospital mortality [29], and our results support this as the ≥ class 2 was also a predictive factor for in hospital mortality by multivariate analysis. Another recent study on RI in STEMI also found a higher Killip class was found with RI, and those patients also showed increased mortality with RI [30]. That study identified that RI patients were more likely to be female as well as older, and more likely to have diabetes mellitus, and hypertension [30]. Our study also identified age, diabetes and hypertension as likely to be higher in the RI group. Increased Killip score and lower LVEF were also significant in RI patients in a study evaluating the in-hospital outcome of patients with acute STEMI [31]. The mean LVEF was also decreased in the RI patients in our study. In terms of the 2-year mortality risk factors the RI group was found to be at much higher risk than the other two groups in this study and the only other predictive factor was age ≥75 years. That was possibly an expected result [32].

We found there were no long-term standardized medication regimens after hospital discharge in the RI group. And dual antiplatelet therapy was used less in hospital in this group. Underuse of antiplatelet therapy, ACE inhibitors, β-blockers and statins might also be related to a reduced survival rate in patients with renal insufficiency as discontinuation of cardiac medication is itself associated with increased risk of mortality [33]. This may be another factor that is related to the high mortality in the RI group.

Renal dysfunction was associated with a 3 fold increased odds of discontinuation of antiplatelet drugs in patients with PCI [34]. Reasons for shorter duration of antiplatelet therapy and discontinuation observed in these studies and ours may include bleeding events, scheduled invasive procedures, psychiatric drug use, unemployment, patient choice and non-adherence and other medical events not specified including earlier mortality. It had been reported AMI patients with decreased GFR may receive less aggressive evidence-based therapies as those normal patients [35].

This study has some limitations as it was a prospective multicenter study with a limited sample size because of the limited number of rural patients. In the RI group the patients were not grouped further to eGFR 30–60 ml/min/1.73 m^2 and eGFR <30 ml/min/1.73 m^2 to provide information on the severity of RI. We also were unable to provide a mean value of eGFR for the groups in this study because some of the raw data was lost, so we had to rely on the grouping ranges for our analysis. We did not include a control group without cardiac disease, to investigate whether these results relating to RI and mortality would be similar in a group of patients without STEMI. In addition, we did not address the question of a relationship between cardiac disease and kidney disease in these patients. Further analysis of more pathophysiological factors such as biomarkers for cardiac damage for example troponin would provide important information on the relationship between cardiac and kidney diseases.

Conclusions

In this real-world prospective multicenter study we found among female rural patients with STEMI after thrombolytic therapy or primary PCI therapy that RI was an independent risk factor for in-hospital and long-term mortality and was associated with poor prognosis. RI could be one of the better indices for clinical risk stratification.

Appendix 1
Details of medication

There were no significant difference in the administration of aspirin, ACEI/ARB, statins, beta -blockers, LWMH and traditional Chinese medicine between the three groups. But clopidogrel and dual antiplatelet therapy were lower in the RI group compared with the Normal group during hospitalization. The patients were followed up at 2 year. We found that clopidogrel, dual antiplatelet therapy, ACEI/ARB, statins, b-blocker were less used,but traditional Chinese medicine were more used in the RI group during follow-up (Appendix 1).

Abbreviations
ACE: angiotensin-converting enzyme; ARB: angiotensin receptor antagonist; BMI: body mass index; CI: confidence intervals; CIN: contrast-induced nephropathy; CKD-EPI: chronic kidney disease epidemiology collaboration; CKMB: creatine kinase MB; Ctni: cardiac troponin I; ECG: electrocardiogram; EF: ejection fraction; eGFR: estimated glomerular filtration rate; GUSTO: global use of strategies to open occluded coronary arteries; HDL: high-density lipoprotein; HR: hazard ratio; IQR: interquartile range; KDIGO: kidney disease: improving global outcomes; LDL: low-density lipoprotein; MACE: major adverse cardiac events; MDRD: modification of diet in renal disease; PCI: percutaneous coronary intervention; RI: renal insufficiency; RMI: recurrent myocardial infarction; Scr: serum creatinine; SD: standard deviation; STEMI: ST-segment elevation acute myocardial infarction; TIMI: thrombolysis in myocardial infarction; TVR: target vessel revascularization; WBC: white blood cell.

Table 5 Medication use

	Normal group (n = 233)	Moderate group (n = 108)	RI group (n = 95)
In hospital			
Aspirin	233	107	95
Clopidogrel	233	108	92
dual antiplatelet therapy	233	107	92
ACEI/ARB	221	101	83
Statins	205	89	77
Beta blockers	209	98	79
Low molecular heparin	230	107	91
Traditional Chinese medicine	157	61	59
At 2-year follow-up			
Aspirin	176	84	55
Clopidogrel	61	29	8
dual antiplatelet therapy	60	29	8
ACEI/ARB	63	3	7
Statins	25	14	9
Beta blockers	155	58	44
Traditional Chinese medicine	81	41	50

Competing interests
The authors declare that they have no competing interests.

Authors' contributions
YG participated in literature search, study design, data collection, data analysis, data interpretation and wrote the manuscript. DMJ, BZ, YJS, LNR and DDF participated in clinical examination and laboratory analysis. GXQ conceived of the study, and participated in its design and coordination and provided the critical revision. All authors read and approved the final manuscript.

Acknowledgements
None.

Funding
None.

Author details
[1]Department of Cardiology, First Affiliated Hospital of China Medical University, Shenyang, Liaoning 110001, China. [2]Department of Cardiology, Dandong Center Hospital, Dandong, Liaoning 118000, China. [3]Department of Cardiology, First Affiliated Hospital, Dalian Medical University, Dalian, Liaoning 116011, China. [4]Department of Geriatric Cardiology, First Affiliated Hospital of China Medical University, Shenyang, Liaoning 110001, China.

References
1. Ojo A. Addressing the global burden of chronic kidney disease through clinical and translational research. Trans Am Clin Climatol Assoc. 2014;125: 229–43. discussion 43–6.
2. Fox CS, Muntner P, Chen AY, Alexander KP, Roe MT, Cannon CP, et al. Use of evidence-based therapies in short-term outcomes of ST-segment elevation myocardial infarction and non-ST-segment elevation myocardial infarction in patients with chronic kidney disease: a report from the National Cardiovascular Data Acute Coronary Treatment and Intervention Outcomes Network registry. Circulation. 2010;121(3):357–65.
3. Task Force on the management of STseamiotESoC, Steg PG, James SK, Atar D, Badano LP, Blomstrom-Lundqvist C, et al. ESC Guidelines for the management of acute myocardial infarction in patients presenting with ST-segment elevation. Eur Heart J. 2012;33(20):2569–619.
4. Said S, Hernandez GT. The link between chronic kidney disease and cardiovascular disease. J Nephropathol. 2014;3(3):99–104.
5. Anavekar NS, McMurray JJ, Velazquez EJ, Solomon SD, Kober L, Rouleau JL, et al. Relation between renal dysfunction and cardiovascular outcomes after myocardial infarction. N Engl J Med. 2004;351(13):1285–95.
6. Masoudi FA, Plomondon ME, Magid DJ, Sales A, Rumsfeld JS. Renal insufficiency and mortality from acute coronary syndromes. Am Heart J. 2004;147(4):623–9.
7. Bae EH, Lim SY, Cho KH, Choi JS, Kim CS, Park JW, et al. GFR and cardiovascular outcomes after acute myocardial infarction: results from the Korea Acute Myocardial Infarction Registry. Am J Kidney Dis. 2012;59(6):795–802.
8. Kim JY, Jeong MH, Ahn YK, Moon JH, Chae SC, Hur SH, et al. Decreased glomerular filtration rate is an independent predictor of In-Hospital Mortality in patients with ST-segment elevation myocardial infarction undergoing Primary percutaneous coronary intervention. Korean Circ J. 2011;41(4):184–90.
9. Choi JH, Kim KL, Huh W, Kim B, Byun J, Suh W, et al. Decreased number and impaired angiogenic function of endothelial progenitor cells in patients with chronic renal failure. Arterioscler Thromb Vasc Biol. 2004;24(7):1246–52.
10. Shlipak MG, Heidenreich PA, Noguchi H, Chertow GM, Browner WS, McClellan MB. Association of renal insufficiency with treatment and outcomes after myocardial infarction in elderly patients. Ann Intern Med. 2002;137(7):555–62.
11. Napoli C, Casamassimi A, Crudele V, Infante T, Abbondanza C. Kidney and heart interactions during cardiorenal syndrome: a molecular and clinical pathogenic framework. Future Cardiol. 2011;7(4):485–97.
12. Gulati M, Shaw LJ, Bairey Merz CN. Myocardial ischemia in women: lessons from the NHLBI WISE study. Clin Cardiol. 2012;35(3):141–8.
13. Pancholy SB, Shantha GP, Patel T, Cheskin LJ. Sex differences in short-term and long-term all-cause mortality among patients with ST-segment elevation myocardial infarction treated by primary percutaneous intervention: a meta-analysis. JAMA Intern Med. 2014;174(11):1822–30.

14. D'Ascenzo F, Gonella A, Quadri G, Longo G, Biondi-Zoccai G, Moretti C, et al. Comparison of mortality rates in women versus men presenting with ST-segment elevation myocardial infarction. Am J Cardiol. 2011;107(5):651–4.

15. Zheng X, Dreyer RP, Hu S, Spatz ES, Masoudi FA, Spertus JA, et al. Age-specific gender differences in early mortality following ST-segment elevation myocardial infarction in China. Heart. 2014;101(5):349–55.

16. Jiang G, Wang D, Li W, Pan Y, Zheng W, Zhang H, et al. Coronary heart disease mortality in China: age, gender, and urban-rural gaps during epidemiological transition. Rev Panam Salud Publica. 2012;31(4):317–24.

17. Mehta RL, Kellum JA, Shah SV, Molitoris BA, Ronco C, Warnock DG, et al. Acute Kidney Injury Network: report of an initiative to improve outcomes in acute kidney injury. Crit Care. 2007;11(2):R31.

18. Levey AS, Stevens LA, Schmid CH, Zhang YL, Castro 3rd AF, Feldman HI, et al. A new equation to estimate glomerular filtration rate. Ann Intern Med. 2009; 150(9):604–12.

19. Kidney Disease: Improving Global Outcomes (KDIGO) Acute Kidney Injury Work Group. KDIGO Clinical Practice Guideline for Acute Kidney Injury. Kidney Int Suppl. 2012;2:1–138.

20. Levine GN, Bates ER, Blankenship JC, Bailey SR, Bittl JA, Cercek B, et al. 2011 ACCF/AHA/SCAI Guideline for Percutaneous Coronary Intervention: a report of the American College of Cardiology Foundation/American Heart Association Task Force on Practice Guidelines and the Society for Cardiovascular Angiography and Interventions. Circulation. 2011;124(23): e574–651.

21. Consultation WHOE. Appropriate body-mass index for Asian populations and its implications for policy and intervention strategies. Lancet. 2004; 363(9403):157–63.

22. Rihal CS, Textor SC, Grill DE, Berger PB, Ting HH, Best PJ, et al. Incidence and prognostic importance of acute renal failure after percutaneous coronary intervention. Circulation. 2002;105(19):2259–64.

23. An international randomized trial comparing four thrombolytic strategies for acute myocardial infarction. The GUSTO investigators. N Engl J Med. 1993; 329(10):673-82.

24. Barrett BJ, Parfrey PS. Clinical practice. Preventing nephropathy induced by contrast medium. N Engl J Med. 2006;354(4):379–86.

25. Liu Y, Gao L, Xue Q, Yan M, Chen P, Wang Y, et al. Impact of renal dysfunction on long-term outcomes of elderly patients with acute coronary syndrome: a longitudinal, prospective observational study. BMC Nephrol. 2014;15:78.

26. Go AS, Chertow GM, Fan D, McCulloch CE, Hsu CY. Chronic kidney disease and the risks of death, cardiovascular events, and hospitalization. N Engl J Med. 2004;351(13):1296–305.

27. Rodrigues FB, Bruetto RG, Torres US, Otaviano AP, Zanetta DM, Burdmann EA. Effect of kidney disease on acute coronary syndrome. Clin J Am Soc Nephrol. 2010;5(8):1530–6.

28. Parikh CR, Coca SG, Wang Y, Masoudi FA, Krumholz HM. Long-term prognosis of acute kidney injury after acute myocardial infarction. Arch Intern Med. 2008;168(9):987–95.

29. de Mello BH, Oliveira GB, Ramos RF, Lopes BB, Barros CB, Carvalho Ede O, et al. Validation of the Killip-Kimball classification and late mortality after acute myocardial infarction. Arq Bras Cardiol. 2014;103(2):107–17.

30. Sabroe JE, Thayssen P, Antonsen L, Hougaard M, Hansen KN, Jensen LO. Impact of renal insufficiency on mortality in patients with ST-segment elevation myocardial infarction treated with primary percutaneous coronary intervention. BMC Cardiovasc Disord. 2014;14:15.

31. Pasha K, Ali MA, Habib MA, Debnath RC, Islam MN. In-hospital outcome of patients with acute STEMI with impaired renal function. Mymensingh Med J. 2011;20(3):425–30.

32. Newell MC, Henry JT, Henry TD, Duval S, Browning JA, Christiansen EC, et al. Impact of age on treatment and outcomes in ST-elevation myocardial infarction. Am Heart J. 2011;161(4):664–72.

33. Ivers NM, Schwalm JD, Grimshaw JM, Witteman H, Taljaard M, Zwarenstein M, et al. Delayed educational reminders for long-term medication adherence in ST-elevation myocardial infarction (DERLA-STEMI): protocol for a pragmatic, cluster-randomized controlled trial. Implement Sci. 2012;7:54.

34. Ferreira-Gonzalez I, Marsal JR, Ribera A, Permanyer-Miralda G, Garcia-Del Blanco B, Marti G, et al. Background, incidence, and predictors of antiplatelet therapy discontinuation during the first year after drug-eluting stent implantation. Circulation. 2010;122(10):1017–25.

14

Lack of "obesity paradox" in patients presenting with ST-segment elevation myocardial infarction including cardiogenic shock

Ibrahim Akin[1,8*†], Henrik Schneider[2†], Christoph A. Nienaber[3], Werner Jung[4], Mike Lübke[4], Andreas Rillig[5], Uzair Ansari[1], Nina Wunderlich[6] and Ralf Birkemeyer[7]

Abstract

Background: Studies have associated obesity with better outcomes in comparison to non-obese patients after elective and emergency coronary revascularization. However, these findings might have been influenced by patient selection. Therefore we thought to look into the obesity paradox in a consecutive network STEMI population.

Methods: The database of two German myocardial infarction network registries were combined and data from a total of 890 consecutive patients admitted and treated for acute STEMI including cardiogenic shock and cardiopulmonary resuscitation according to standardized protocols were analyzed. Patients were categorized in normal weight ($\leq$24.9 kg/m^2), overweight (25-30 kg/m^2) and obese (>30 kg/m^2) according to BMI.

Results: Baseline clinical parameters revealed a higher comorbidity index for overweight and obese patients; 1-year follow-up comparison between varying groups revealed similar rates of all-cause death (9.1 % vs. 8.3 % vs. 6.2 %; p = 0.50), major adverse cardiac and cerebrovascular [MACCE (15.1 % vs. 13.4 % vs. 10.2 %; p = 0.53)] and target vessel revascularization in survivors [TVR (7.0 % vs. 5.0 % vs. 4.0 %; p = 0.47)] with normal weight when compared to overweight or obese patients. These results persisted after risk-adjustment for heterogeneous baseline characteristics of groups. An analysis of patients suffering from cardiogenic shock showed no impact of BMI on clinical endpoints.

Conclusion: Our data from two network systems in Germany revealed no evidence of an "obesity paradox"in an all-comer STEMI population including patients with cardiogenic shock.

Keywords: Coronary stent, Obesity paradox, Mortality, Cardiogenic shock

Background

Obesity and associated disorders like hypertension, hyperlipidemia and diabetes are linked to increased morbidity and mortality among a Western population [1, 2]. This patient cohort is also at greater risk to develop coronary artery disease [2]. Population-based registry data revealed that 43 % and 24 % of coronary revascularizations were carried out in overweight and obese patients, respectively

[3]. However, despite evidence of a positive correlation between obesity and increased cardiovascular morbidity, previous studies have described an "obesity paradox" in patients undergoing coronary revascularization either by interventional (PCI) or surgical (CABG) strategies, reporting a protective effect of obesity in terms of postoperative mortality. The first description of this phenomenon was done by Gruberg et al. 12 years ago [4]. Although the impact of obesity on clinical outcomes after elective PCI has been subsequently investigated in several studies, the issue remains controversial. Thus, there is insufficient data in unselected populations suffering from acute coronary syndrome (ACS), which is additionally associated with a complex thrombogenic and proinflammatory status [5–10]. Our current analysis compares clinical outcomes after PCI

* Correspondence: Ibrahim.akin@med.uni-rostock.de
†Equal contributors
[1]Universitätsmedizin Mannheim, Mannheim, Germany
[8]Medical Faculty Mannheim, University Heidelberg, Theodor-Kutzer Ufer 1-3, 68167 Mannheim, Germany
Full list of author information is available at the end of the article

between consecutive normal weight, overweight and obese patients diagnosed with an ST-segment elevation myocardial infarction (STEMI) including patients with cardiogenic shock.

Methods

Network structures

Both myocardial infarction networks, which were the first networks in Germany, aim at coronary reperfusion therapy with primary PCI as the treatment prerogative for all presumed STEMI patients according to a uniform, regional treatment protocol patterned for a 24 h/7days week in a single interventional centre.

"Network A", located in northeastern Germany constituted a mixed urban and rural catchment area with an approximate population of 415,000 inhabitants and was spread across a 60 km radius from its centre. At the time of collecting data, there were eight hospitals in the network area, with a lone high-volume interventional facility functioning as a 24 h/7days primary PCI service point. Emergency Medical Services (EMS) transferred suspected STEMI patients to the emergency department of the nearest hospital without prior announcement. Upon arrival of the patient, local emergency departments alarmed the interventional cardiology team and organized the direct transfer of the patient to the cathlab.

"Network B", located in southwestern Germany, constituted a rural catchment area with approximately 350,000 inhabitants and was spread across a 35 km radius from its centre. At the time of data collection there were six hospitals in this network area, with a lone high-volume interventional facility functioning as a 24 h/7days primary PCI service point.

Trained personnel at all collection points supported both Network structures. All STEMI patients, irrespective of cardiogenic shock or preceding cardiopulmonary resuscitation were intended for primary PCI through femoral access.

Primary PCI protocol

All provisionally diagnosed STEMI patients were treated with 250–500 mg Aspirin intravenously and received a weight adjusted unfractionated dose of Heparin (70 IU/kg) by EMS. The loading dose of clopidogrel (600 mg) was mostly administered before the PCI. In few cases, this was administered immediately after the procedure.

When treating patients in shock, interventional cardiologists were encouraged to treat all presumed hemodynamically relevant non-target lesions. Thrombectomy, periprocedural GPIIb/IIIa blockers (predominantly abciximab) and drug-eluting stents (DES) were utilized at the discretion of the operator. The full anticoagulant dosing of heparin was stopped after PCI, unless there was a high risk of thromboembolism (eg. atrial fibrillation or mechanical heart valves).

Study population

Consecutive STEMI patients admitted for primary PCI were prospectively included in their respective registries, in network A from 2001 to 2003 and in network B from 2005 to 2007.

Definitions

These were based on parameters defined by the World Health Organization (WHO) and the National Heart, Lung and Blood Institute. The patient population was classified into normal weight (body mass index [BMI] 18.5 - 24.9 kg/m^2), overweight (BMI 25–30 kg/m^2) and obese group (>30 kg/m^2) [11, 12]. STEMI was diagnosed by the presence of chest pain lasting > 20 min and of significant ST-segment elevation (≥ 0.1 mV in two adjacent leads if leads I-III, aVF, aVL, V4-V6, and ≥ 0.2 mV in leads V1-V3), as in the first recorded electrocardiogram (ECG). Patients with persistent angina and presumably new left bundle branch block (LBBB) were included in the registry if myocardial infarction (MI) was subsequently confirmed. Cardiogenic shock was defined clinically by the presence of hypotension (systolic blood pressure < 90 mmHg for >30 min or need for vasopressors to maintain systolic blood pressure >90 mmHg) and tachycardia (heart rate >90 beats/min) with evidence of end-organ hypoperfusion [13]. Thrombolysis In Myocardial Infarction (TIMI) flow grades were assessed in the culprit vessel before and after the PCI procedure. Major bleeding was defined according to the TIMI major bleeding definition as intracerebral bleeding, bleeding requiring surgical intervention, bleeding requiring transfusion or loss of more than 5 g/% haemoglobin [14]. As indicators of guideline adherent therapy we analyzed pre- and in-hospital delays, procedural success of primary PCI, stent use, peri-interventional antiplatelet management, medication at discharge and medication at 12 months [15]. Procedural success was defined as residual stenosis < 30 % of the culprit lesion. For outcomes we analyzed mortality, re-infarction rate, target lesion revascularization (TLR) and target vessel revascularization (TVR) up to 12 months. TVR included repeat procedures, either PCI or CABG, in the target vessel. The composite of these events was defined as the major adverse cardiac and cerebrovascular events (MACCE) including death, MI, TVR and stroke. Patients were discouraged to undergo routine angiography for follow-up; therefore, all re-interventions can be counted as clinically driven. Stent thrombosis (ST) was classified according to the definition proposed by the Academic Research Consortium (ARC) [16].

Data collection and follow-up

All patients diagnosed with STEMI were cataloged in a dedicated database. The procedure for follow-up usually included telephone interviews and subject-based questionnaires at the time frame of 6 and 12 months. A descriptive follow-up concerning mortality was obtained from state registries. The local ethics committees in Rostock (Medical Faculty of University Rostock, Germany) and Freiburg (Albert-Ludwigs-University Freiburg, Germany) approved the registries. All patients included in this study gave pre-emptive informed consent for the extension of our routine follow-up.

Statistical methods

Data was analyzed according to established standards of descriptive statistics. Categorical variables were compared by chi^2 test. Continuous variables were reported as mean ± standard deviation or median with interquartile ranges. For comparisons, the t test, the two-tailed Mann–Whitney U test and ANOVA model was used where appropriate. Odds ratios (OR) and 95 % confidence intervals (CI) were provided where appropriate. A p value of less than 0.05 was considered significant. A multivariate logistic regression analysis (stepwise backward model) including sex, age, diabetes, hypertension, smoking, renal failure, cardiogenic shock, resuscitation, stent type and impaired ejection fraction (<45 %) at discharge with normal weight as a fixed parameter was performed to determine independent factors predicting 12-month mortality and MACCE. The final logistic model for 12-month mortality with the independent variables age, diabetes and impaired ejection fraction (<45 %) at discharge showed a good predictive value (C-statistic = 0.84), and good calibration characteristics using the Hosmer-Lemeshow test (p = 0.90). Mortality and MACE at 12 months was adjusted for the above-mentioned variables. One-year survival was demonstrated by Kaplan-Meier curves and compared by log-rank test.

Results

Baseline characteristics and procedural outcomes

Our analysis is based on the 890 patients diagnosed with STEMI between 2001 and 2007 in this prospective study at the two participating centers. Patients were categorized as normal weight (n = 263), overweight (n = 432) and obese (n = 195) with a mean BMI of 23.2 ± 1.72 kg/m^2 27.2 ± 1.32 kg/m^2, and 32.9 ± 2.83 kg/m^2, respectively. Obese patients were younger than overweight and normal weight patients (65.7 ± 12.87 vs. 62.8 ± 11.70 vs. $60.4 \pm$

11.67; p < 0.0001) and had a higher comorbidity index with higher rates of diabetes (13.3 % vs. 19.5 % vs. 27.2 %; p < 0.006), and arterial hypertension (48.7 % vs. 63.9 % vs. 73.9 %; p < 0.0001), but with lower rates of impaired renal function (29.3 % vs. 18.7 % vs. 11.5 %; p < 0.0001) (Table 1).

Data pertaining to pre-hospital and intra-hospital time intervals were also not different between groups. However we observed that normal weight and overweight patients suffered more often from cardiogenic shock (9.9 % vs. 11.1 % vs. 5.1 %; p = 0.02) and had a higher calculated Grace Score (100.6 ± 16.18 vs. 87.2 ± 12.56 vs. 74.2 ± 10.14; p = 0.02) (Table 2).

Approximately half of all patients included in this study had a multivessel coronary artery disease with no significant difference in the distribution of dual-vessel, triple-vessel and left-main vessel disease as well as treated target vessel (Table 2). Primary PCI, being performed through femoral access in all patients, with implantation of nearly 1.4 ± 0.9 stents per patient was carried out as a single

Table 1 Baseline demographics of patients presenting with STEMI

	BMI			p Trend
	≤24.9	25-30	>30	
Patients (n)	263	432	195	<0.0001
Mean BMI, kg/m^2 (SD)	23.2 (1.7)	27.2 (1.3)	32.9 (2.8)	0.11
Male (%)	73.0	79.9	75.9	
Age (SD), y	65.7 (12.8)	62.8 (11.7)	60.4 (11.7)	<0.006
Diabetes (%)				0.59
NIDDM	13.3	19.3	26.7	
IDDM	0	0.2	0.5	
Hypercholesterinemia (%)	45.2	45.8	49.7	<0.0001
Renal insufficiency (%)	29.3	18.7	11.5	<0.0001
Hypertension (%)	48.7	63.9	73.9	<0.0001
Smoking (%)				
Current	42.9	37.5	46.7	0.48
Previous myocardial infarction (%)	11.0	9.5	7.7	0.72
Previous PCI (%)	9.1	7.4	7.7	0.90
Previous CABG (%)	1.5	1.9	2.1	0.92
Previous stroke (%)	4.6	3.9	4.1	
Ejection fraction				0.88
>55 % (%)	32.5	30.7	36.1	
45-55 % (%)	33.5	37.9	36.2	
30-44 % (%)	28.4	25.8	22.0	
<30 % (%)	5.6	5.6	5.7	

Legend
BMI Body mass index, CAD Coronary artery disease, PCI Percutaneous coronary intervention, NIDDM Non-insulin dependent diabetes mellitus, IDDM Insulin-dependent diabetes mellitus, CABG Coronary artery bypass grafting

Table 2 Descriptive morphology of coronary artery disease in patients stratified according to body weight

	BMI			p Trend
	≤24.9	25-30	>30	
Vessel Disease (%)				
Single	47.1	48.0	50.5	0.78
Dual	28.8	28.4	29.4	
Triple	22.6	21.5	19.6	
Left main stenosis (%)	2.5	3.0	1.0	
Target vessel (%)				
LAD	48.1	44.0	47.2	0.55
LCX	16.5	16.7	11.4	
RCA	34.6	37.4	40.4	
LMCA	0.8	1.9	0.5	
Bypass graft	0	0	0.5	
TIMI-flow (%)				
0	62.0	55.8	65.6	0.65
1	8.2	8.4	8.3	
2	12.7	16.8	13.5	
3	17.1	19.0	12.6	
Grace score (%)	100.6 (87.6)	87.2 (77.6)	74.2 (53.8)	0.02
CPR (%)	9.1	8.1	5.1	0.25
Cardiogenic shock (%)	9.9	11.1	5.1	0.02
Fibrinolysis prior PCI (%)	1.1	1.2	2.6	0.35
Pain-to-door time, min (SD)	212.2 (164.0)	212.5 (154.6)	213.6 (165.2)	0.99
Door-to-lab time, min (SD)	30.2 (67.9)	27.9 (46.5)	26.0 (46.3)	0.73
Lab-to-balloon time, min (SD)	30.8 (15.21)	31.4 (16.5)	32.6 (15.6)	0.67

Legend
LAD Left anterior descending coronary artery, LCX Left circumflex coronary artery, RCA Right coronary artery, LMCA Left main coronary artery, TIMI Thrombolysis in myocardial infarction, CPR cardiopulmonary resuscitation

vessel PCI in more than 90 % of cases without any change in strategy between groups. Use of DES was predominant in the study population. Normal weight patients presented more often with smaller vessel diameter (Table 3). Although anatomical and procedural characteristics including periprocedural complications were comparable the use of GP IIb/IIIa was more frequent in obese patients (81.3 % versus 85.7 % versus 94.3 %; p = 0.01).

In-hospital follow-up

The overall in hospital mortality rate was 5.3 % in the normal weight, 4.4 % in the overweight, and 3.1 % in obese groups (p = 0.51). Similarly, rates of MI, stroke and bleeding complications as well as need for repeat urgent

revascularization and resuscitation was low with no differences between subsets (Table 4).

One-year follow-up

At one-year follow-up no significant differences were noted between groups with respect to the incidence of MACCE-free survival and TVR-free survival. Similarly, no differences were noted in the rates of overall death, MI, stroke, and definite ST (Table 4, Fig. 1). The use of antiplatelet and anticoagulation treatment was not different between groups.

Subsequent risk-adjustment and multivariate analysis revealed no impact of overweight and obesity on clinical events. Predictors for one-year mortality were the presence of diabetes (OR 2.79; 95 % CI 1.50-5.19), age (OR 1.10; 95 % CI 1.06-1.14) and impaired left ventricular ejection fraction defined as < 45 % (OR 3.82; 95 % CI 2.05-7.13) without any impact of increasing BMI (OR 1.03; 95 % CI 0.62-1.42). Similarly, predictors for MACCE at follow-up were increasing age (OR 1.03; 95 % CI 1.01-1.06), while the use of a DES had protective effects (OR 0.44; 95 % CI 0.24-0.82) without impact of BMI (OR 0.91; 95 % CI 0.63-1.31).

An exclusion of lean patients (BMI < 18.5 kg/m^2; n = 5) from the normal weight group did not change abovementioned intrahospital and follow-up results with similar event rates in all three groups.

Additionally, a separate analysis of patients suffering from cardiogenic shock (26 versus 48 versus 8) did not show any differences between groups with a mean intrahospital and one-year follow-up mortality rate of up to 26 % and 31 %, respectively.

Discussion

In Europe, the prevalence of obesity ranges from 4.0 to 36.5 % [17] and it is also well known that obesity acts as an independent cardiovascular risk factor for the development of coronary artery disease as well as general atherosclerosis and is associated with increased overall morbidity and mortality [18, 19]. There is evidence that this increased risk is mediated through obesity-related co-morbidities such as diabetes mellitus, hyperlipidemia, hypertension, increased insulin resistance, enhanced free fatty acid turnover, and promotion of systemic inflammation [20]. However, despite this correlation there is an assumption of an inverse correlation of obesity with mortality post PCI and less pronounced with a smaller need for repeat revascularisation. This has been described as the "obesity paradox" [10, 21]. An analysis of 9,633 patients being stratified in normal weight (n = 1,923), overweight (n = 4,813) and obese (n = 2,897) undergoing PCI revealed a higher incidence of major in-hospital complications, including cardiac death (1.0 % vs. 0.7 % vs.

Table 3 Procedural characteristics of patients receiving coronary intervention

	BMI			p Trend
	≤24.9	25-30	>30	
Primary PCI performed				
Single vessel PCI (%)	90.8	89.7	96.9	0.30
Multivessel PCI (%)	4.6	5.9	1.0	
Staged PCI (%)	23.2	21.8	24.7	
Stent details				
Number of implanted stents (SD)	1.4 (0.9)	1.4 (0.9)	1.5 (1.0)	0.82
Drug-eluting stents (%)	63.8	61.3	62.9	0.61
Diameter (mm)	3.0 (2.75-3.00)	3.0 (2.80-3.00)	3.0 (2.80-3.50)	0.030
Length (mm)	24.0 (20.0-35.0)	24.0 (20.0-38.0)	24.0 (22.0-36.0)	0.47
Postprocedural TIMI III (%)	84.1	82.3	82.3	0.29
Periprocedural complication (%)				
No-reflow	0	2.0	3.0	0.12
Complete AV-block	3.0	2.0	0	0.18
CPR	1.0	3.0	2.0	0.66
Stroke / TIA	1.0	0	0	0.74
Death	0	0	1.0	0.46
No complication during incex PCI	94.0	95.0	94.0	0.94
GP IIb/IIIA antagonist (%)	81.3	85.7	94.3	0.01

Legends

TIMI Thrombolysis in myocardial infarction, *GP* Glycoprotein, *PCI* percutaneous coronary intervention, *AV* atrioventricular node, *CPR* cardiopulmonary resuscitation, *TIA* transient cerebral ischemic attack

0.4 %; p = 0.001) in normal weight than overweight and obese patients despite similar periprocedural data. This was driven by overall mortality (10.6 % vs. 5.7 % vs. 4.9 %; p < 0.0001). Cardiac mortality (4.8 % versus 3.3 % versus 2.5 %; p < 0.0001) was also significantly higher in normal weight patients; whereas rates of MI and TVR were similar [10]. A large meta-analysis including 250,152 patients with established coronary artery disease and a mean follow-up of 3.8 years supported these findings with increased relative risk for overall mortality [RR 1.37 (95 % CI 1.32-1.43)], and cardiovascular mortality [RR 1.45 (1.16-1.81)] after revascularization in normal weight patients [22]. These results persisted even after adjustment for potential confounders, including age, arterial hypertension, diabetes, and left ventricular function. Another analysis on patients with established coronary artery disease undergoing medical, interventional or surgical treatment showed an "obesity paradox" after revascularisation irrespective of the chosen strategy. In the whole cohort patients who were overweight or obese were more likely to undergo revascularization procedures compared with those with normal BMI, despite having lower risk coronary anatomy [23]. The underlying mechanism of the "obesity paradox" is speculative. Obesity is associated with lower levels of plasma renin, epinephrine and high serum levels of low-density lipoproteins that bind circulating lipopolysaccharides [24]. Coronary vessel diameters, as confirmed in out-patient cohorts, have been shown to correlate with the increase in body weight; thus a smaller coronary artery size in normal weight and lean patients could theoretically influence periprocedural outcome [25]. The relationship between obesity and survival is characterized in the literature by a J- or U-shaped curve with increasing mortality in the very lean or severely obese group [26, 27]; however, after adjustment for smoking and concurrent illness, the relationship has always been linear [28, 29]. Contrasting with these findings our analysis of high-risk all-comers STEMI population including patients with cardiogenic shock does not support the presence of an "obesity paradox". Although there is a trend for better one-year survival in obese patients, this difference did not reach statistical significance. However, with access site being femoral there might be more bleeding events in obese patients, which could be avoided by radial access. Nevertheless, we think that the term "obesity paradox" might predominantly reflect different degrees of bias that cannot be completely corrected for by statistical means. Inherent bias in all obesity analyses result from the fact that overweight and obese

Table 4 In-hospital and 1-year clinical follow-up of patients receiving stent implantation

	In-hospital follow-up			
	BMI			p Trend
	≤24.9	25-30	>30	
Death (%)	5.3	4.4	3.1	0.51
Myocardial infarction (%)	0.6	0	2.0	0.09
Stroke (%)	1.0	0	0	0.45
Repeat urgent revascularization (%)				
PCI	1.0	0	2.0	0.31
CABG	1.0	0	0	0.35
CPR (%)	2.0	2.0	0	0.41
Complete AV-block (%)	1.0	0	1.0	0.25
Aneurysma spurium (%)	1.0	2.0	0	0.43
Bleeding (%)				
Major	1.9	3.4	1.0	0.37
Minor	6.9	7.3	3.1	0.33
Insignificant	17.6	14.2	13.3	0.56
Triple antiplatelet therapy (%)	14.5	9.4	10.6	0.27
One-year follow-up				
Death (%)	9.1	8.3	6.2	0.50
Myocardial infarction (%)	5.7	4.7	5.1	0.92
Stroke (%)	0	1.3	1.0	0.37
MACCE (%)	15.1	13.4	10.2	0.53
TVR (%)	7.0	5.0	4.0	0.47
Definite ST according ARC (%)	4.0	2.0	1.0	0.26
ASS	70.6	69.0	74.4	0.66
Clopidogrel	46.9	37.6	48.9	0.13
Oral anticoagulation (%)	4.2	8.5	5.6	0.24

Legends

PCI Percutaneous coronary intervention, *CABG* Coronary bypass graft, *CPR* Cardiopulmonary resuscitation, *MACCE* Major adverse cardiac and cerebrovascular event, *TVR* Target vessel revascularization, *ST* Stent thrombosis, *ARC* Academic Research Consortium

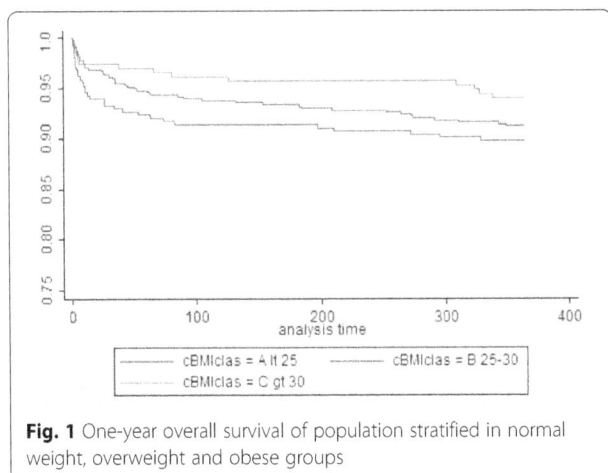

Fig. 1 One-year overall survival of population stratified in normal weight, overweight and obese groups

patients are usually younger and have larger culprit coronary vessel diameters than normal weight counterparts. In general younger patients have better clinical outcomes after acute MI regardless of reperfusion modality [30, 31]. Additionally, the presence of co-morbidities in obese and overweight younger patients usually leads to more aggressive therapy of cardiovascular risk factors likely to improve outcomes despite obesity [30, 31]. In a study of 130,139 patients hospitalized for coronary artery disease, higher BMI was associated with increased use of standard medical therapies such as aspirin, beta-blockers, renin-angiotensin inhibitors, and lipid lowering therapy, and an increased likelihood of undergoing diagnostic catheterization and revascularization [32, 33]. The all-comer design of our registry with the majority of patients having had no established coronary artery disease before the index STEMI reduces the influence of potential confounders. Especially promotion of primary PCI in shock patients and after resuscitation (significantly more frequent in obese and overweight patients) avoided a severe pre-selection bias. Another point of discussion with respect to the obesity paradox is that underweight patients may receive standard anti-coagulation doses that are too high for their body size, making them more prone to post-procedural bleeding complications, which could be ruled out in our cohort by weight-adjusted doses [3, 5]. In addition obesity was found to correlate with higher levels of factor VII, VIII, fibrinogen and plasminogen activator inhibitor-1, which were all associated with increased risk of thrombosis [34]. Accordingly prospective investigations have shown that overweight and obese patients were more likely to suffer from suboptimal platelet response to clopidogrel and aspirin treatment [35, 36]. In our cohort the use of GP IIb/IIIa inhibitor was high facing the nature of exclusively high-risk STEMI patients. Furthermore obesity as well as STEMI is considered a low-grade inflammatory state, as demonstrated by increased levels of the pro-inflammatory cytokines interleukin-6 and tumor necrosis factor-alpha, and acute phase proteins such as C-reactive protein [37]. This proinflammatory state may also directly and indirectly cause thrombosis by oxidative stress and endothelial dysfunction [38]. Such findings could not be confirmed in our real-world setting with similar rates of stent thrombosis in all subsets. Since low BMI may be a marker of severe systemic illness [18, 39], we defined in a separate analysis the normal-weight group from 18.5 kg/m^2-24.9 kg/m^2 and excluded 5 extremely underweight patients. However, this did not change the previous findings with lack of an "obesity paradox". A separate analysis of patients with cardiogenic shock, which is associated with a prothrombic situation and systemic inflammation, also revealed no statistical differences in clinical endpoints for all three groups.

Study limitation

The present study is an observational non-randomized study in which patients were stratified according to their BMI at index-PCI. Thus, we had no information on intended or unintended weight change, as well as on variables like physical inactivity and socioeconomic factors which may have influenced the results. BMI is not as well correlated to cardiovascular disease and death as waist circumference and waist-to-hip ratio, which, however, were unavailable in our registries. Another limitation of our analysis is the length of follow-up and small sample size that might result in lack of power for meaningful conclusions but is reliable enough for hypothesis generation. An extended follow-up may result in a cumulative detrimental effect of obesity and may even manifest as increased late mortality and confirm the negative correlation of obesity with clinical outcomes even in a setting of coronary revascularization. Additionally the access site during PCI was femoral. With use of radial access site, bleeding events might be reduced in overweight and obese patients, which might result in better clinical outcomes as bleeding events correlate with overall mortality and myocardial infarction rate.

Conclusions

Data from our all-comer network registry does not confirm the evidence of the "obesity paradox" during short and long term follow-up in patients suffering from STEMI including patients with cardiogenic shock. With respect to the limitations of available data prospective large-scale studies with long-term follow-up focusing on more reliable parameters reflecting the body fat are needed to reveal the phenomenon of the obesity paradox.

Abbreviations

ACS: Acute coronary syndrome; ARC: Academic Research Consortium; BMI: Body mass index; CABG: Coronary artery bypass surgery; CI: Confidence interval; DES: Drug eluting stent; ECG: Electrocardiogram; EMS: Emergency medical service; LBBB: Left bundle branch block; MACCE: Major adverse cardiac and cerebrovascular events; MI: Myocardial infarction; OR: Odds ratio; PCI: Percutaneous coronary intervention; ST: Stent thrombosis; STEMI: ST elevation myocardial infarction; TIMI: Thrombolysis In Myocardial Infarction; TLR: Target lesion revascularization; TVR: Target vessel revascularization; WHO: World Health Organisation.

Competing interests

The authors declare that they have no competing interests.

Authors' contributions

IA, HS, CAN, WJ, ML, AR, UA, NW, RB participate in treating the patients during intervention/ICU and acquisition of data. IA and RB wrote the manuscript. RB performed the statistical analyses. All authors read and approved the final manuscript.

Author details

[1]Universitätsmedizin Mannheim, Mannheim, Germany. [2]Universitätsklinikum Rostock und Hanseklinikum Wismar, .Rostock, .Germany. [3]Universitätsklinikum Rostock, .Rostock, .Germany. [4]Schwarzwald-Baar Klinikum Villingen-Schwenningen, .Villingen-Schwenningen, .Germany. [5]Asklepios Klinikum St. Georg Hamburg, .Hamburg, Germany. [6]Universitätsklinikum Rostock und Kardiovaskuläres Zentrum Darmstadt, Darmstadt, Germany. [7]Universitätsklinikum Rostock und Herzklinik Ulm, Ulm, Germany. [8]Medical Faculty Mannheim, University Heidelberg, Theodor-Kutzer Ufer 1-3, 68167 Mannheim, Germany.

References

1. Garrison RJ, Higgins MW, Kannel WB. Obesity and coronary heart disease. Curr Opin Lipidol. 1996;4:199–202.
2. Lakka HM, Laaksonen DE, Lakka TA, Nishkanen LK, Kumpusalo E, Tuomilehto J, et al. The metabolic syndrome and total and cardiovascular disease mortality in middle-aged men. JAMA. 2002;288:2709–16.
3. Minutello RM, Chou ET, Hong MK, Bergman G, Parikh M, Iacovone F, et al. Impact of body mass index on in-hospital outcomes following percutaneous coronary intervention (report from the New York State Angioplasty Registry). Am J Cardiol. 2004;93:1229–32.
4. Gruberg L, Weissman NJ, Waksman R, Fuch S, Deible R, Pinnow EE, et al. The impact of obesity on the short-term and long-term outcomes after percutaneous coronary intervention: the obesity paradox? J Am CollCardiol. 2002;39:578–84.
5. Powell BD, Lennon RJ, Lerman A, Bell MR, Berger PB, Higano ST, et al. Association of body mass index with outcome after percutaneous coronary intervention. Am J Cardiol. 2003;91:472–6.
6. Ellis SG, Elliott J, Horrigan M, Raymond RE, Howell G. Low-normal or excessive body mass index: newly identified and powerful risk factors for death and other complications with percutaneous coronary intervention. Am J Cardiol. 1996;78:642–6.
7. Gurm HS, Brennan DM, Booth J, Tcheng JE, Lincoff AM, Topol EJ. Impact of body mass index on outcome after percutaneous coronary intervention (the obesity paradox). Am J Cardiol. 2002;90:42–5.
8. Niedziela J, Hudzik B, Niedziela N, Gasior M, Gierlotka M, Wasilewski J, et al. The obesity paradox in acute coronary syndrome: a meta-analysis. Eur J Epidemiol. 2014;29:801–12.
9. Li Y, Wu C, Sun Y, Jiang D, Zhang B, Ren L, et al. Obesity paradox: clinical benefits not observed in obese patients with ST-segment elevation myocardial infarction: a multicenter, prospective, cohort study of the northern region of China. Int J Cardiol. 2013;168:2949–50.
10. Kosuge M, Kimura K, Kojima S, Sakamoto T, Ishihara M, Asada Y, et al. Impact of body mass index on in-hospital outcomes after percutaneous coronary intervention for ST segment elevation acute myocardial infarction. Circ J. 2008;72:521–5.
11. HealthOrganization W. Obesity: Preventing and Managing the Global Epidemic. Report of a WHO Consultation on Obesity, June 3–5, 1997. WHO Technical Series No. 894. Geneva, Switzerland: World Health Organization; 2000.
12. National Institutes ofHealth. Clinical guidelines on the identification, evaluation, and treatment of overweight and obesity in adults-the evidence report. Obes Res. 1998;6:51S–209S.
13. The GUSTO Investigators. An interventional randomized trial comparing four thrombolytic strategies for acute myocardial infarction. N Engl J Med. 1993;329:673–82.
14. Serebruany VL, Atar D. Assessment of bleeding events in clinical trials–proposal of a new classification. Am J Cardiol. 2007;99:288–90.
15. Steg PG, James SK, Atar D, Badano LP, Blömstrom-Lundqvist C, Borger MA, et al. ESC Guidelines for the management of acute myocardial infarction in patients presenting with ST-segment elevation. Eur Heart J. 2012;33:2569–619.
16. Cutlip DE, Windecker S, Mehran R, Boam A, Cohen DJ, van Es GA, et al. Clinical end points in coronary stent trials: a case for standardized definitions. Circulation. 2007;115:2344–51.
17. Berghofer A, Pischon T, Reinhold T, Apovian CM, Sharma AM, Willich SN. Obesity prevalence from a European perspective: a systematic review. BMC Public Health. 2008;8:200.
18. Calle EE, Thun MJ, Petrelli JM, Rodriguez C, Heath Jr CW. Body-mass index and mortality in a prospective cohort of U.S. adults. N Engl J Med. 1999;341:1097–105.

19. Must A, Spadano J, Coakley EH, Field AE, Colditz G, Dietz WH. The disease burden associated with overweight and obesity. JAMA. 1999;282:1523–9.

20. Pi-Sunyer FX. The obesity epidemic: pathophysiology and consequences of obesity. Obes Res. 2002;10 suppl 2:97–104.

21. Oreopoulos A, Padwal R, Norris C, Pretorius V, Kalantar-Zadeh K. Effect of obesity on short- and long-term mortality post coronary revascularization: a meta-analysis. Obesity. 2008;16:442–50.

22. Romero-Corral A, Montori VM, Somers VK, Korinek J, Thomas RJ, Allison TG, et al. Association of body weight with total mortality and and with cardiovascular events in coronary artery disease: a systematic review of cohort studies. Lancet. 2006;368:666–78.

23. Oreopoulos A, McAlister FA, Kalantar-Zadeh K, Padwal R, Ezekowitz JA, Sharma AM, et al. The relationship between body mass index, treatment, and mortality in patients with established coronary artery disease: a report from APPROACH. Eur Heart J. 2009;30:2584–92.

24. Mohamed-Ali V, Goodrick S, Bulmer K, Holly JM, Yudkin JS, Coppack SW. Production of soluble tumor necrosis factor receptors by human subcutaneous adipose tissue in vivo. Am J Physiol. 1999;277:E971–5.

25. Schunkert MD, Harrell L, Palacios IF. Implications of small reference vessel diameter in patients undergoing percutaneous coronary revascularization. J Am CollCardiol. 1999;34:40–8.

26. Manson JE, Willett WC, Stampfer MJ, Colditz GA, Hunter DJ, Hankinson SE, et al. Body weight and mortality among women. N Engl J Med. 1995;333:677–85.

27. Harris T, Cook EF, Garrison R, Higgins M, Kannel W, Goldman L. Body mass index and mortality among non-smoking older persons: the Framingham Heart Study. JAMA. 1988;259:1520–4.

28. Lee IM, Manson JE, Hennekens CH, Paffenbarger Jr RS. Body weight and mortality: a 27-year follow-up of middle-aged men. JAMA. 1993;270:2823–8.

29. Adams KF, Schatzkin A, Harris B, Kipnis V, Mouw T, Ballard-Barbash R, et al. Overweight, obesity, and mortality in a large prospective cohort of persons 50 to 71 years old. N Engl J Med. 2006;355:763–78.

30. Holmes Jr DR, White HD, Pieper KS, Ellis SG, Califf RM, Topol EJ. Effect of age on outcome with primary angioplasty versus thrombolysis. J Am CollCardiol. 1999;33:412–9.

31. Halkin A, Singh M, Nikolsky E, Grines CL, Tcheng JE, Garcia E, et al. Prediction of mortality after primary percutaneous coronary intervention for acute myocardial infarction. The CADILLAC risk score. J Am CollCardiol. 2005;45:1397–405.

32. Niraj A, Pradahan J, Fakhry H, Veeranna V, Afonso L. Severity of coronary artery disease in obese patients undergoing coronary angiography: 'obesity paradox' revisited. Clin Cardiol. 2007;30:391–6.

33. Steinberg BA, Cannon CP, Hernandez AF, Pan W, Peterson ED, Fonarow GC. Medical therapies and invasive treatments for coronary artery disease by body mass: the 'obesity paradox' in the Get with the Guidelines database. Am J Cardiol. 2007;100:1331–5.

34. Reiner A, Siscovick D, Rosendaal F. Hemostatic risk factors and arterial thrombotic disease. Thromb Haemost. 2001;85:584–95.

35. Angiolillo DJ, Fernandez-Ortiz A, Bernardo E, Ramirez C, Sabate M, Hernandez-Antolin R. Platelet aggregation according to body mass index in patients undergoing coronary stenting: should clopidogrel loading-dose be weight adjusted? J Invasive Cardiol. 2004;16:169–74.

36. Sibbing D, von Beckerath O, Schömig A, Kastrati A, von Beckerath N. Impact of body mass index on platelet aggregation after administration of a high dose of 600 mg of clopidogrel before percutaneous coronary intervention. Am J Cardiol. 2007;100:203–5.

37. Panagotiakos DB, Pitsavos C, Yannakoulia M, Chrysohoou C, Stefanadis C. The implication of obesity and central fat on markers of chronic inflammation: the ATTICA study. Atherosclerosis. 2005;183:308–15.

38. Sonnenberg G, Kraower G, Kissebah A. A novel pathway to the manifestation of metabolic syndrome. Obes Res. 2004;12:180–6.

39. Tremblay A, Bandi V. Impact of body mass index on outcomes following critical care. Chest. 2003;123:1202–7.

15

Aspiration thrombectomy prior to percutaneous coronary intervention in ST-elevation myocardial infarction

Regina El Dib[1,2], Frederick Alan Spencer[3*], Erica Aranha Suzumura[4], Huda Gomaa[5], Joey Kwong[6], Gordon Henry Guyatt[7,8] and Per Olav Vandvik[9,10]

Abstract

Background: Trials of aspiration thrombectomy (AT) prior to primary percutaneous intervention (PCI) in patients with ST-segment elevation MI (STEMI) have shown apparently inconsistent results and therefore generated uncertainty and controversy. To summarize the effects of AT prior to PCI versus conventional PCI in STEMI patients.

Methods: Searches of MEDLINE, EMBASE and CENTRAL to June 2015 and review of reference lists of previous reviews. We included randomized controlled trials (RCTs) comparing AT prior to PCI with conventional PCI alone. Pairs of reviewers independently screened eligible articles; extracted data; and assessed risk of bias. We used the GRADE approach to rate overall certainty of the evidence.

Results: Among 73 potential articles identified, 20 trials including 21,660 patients were eligible; data were complete for 20,866 patients. Moderate-certainty evidence suggested a non statistically significant decrease in overall mortality (risk ratio (RR) 0.89, 95 % confidence interval, 0.78 to 1.01, risk difference (RD) 4/1,000 over 6 months), no impact on recurrent MI (RR 0.94, 95 % CI, 0.79 to 1.12) or major bleeding (RR 1.02, 95 % CI, 0.78 to 1.35), and an increase in stroke (RR 1.56, 95 % CI, 1.09 to 2.24, RD 3/1,000 over 6 months).

Conclusions: Moderate certainty evidence suggests aspiration thrombectomy is associated with a possible small decrease in mortality (4 less deaths/1000 over 6 months) and a small increase in stroke (3 more strokes/1000 over 6 months). Because absolute effects are very small and closely balanced, thrombectomy prior to primary PCI should not be used as a routine strategy.

Keywords: Myocardial infarction, Aspiration thrombectomy, GRADE, Systematic review, Meta-analysis

Background

In patients with ST-segment elevation myocardial infarction (STEMI), primary percutaneous coronary intervention (PCI) rapidly restores myocardial flow resulting in decreased infarct size and decreased mortality compared to thrombolysis or conservative medical management [1]. Some patients may, however, experience distal embolization of thrombus and plaque debris with failure to adequately restore distal microcirculatory flow. This "no reflow" phenomenon is associated with an increase in infarct size and lower survival [2].

Randomized clinical trials (RCTs) comparing aspiration or mechanical thrombectomy prior to primary PCI to PCI alone have shown improvement in markers of myocardial reperfusion (e.g. "myocardial blush", ST-segment resolution post procedure) [3]. A recent meta-analysis of 20 RCTs addressing patient-important outcomes and including over 11,000 patients reported that aspiration thrombectomy prior to primary PCI was associated with a reduction in major coronary adverse events and 1-year mortality [4]. A more recent meta-analysis including 26 RCTs, reported a different conclusion: aspiration thrombectomy did not

* Correspondence: fspence@mcmaster.ca
[3]Division of Cardiology, Department of Medicine, McMaster University, St. Joseph's Healthcare - 50 Charlton Avenue East, Hamilton, Ontario, Canada
Full list of author information is available at the end of the article

improve clinical outcomes [5]. Neither of these meta-analyses included the recently published Trial of Routine Aspiration Thrombectomy with PCI versus PCI Alone in Patients with STEMI (TOTAL), which randomized over 10,000 patients [6].

We therefore undertook a systematic review of all RCTs comparing aspiration thrombectomy prior to PCI *versus* PCI alone in patients with STEMI, focusing on patient-important outcomes. As composite endpoints varied between trials and can produce misleading results [7, 8], we focused on individual endpoints of overall mortality, recurrent MI, stroke, and major bleeding.

Methods

This review adheres to the Preferred Reporting Items for Systematic Reviews and Meta-analyses (PRISMA) Statement [9]; the Quality of Reporting of Meta-analyses QUOROM [10]; and the Cochrane Handbook for Systematic Reviews of Interventions [11].

Eligibility criteria

We included RCTs that compared aspiration thrombectomy prior to PCI with conventional PCI in patients with STEMI, included any one of the following patient-important outcomes: overall mortality, cardiovascular (CV) mortality, myocardial infarction (MI), stroke (including ischemic and hemorrhagic stroke) and, non-fatal extracranial major bleeding, and followed patients for at least 30 days. We excluded studies reported only as conference abstracts.

Data source and searches

A previous review with similar inclusion criteria identified studies up to December 2013 [5]. Using Medical Subject Headings (MeSH) based on the terms "thrombectomy," "thrombus aspiration," "thromboaspiration," "infarction," and "myocardial infarction" (Appendix Table 1) we replicated the search strategy of that review [5] for Medline, EMBASE, and Cochrane Controlled Trials Register (CENTRAL) from January 1, 2014 to June 26, 2015. We also reviewed reference lists of relevant review articles [4, 5, 12] and primary studies.

Selection of studies

Teams of two reviewers independently screened all titles and abstracts identified by the literature search, obtained full-text articles of all potentially eligible studies, and evaluated these studies for eligibility criteria.

Data extraction and risk of bias assessment

Three pairs of reviewers independently extracted the following data using a pre-standardized data extraction form: characteristics of the study design; participants; interventions; outcomes event rates and follow-up.

Reviewers independently assessed risk of bias by using a modified version of the Cochrane Collaboration's tool for assessing risk for bias tool [13] (http:/distillercer.com/resources/) [14] that includes nine domains: adequacy of sequence generation, allocation sequence concealment, blinding of participants and caregivers, blinding of data collectors, blinding for outcome assessors, blinding of data analysts, incomplete outcome data, selective outcome reporting, and the presence of other potential sources of bias not accounted for in the previously cited domains [14]. For incomplete outcome data we stipulated as low risk of bias loss to follow-up of less than 10 % and a difference of less than 5 % in missing data in intervention and control groups.

Certainty of evidence

The reviewers used the Grading of Recommendations Assessment, Development and Evaluation (GRADE) methodology to rate certainty of the evidence for each outcome as high, moderate, low, or very low [15]. Detailed GRADE guidance was used to assess overall risk of bias [16], imprecision [17], inconsistency [18], indirectness [19] and publication bias [20], and summarized results in an evidence profile. We assessed publication bias through visual inspection of funnel plots for 10 or more studies.

For decisions regarding eligibility, risk of bias assessment, and data abstraction, reviewers resolved disagreement through discussion with third party adjudication if necessary.

Data synthesis and statistical analysis

We chose six months as a follow-up time that represented duration important to patients, sufficient to include most events that would likely be influenced by thrombectomy, and would include relatively few events that would not be potentially influenced by thrombectomy. For meta-analyses we used six months data if available; and otherwise we chose the time point closest to six months, but preferring 1-year over 30 days.

We calculated pooled risk ratios (RRs) and associated 95 % confidential intervals (CIs) using random-effects models with statistical method of Mantel-Haenszel. Absolute effects and 95 % CI were calculated by multiplying pooled RRs and 95 % CI by baseline risk estimates derived from the TOTAL study (the most recent and largest of the included RCTs) [6]. We addressed variability in results across studies by using I^2 statistic and the P value obtained from the Cochran chi square test. Our primary analyses were based on eligible patients who had reported outcomes for each study (complete case analysis). For overall mortality we used all-cause mortality when available. For studies that did not present all-cause mortality we used cardiovascular mortality. We assessed publication bias through visual inspection of funnel plots for outcomes addressed in 10 or more studies. Review Manager (RevMan) provided the software for all analyses (version 5.3; Nordic Cochrane Centre, Cochrane) [21].

We also performed a meta-regression with a fixed-effect model using restricted estimated maximum likelihood with an observed log-odds ratio to predict whether mortality and recurrent myocardial infarction rates changed significantly by mean age. Meta-regression analysis was performed using Stata-13 (StataCorp LP, College Station, TX).

Results

Selection of titles

Our search strategy focusing on publications since the last review identified 103 unique citations (Fig. 1).

After title and abstract screening, we assessed the full-text version of 38 relevant citations. In addition, we identified 42 potentially eligible publications included in previous systematic reviews, six [6, 22–26] of which were also identified in our search strategy. Thereafter, we assessed eligibility of 74 unique publications and excluded 49 studies (Fig. 1). As a result, we included 25 publications documenting 20 randomized controlled trials [6, 25–48] involving 21,660 participants. Two studies [28, 35] and one updated follow-up [46] were not included in any of the previous reviews.

Study characteristics

Ten studies [26, 27, 29, 31–34, 39–41, 43–46] were conducted largely in Europe (Table 1). Sample size ranged from 56 [35] to 10,732 [6] patients of whom a majority were males with mean ages typically in the early 60s. Studies included adult STEMI patients typically with symptoms lasting >30 min but <12 hours, and cumulative ST-segment elevation of

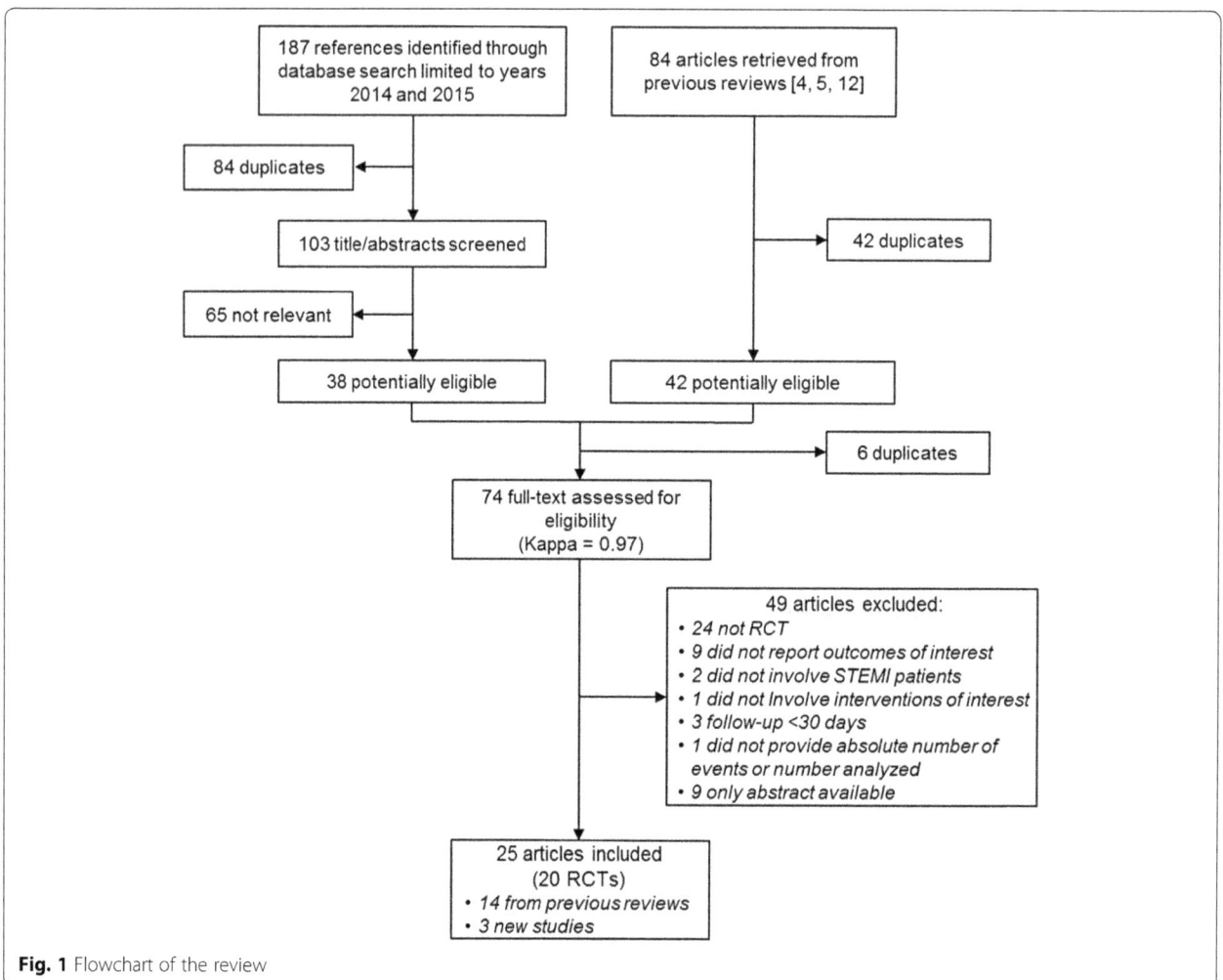

Fig. 1 Flowchart of the review

Table 1 Study characteristics

Author, year	Location	No. patient	Mean age (SD)	No. male (%)	Inclusion criteria	Exclusion criteria	Follow-up time (months)	Outcomes evaluated
ADMIT [28]	Haifa, Israel	100	I = 57.5 (12.4) C = 57.2 (12.1)	86 (86.0)	Admission <12 hours of onset of symptoms of STEMI, regardless of the initial TIMI flow	Inability to consent; known allergy to either aspirin or clopidogrel; life expectancy <6 months; cardiogenic shock	6 months	Quality of epicardial and microcirculation perfusion; LV function; ischemic mitral regurgitation; MACE (death, recurrent MI, TVR)
Bulum 2012 [29]	Zagreb, Croatia	60	I = 54.3 (9.7) C = 58.5 (8.6)	47 (78.3)	Symptoms suggesting acute myocardial ischemia of >20 min, time from symptom onset of <12 hours, and ST-segment elevation >0.1 mV in >2 contiguous ECG leads	Need for rescue PCI after failed thrombolysis; cardiogenic shock; triple-vessel disease; significant LMCA stenosis; previous PCI of an IRA; previous CABG; life expectancy <6 months	6 months	Referent vessel diameter; minimal lumen diameter; lesion length; percentage of diameter stenosis; MACE (death, recurrent MI, stroke, TLR)
Chao 2008 [30]	Taipei City, Taiwan	74	I = 60 (13) C = 62 (11)	63 (85.1)	STEMI (typical chest pain >30 min with new ST-segment elevation ≥0.1 mV in >2 contiguous leads on a 12-lead ECG), <12 hours after onset, and eligible for primary PCI	Killip IV hemodynamic status; ventricular tachyarrhythmias; previous CABG or significant LMCA lesion; culprit vessel diameter <2 mm; existing TIMI 3 flow without visible thrombus in IRA	6 months	Angiographic differences in TIMI and MBG (post PCI - baseline); MACE (death, stroke, non-fatal recurrent MI, TVR)
De Luca 2006 [31]	Rome, Italy	76	I = 66.7 (14.1) C = 64.6 (12.5)	48 (63.2)	Anterior STEMI, >18 years old, and have an identifiable thrombus on IRA at coronary angiography	Previous MI or CABG; triple-vessel disease; severe valvar disease; TIMI 2 or 3 flow at the time of initial angiography; unsuccessful PCI defined as no antegrade flow or >50 % residual stenosis in the IRA	6 months	LV remodeling; MACE (death, recurrent MI, hospitalization for HF)
EXPIRA [32, 33]	Rome, Italy	175	I = 66.7 (14.1) C = 64.6 (12.5)	105 (60.0)	First STEMI, <9 hours from symptoms onset, IRA ≥2.5 mm in diameter, thrombus score ≥ 3, TIMI flow ≤1, and >18 years old	Previous PCI on IRA; previous CABG; cardiogenic shock; triple-vessel disease; LMCA disease; severe valvular disease; thrombolysis; contraindication to glycoprotein IIb/IIIa inhibitors	9 months	Final MBG ≥2; rate of 90-min ST-segment resolution >70 %; MACE (cardiac death, recurrent MI, TVR); stent thrombosis
EXPORT [34]	24 centres in India and Europe	249	I = 59.2 (12.8) C = 61.2 (12.9)	202 (81.1)	>18 years old, STEMI <12 hours of symptom onset, ST-segment elevation ≥2 mm in ≥2 contiguous leads, visual reference vessel diameter >2.5 mm, and with TIMI flow of 0 or 1 before placing the wire in the IRA	Cardiogenic shock; cardiac arrest prior to intervention; pre-catheterization therapy with lytic agents, or with glycoprotein IIb/IIIa inhibitors, or with pacemakers; life expectancy <1 year; current participation in other investigations	1 month	Reperfusion (rate of ST-segment resolution >50 % at 60 minutes postprocedure or MBG 3 immediately postprocedure); magnitude of ST-segment resolution; improvement in TIMI flow; corrected TIMI frame count; MACE (death, recurrent MI, emergent CABG, TLR or TVR, stroke); rate of distal embolization; rate of required bailout techniques (rescue use of the aspiration catheter, distal protection, or glycoprotein IIb/IIIa inhibitors)
IMPACT [35]	Cambridge, UK	56	I = 64.9 (11.2) C = 67.2 (11.6)	31 (55.3)	>18 and <90 years old, ability to give informed consent, STEMI (ST-segment elevation ≥2 mm in ≥2 contiguous chest leads or ≥1 mm in ≥2 contiguous limb leads) or new LBBB, chest pain for <12 hours, restoration of at least TIMI 1 flow after the wire crossed the occlusion	Cardiogenic shock; previous MI in the IRA territory; unfavourable anatomy (LMCA occlusion or distal vessel occlusion); severe asthma or bradycardia precluding use of adenosine; women of childbearing age; life expectancy <3 months	6 months	Index of microcirculatory resistence; MACE (all-cause death or MI)

Table 1 Study characteristics (Continued)

					Inclusion criteria	Exclusion criteria	Follow-up	Outcomes
INFUSE-AMI [36, 37]	37 sites in 6 countries	452	I = 61 (NR) C = 60 (NR)	334 (73.9)	≥18 years old, STEMI with ≥1 mm of ST-segment elevation in ≥2 contiguous leads in V1 through V4 or new LBBB with anticipated symptom onset to device time of ≤5 hours	Prior MI, CABG or LAD stenting; contraindications to study medications, contrast or CMRI; creatinine clearance <30 mL/min per 1.73 m² or dialysis; platelet count <100,000 or >700,000 cells/mm³; hemoglobin <10 g/dL; recent major bleeding; bleeding diathesis; current warfarin use; intracranial disease, stroke or TIA within 6 months or any neurological defect; cardiogenic shock; prior fibrinolysis or glycoprotein IIb/IIIa inhibitors for the present admission; any comorbid likely to interfere with protocol compliance or associated with <1 year survival	12 months	Infarct size measured as a percentage of LV mass at 30 days. MACE (death, recurrent MI, new-onset severe HF, re-hospitalization for HF, stroke, clinically driven TVR)
ITTI [38]	Kaohsiung City, Yun-Lin Branch, Taiwan	100	I = 60.4 (11.9) C = 56.5 (11.9)	86 (86.0)	≥18 years old, continuous chest pain ≥30 min, ST-segment elevation >0.1 mV in ≥2 contiguous leads on a 12-lead ECG	Cardiogenic shock (systolic BP > 80 mmHg or need for inotropic agent); history of bleeding tendency, major operation within 6 weeks; hepatic or renal insufficiency; contraindication to tirofiban use	6 months	Occurrence of MBG 3; complete ST-segment resolution; procedure time; occurrence of no-reflow; CK-MB peak and time to peak; TIMI flow and corrected TIMI frame count; MACE (death, recurrent MI, TLR, stroke)
Kaltoft 2006 [39]	Aarhus, Denmark	215	I = 65 (11) C = 63 (13)	168 (78.1)	STEMI, symptoms lasting >30 min but <12 hours, and cumulative ST-segment elevation of ≥2 mV in ≥2 contiguous leads	LBBB; MI within the previous 30 days; fibrinolytic treatment; previous CABG; previous LCA stenosis; need for mechanical ventilation; severe HF treated with intra-aortic balloon pump	1 month	Myocardial salvage estimated by 99mTc-sestamibi SPECT; final infarct size; markers of effective reperfusion (TIMI flow, corrected TIMI frame count, ST-segment resolution immediately, 90 min and 6 hours after PCI); release of TnT; distal embolization visible at the end of PCI; total procedure time; MACE (death, recurrent MI, disabling stroke); LVEF after 30 days; technical success of the thrombectomy
Liistro 2009 [40]	Arezzo, Italy	111	I = 64 (11) C = 65 (11)	86 (77.5)	STEMI with symptoms lasting >30 minutes and <12 hours, ST-segment elevation >0.1 mV in ≥2 leads on the ECG	Contraindication to the use of platelet glycoprotein IIb/IIIa inhibitors; rescue PCI after thrombolysis; previous MI; absence of optimal echocardiographic apical view; life expectancy <6 months; lack of informed consent	6 months	Rate of ST-segment resolution ≥70 %; TIMI 3 grade flow; corrected TIMI frame count; myocardial contrast echocardiography score index; absence of persistent ST-segment deviation; time course of wall-motion score index; LVEF; LV volume; death; recurrent MI; LV failure; new revascularization
REMEDIA [41]	Rome, Italy	99	I = 61 (13) C = 60 (13)	83 (83.3)	<12 hours of onset of STEMI referred for primary or rescue PCI	No angiographic exclusion criteria were adopted	1 month	MBG ≥2; rate of ST-segment resolution ≥70 %; peak CK-MB; direct stenting rate; distal embolization rate (abrupt "cutoff" occlusion of a distal branch); composite of distal embolization, slow-flow (TIMI flow grade 2), no-reflow (TIMI flow grade 0 to 1); death; recurrent MI; stroke; TLR; any major adverse event

Table 1 Study characteristics *(Continued)*

Study	Location	N	Age	Male n (%)	Inclusion criteria	Exclusion criteria	Follow-up	Outcomes
Shehata 2014 [25]	Cairo, Egypt	100	I = 60.32 (9.2) C = 59.4 (7.4)	64 (64)	Diabetic patients suffering from acute STEMI, symptoms lasting >30 minutes and <12 hours before admission, and ST-segment elevation of >0.1 mV in ≥2 leads	Need for rescue PCI after thrombolysis; prior history of unstable angina or MI; prior PCI CABG; congenital heart disease or any myocardial disease apart from ischemia; limited life expectancy due to coexistent disease	8 months	In-stent restenosis (angiographic luminal diameter stenosis by >50 % in quantitative coronary angiography); MACE (death due to cardiac cause, nonfatal MI, TLR)
Sim 2013 [42]	Gwangju, Republic of Korea	86	I = 63 (NR) C = 60(NR)	59 (71.1)	STEMI with onset of symptoms <12 hours, coronary artery lesions with visible thrombus, ability to undergo a complete CCT examination (Killip I and II) with the ability to perform a 15-second breath-hold	Previous MI or CABG; cardiogenic shock; LMCA disease; severe valvular heart disease; unsuccessful PCI (post-PCI TIMI flow <2 or ≥50 % residual stenosis in IRA); rescue or facilitated PCI; contraindication to glycoprotein IIb/IIIa inhibitors	12 months	Infarct size at 2 months; markers of myocardial reperfusion (TIMI flow, MBG, ST-segment resolution rate at 90 min); LV function and volumes at 2 months; MACE (cardiac death, MI, TVR)
TAPAS [43, 44]	Groningen, The Netherlands	1071	I = 63 (13) C = 63 (13)	755 (70.5)	STEMI, symptoms >30 minutes and <12 hours, and ST-segment elevation of ≥0.1 mV in ≥2 leads	Rescue PCI after thrombolysis; life expectancy <6 months; lack of informed consent	1 month	Rate of post-procedural MBG of 0; rate of TIMI flow grade of 3; complete resolution of ST-segment elevation; absence of persistent ST-segment deviation; TVR; recurrent MI; death
TASTE [26, 27]	29 centers in Sweden, 1 center in Iceland and 1 in Denmark	7244	I = 66.5 (11.5) C = 65.9 (11.7)	5424 (74.9)	STEMI, chest pain for >30 minutes and <24 hours, ST-segment elevation in ≥2 contiguous leads (≥0.2 mV in lead V2 or V3 or ≥0.1 mV in other leads) or a presumably new LBBB, and a corresponding culprit-artery lesion on angiography	Need for emergency CABG; inability to provide oral informed consent; <18 years old; previously randomized in the study	12 months	MACE (all-cause mortality; rehospitalization for MI; stent thrombosis); TVR; TLR; complications of PCI, stroke or neurologic complications, HF and length of stay during index hospitalization
TOTAL [6]	87 hospitals in 20 countries	10732	I = 61.0 (11.8) C = 65.0 (11.9)	7797 (72.6)	Symptoms of MI lasting for ≥30 min, definite ECG changes indicating STEMI, referred for PCI for presenting symptoms, randomized within 12 hours of symptoms onset and before diagnostic angiography, Informed consent	≤18 years old; prior CABG; life expectancy <6 months due to noncardiac condition; treatment with fibrinolytic therapy for qualifying index STEMI event	6 months	MACE (cardiovascular death, recurrent MI, cardiogenic shock, HF NYHA class IV); stroke
TROFI [45, 46]	5 european centres	141	I = 61.1 (11.8) C = 60.9 (12.7)	102 (72.3)	≥18 years old, STEMI documented with ≥2 mm ST-segment elevation in ≥2 contiguous leads prior to PCI, presenting in the cath lab <12 hours after the onset of symptoms lasting ≥20 min and having an angiographically visible stenosis (>30 %) or TIMI ≤ II in a single de novo, native, previously unstented vessel	Pregnancy; known intolerance to aspirin, clopidogrel, heparin, stainless steel, limus drugs, contrast material; diameter stenosis <30 % in the target lesion; multi-vessel CAD; unprotected LMCA stenosis >30 %; distal vessel occlusion; severe tortuous, calcified or angulated anatomy that would result in sub-optimal imaging or excessive risk of complication from insertion of catheter; fibrinolysis prior to PCI; platelet <100,000 cells/μl coagulopathy or active bleeding or chronic anticoagulation therapy; cardiogenic shock; significant comorbidities precluding follow-up as judged by investigators; major planned surgery requiring discontinuation of antiplatelets; proximal RCA stenosis (>30 %) if the IRA is mid or distal-RCA	12 months	Minimum flow area immediately after PCI assessed by OFDI; MACE (cardiac death, recurrent MI in the territory of IRA, clinically driven TVR)

Table 1 Study characteristics (Continued)

Study	Location	No.	Age, mean (SD)	n (%)	Inclusion criteria	Exclusion criteria	Follow-up	Outcomes
VAMPIRE [47]	23 hospitals in Japan	355	I = 63.2 (10.6) C = 63.5 (9.9)	281 (79.1)	≥21 years old, STEMI symptom >30 min but <24 hours, ST-segment elevation ≥2 mm in ≥2 contiguous leads or with a presumably new LBBB	Primary thrombolysis prior to randomization; cardiogenic shock; history of cardiac arrest; history of CABG; chronic renal failure (Cr >2.0 mg/dl) or hemodialysis; LMCA disease; target vessel <2.5 mm or >5 mm in diameter	8 months	Incidence of slow flow or no reflow during primary PCI (TIMI flow grade <3 not attributable to dissection, occlusive thrombus, or epicardial spasm); coronary flow and myocardial perfusion immediately after PCI (assessed by TIMI flow grade, corrected TIMI frame count and MBG); magnitude of ST-segment resolution, peak CK and CK-MB; angiographic in-stent late lumen loss; LV function; brain natriuretic peptide; MACE (death, recurrence MI, TLR)
Yin 2011 [48]	Dalian, China	164	I = 63.1 (12.9) C = 62.9 (9.5)	120 (73.2)	STEMI patients who had PCI	Not reported	12 months	Thrombus score; periprocedural no-reflow; TIMI frame count; lumen diameter; stent length; 1-week post-procedural ejection fraction; post-procedural angina; recurrent MI; death

SD standard deviation, no. number, I intervention group, C control group, STEMI ST-segment elevation myocardial infarction, TIMI thrombolysis in myocardial infarction, LV left ventricular, MACE major adverse cardiac events, MI myocardial infarction, TVR target vessel revascularization, ECG electrocardiogram, PCI percutaneous coronary intervention, LMCA left main coronary artery, IRA infarct-related artery, CABG coronary artery bypass grafting, TLR target lesion revascularization, MBG myocardial blush grade, HF heart failure, LBBB left bundle branch block, NR not reported, LAD left anterior descending, CMRI cardiac magnetic resonance imaging, TIA transient ischemic attack, SPECT single-photon emission computed tomography, TnT troponin T, LVEF left ventricular ejection fraction, CK-MB creatine kinase myocardial band, CCT cardiac computed tomography, NYHA New York Heart Association, CAD coronary artery disease, OFDI optical frequency domain imaging, RCA right coronary artery

>0.1 mV in ≥2 leads. Some studies excluded life expectancy < 6 months [6, 28, 29]; cardiogenic shock [28, 29, 32, 33, 35–38, 45–47]; previous CABG or MI or significant left main coronary lesion [6, 25, 29–33, 35–37, 39, 40, 42, 45–47]; pre-catheterization therapy with lytic agents [34]; severe asthma or bradycardia precluding use of adenosine [35]; dialysis; platelet count <100,000 or >700,000 cells/mm3; hemoglobin <10 g/dL [36, 37]; severe HF treated with intra-aortic balloon pump [39]; contraindication or prior use of platelet glycoprotein IIb/IIIa inhibitors [32–34, 40, 42]; rescue or facilitated PCI [42–44]; need for emergency CABG [26, 27]; pregnancy [45, 46]; and major planned surgery requiring discontinuation of antiplatelets agents [45, 46]. Follow-up time ranged from 30 to 360 days.

Table 2 Study protocol used as preprocedure reported by the included studies

Author, year	Different regimens of anti-aggregation/anticoagulation used
ADMIT [28]	Oral aspirin 300 mg as a loading dose (or only 100 mg if the patient was on aspirin therapy) continued by 100 mg/day indefinitely, 600 mg clopidogrel loading dose continued by 75 mg/day for one year and IV 60 mg/ kg unfractionated heparin as loading dose to keep activating clotting time during procedure > 250 second.
Bulum 2012 [29]	300 mg of aspirin and 600 mg of clopidogrel and a weight-adjusted dose of unfractionated heparin; the usage of glycoprotein IIb/IIIa inhibitor (eptifibatide) was left to the discretion of the operator.
Chao 2008 [30]	Aspirin 300 mg and clopidogrel 300 mg were given as loading dose, with intravenous heparin 70– 100 U/kg to achieve activated clotting time (ACT) > 200 s prior to intervention.
De Luca 2006 [31]	Aspirin 300 mg orally and heparin 8000 IU intravenously before the procedure and abciximab as a 0.25 mg/kg bolus and 0.125 mg/kg/min intravenous infusion immediately before the revascularisation and continued for 12 hours.
EXPIRA [32, 33]	Aspirin 300 mg, intravenous heparin, abciximab at a standard dose, and clopidogrel 300 mg before the revascularization.
EXPORT [34]	The choice of medication during the procedure such as aspirin, heparin, clopidogrel, and glycoprotein IIb/IIIa inhibitors was also at the investigator's discretion, and were administrated according to standard hospital procedure.
IMPACT [35]	Aspirin 300 mg and clopidogrel 600 mg preloading in the ambulance and anticoagulated with a heparin bolus (70–100 U/kg) after arterial sheath insertion to achieve an activated clotting time (ACT) >250 s. Adjunctive pharmacotherapy, including abciximab and bivalirudin, was given at the operator's discretion.
INFUSE-AMI [36, 37]	Patients undergoing primary PCI received bivalirudin anticoagulation.
ITTI [38]	Aspirin (300 mg loading followed by 100 mg daily) and clopidogrel (300 mg loading followed by 75 mg daily) and unfractionated heparin 100 IU/kg.
Kaltoft 2006 [39]	Aspirin 300 mg orally or intravenously, clopidogrel 300 mg orally, and unfractionated heparin 10 000 IE intravenously. During the intervention, all patients were treated with abciximab.
Liistro 2009 [40]	Aspirin (a loading dose of 500 mg), heparin (70 IU/kg), and clopidogrel (a loading dose of 600 mg). All patients also received the glycoprotein IIb/IIIa inhibitor abciximab with an intravenous procedural bolus of 0.25 mg/kg followed by a continuous intravenous infusion of 0.125 µg/kg/min for 12 hours and postprocedural infusion without heparin.
REMEDIA [41]	Heparin (initial weight-adjusted IV bolus then further boluses administered with the aim of obtaining an activated clotting time of 250 to 300 s in patients treated with abciximab and > 300 s in the remaining subjects) and with double antiplatelet therapy with aspirin and clopidogrel (loading dose of 300 mg followed by 75 mg/day) for at least four weeks. Unless contraindicated, abciximab (0.25 mg/kg bolus plus infusion of 0.125 µg/kg/min for 12 h) was intravenously administered in all patients undergoing primary PCI, whereas in those with failed thrombolysis, abciximab use was left to the operator's discretion.
Shehata 2014 [25]	Aspirin (a loading dose of 500 mg), heparin (70 IU/kg), and clopidogrel (a loading dose of 600 mg). All patients also received the glycoprotein IIb/IIIa inhibitor abciximab with an intravenous procedural bolus of 0.25 mg/kg followed by a continuous intravenous infusion of 0.125 g/kg/min for 12 hours and postprocedural infusion without heparin.
Sim 2013 [42]	Aspirin 300 mg, clopidogrel 600 mg, intravenous unfractionated heparin and nitroglycerin. Oral atenolol 50–100 mg was given to optimize heart rate ≤ 65 beats per minute prior to CT scan, unless contraindicated.
TAPAS [43, 44]	Aspirin (a loading dose of 500 mg), heparin (5000 IU), and clopidogrel (a loading dose of 600 mg). Patients also received the glycoprotein IIb/IIIa inhibitor abciximab, with the dose based on body weight, unless contra-indicated, and additional heparin, with the dose based on the activated clotting time.
TASTE [26, 27]	Patients received the following procedure-related medication: bivalirudin, clopidogrel or ticlopidine, acetylsalicylic acid, ticagrelor, prasugrel, heparin, low-molecular-weight heparin, and glycoprotein IIb/IIIa blocker. The use of platelet inhibitors or anticoagulants was left to the discretion of the treating physician.
TOTAL [6]	Unfractionated heparin; bivalirudin; enoxaparin and; glycoprotein IIb/IIa inhibitor.
TROFI [45, 46]	Heparin in ambulance.
VAMPIRE [47]	Aspirin and intravenous heparin boluses were administered during the procedure to maintain an activated clotting time ≥ 300 s.
Yin 2011 [48]	Aspirin 300 mg and clopidogrel 300 mg prior to angiography.

IV: intravenous

Twelve studies [25, 28–30, 34, 35, 38–44] used aspirin and clopidogrel as a preprocedure antithrombotic therapy; some of them [6, 25–30, 32–35, 38, 39, 41–47] also used intravenous heparin; seven of them had all patients were treated with abciximab [25, 31, 35, 39, 40, 41, 43, 44] and; one of them [42] also used nitroglycerin (Table 2).

The choice of medication during the procedure such as aspirin, heparin, clopidogrel, and glycoprotein IIb/IIIa inhibitors was at the investigator's discretion in one of the included studies [34]. The patients in one further trial [26, 27] received the following procedure-related medication: bivalirudin, clopidogrel or ticlopidine, acetylsalicylic acid, ticagrelor, prasugrel, heparin, low-molecular-weight heparin, and glycoprotein IIb/IIIa blocker, while in other one [6] patients received unfractionated heparin; bivalirudin; enoxaparin and; glycoprotein IIb/IIa inhibitor (Table 2). Patients in TROFI trial [45, 46] received only heparin in ambulance and, in VAMPIRE trial [47] aspirin and intravenous heparin boluses were administered during the procedure to maintain an activated clotting time ≥ 300 s.

Risk of bias assessment

A possibly important limitation with respect to risk of bias was lack of blinding for caregivers. A number of studies, including the larger ones, blinded the adjudicators of outcome. Follow-up was largely satisfactory: 14 trials lost less than 10 % of patients to follow-up (Table 3 and Fig. 2).

Table 3 Risk of bias assessment

Author, year	Randomization sequence adequately generated?	Allocation adequately concealed?	Blinding of patients and caregivers?	Blinding of data collectors?	Blinding of adjudicators of outcome?	Blinding of data analysts?	Infrequent missing outcome data?[a]	Free of suggestion of selective outcome reporting?	Free of other problems that could put it at a risk of bias?
ADMIT (28)	Yes	Yes	No	Probably no	Probably yes	Probably no	Yes	Yes	Yes
Bulum 2012 (29)	Probably no	Probably no	No	No	No	No	Yes	Yes	Yes
Chao 2008 (30)	Probably yes	Probably no	No	No	No	No	Yes	Probably yes	Yes
De Luca 2006 (31)	Probably no	Probably no	No	Probably no	Probably no	Probably no	No	Yes	Yes
EXPIRA (32, 33)	Probably yes	Probably no	No	No	Yes	No	Probably yes	Probably yes	Probably yes
EXPORT (34)	Yes	Yes	No	No	Yes	No	Yes	Probably no	Probably yes
IMPACT (35)	Probably no	Probably no	No	Probably no	Probably no	Probably no	No	No	Yes
INFUSE-AMI (36, 37)	Yes	Probably no	No	Probably no	Yes	Probably no	Yes	Yes	No
ITTI (38)	Yes	Probably no	No	Probably no	Probably yes	Probably no	Yes	Yes	Yes
Kaltoft 2006 (39)	Yes	Yes	No	Probably no	Probably no	Probably no	Yes	Yes	Yes
Liistro 2009 (40)	Yes	Probably no	No	No	Probably yes	No	Probably yes	Yes	Yes
REMEDIA (41)	Yes	Probably yes	No	No	No	No	Probably yes	Yes	Probably yes
Shehata 2014 (25)	Yes	Yes	No	Probably no	Yes	Probably no	Yes	Yes	Yes
Sim 2013 (42)	Probably no	Probably no	No	No	No	No	Yes	Probably no	Yes
TAPAS (43, 44)	Yes	Probably yes	No	No	Yes	No	Yes	Yes	Yes
TASTE (26, 27)	Yes	Yes	No	No	No	Probably no	Yes	Yes	Yes
TOTAL (6)	Yes	Yes	No	Probably no	Yes	Probably yes	Yes	Yes	Probably no
TROFI (45, 46)	Yes	Yes	No	No	Yes	Probably no	Yes	Yes	Yes
VAMPIRE (47)	Probably yes	Probably no	No	No	Yes	No	No	Yes	Probably yes
Yin 2011 (48)	No	No	No	No	No	No	No	No	Probably no

[a]Defined as less than 10 % loss to outcome data or difference between groups less than 5 % and those excluded are not likely to have made a material difference in the effect observed

All answers as: yes (low risk of bias), probably yes, probably no, no (high risk of bias)

Outcomes

Appendix Table 2 presents the mortality data by individual study and Appendix Table 3 presents individual study outcome data for recurrent MI, stroke, and bleeding.

Overall mortality

In 20 trials [6, 25–48] that addressed overall mortality, 457 of 10,433 (4.4 %) patients died in the control arm compared to 403 of 10,433 (3.9 %) in the aspiration PCI arm (relative risk (RR) 0.89, 95 % CI 0.78 to 1.01; $I^2 = 0$ %; risk difference (RD) 4/1,000 over 6 months; moderate certainty) (Fig. 3). Certainty in evidence was rated down to moderate because of imprecision and unblinding of caregivers in all included studies (Table 4).

Recurrent myocardial infarction

In 17 trials [6, 25–29, 31–34, 36–41, 43–48], 246 of 10,331 (2.4 %) patients suffered a recurrent MI in the control arm compared to 229 of 10,331 (2.2 %) in the aspiration PCI arm (RR 0.94, 95 % CI 0.79 to 1.12; $I^2 = 0$ %; RD 1/1,000 over 6 months; moderate certainty) (Fig. 4). Certainty in evidence was rated down to moderate because of imprecision, lack of blinding of caregivers in all included studies and inadequate or unreported blinding of outcome adjudicators in some studies [26, 27, 29, 31, 39, 41, 48] (Table 4).

Stroke

In 8 trials [6, 26, 27, 29, 36–39, 41, 45, 46], 77 of 9,185 (0.8 %) patients that underwent aspiration PCI use had a stroke compared to 48 of 9,162 (0.5 %) in the PCI alone (RR 1.56, 1.09 to 2.24; $I^2 = 0$ %; RD 3/1,000 over 6 months; moderate certainty) (Fig. 5). Certainty in evidence was rated down to moderate because of imprecision, lack of blinding of caregivers in all included studies and inadequate or unreported blinding of outcome adjudicators in some studies [26, 27, 29, 39, 41] (Table 4). We intended to evaluate non-fatal stroke, but data was not available in sufficient number of studies to provide a useful comparison.

Major bleeding

In 4 trials [6, 36–38, 43, 44], 99 of 5823 (1.7 %) patients presented major bleeding in the control arm compared to 101 of 5,832 (1.7 %) in the aspiration PCI arm (RR 1.02, 0.78 to 1.35; $I^2 = 0$ %; RD 0/1,000 over 6 months; moderate certainty) (Fig. 6). Certainty in evidence was rated down to moderate because of imprecision and lack of blinding of caregivers in all included studies (Table 4).

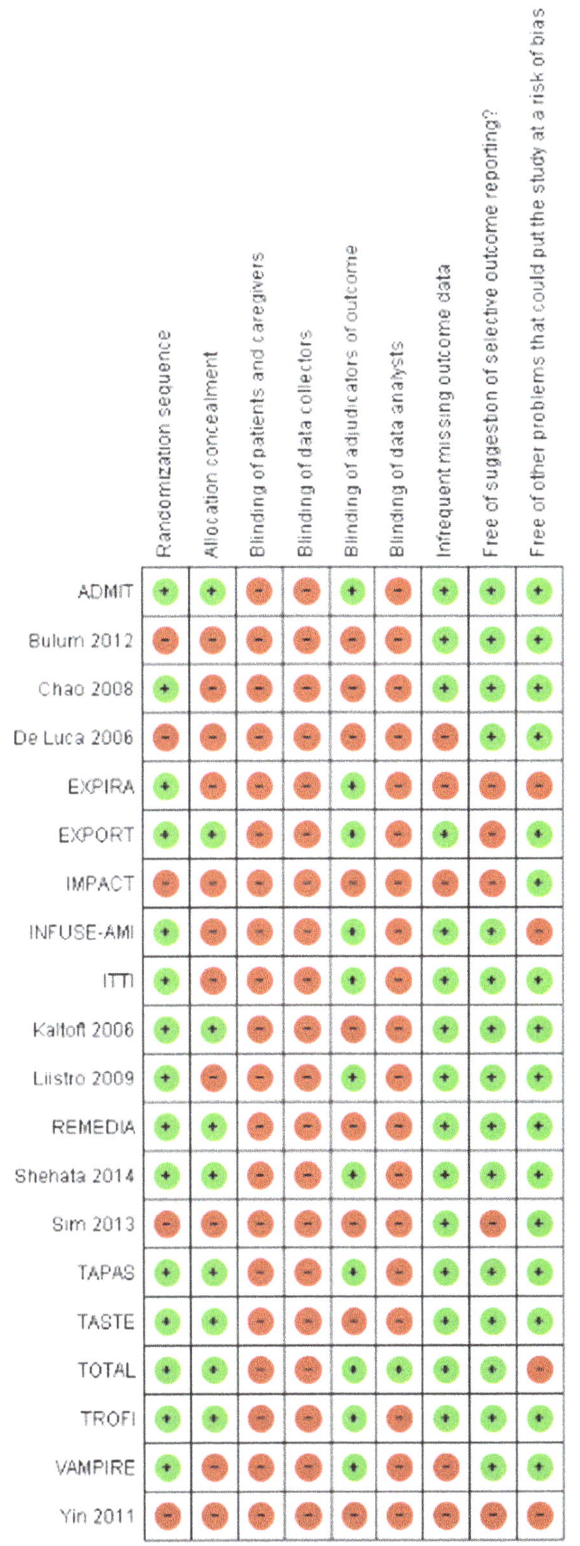

Fig. 2 Risk of bias assessment

Study or Subgroup	Aspiration PCI Events	Total	Conventional PCI Events	Total	Weight	Risk Ratio M–H, Random, 95% CI
ADMIT	4	41	2	43	0.6%	2.10 [0.41, 10.84]
Bulum 2012	0	30	0	30		Not estimable
Chao 2008	1	37	0	37	0.2%	3.00 [0.13, 71.34]
De Luca 2006	0	35	2	38	0.2%	0.22 [0.01, 4.36]
EXPIRA	0	88	4	87	0.2%	0.11 [0.01, 2.01]
EXPORT	3	120	5	129	0.9%	0.65 [0.16, 2.64]
IMPACT	1	20	1	21	0.2%	1.05 [0.07, 15.68]
INFUSE–AMI	11	222	15	207	3.0%	0.68 [0.32, 1.45]
ITTI	1	52	0	48	0.2%	2.77 [0.12, 66.49]
Kaltoft 2006	0	108	1	107	0.2%	0.33 [0.01, 8.02]
Liistro 2009	1	55	0	56	0.2%	3.05 [0.13, 73.38]
REMEDIA	3	48	3	48	0.7%	1.00 [0.21, 4.71]
Shehata 2014	0	48	1	46	0.2%	0.32 [0.01, 7.65]
Sim 2013	1	43	0	43	0.2%	3.00 [0.13, 71.65]
TAPAS	25	530	41	530	7.4%	0.61 [0.38, 0.99]
TASTE	191	3621	202	3623	46.5%	0.95 [0.78, 1.15]
TOTAL	157	5033	174	5030	38.2%	0.90 [0.73, 1.11]
TROFI	0	59	1	61	0.2%	0.34 [0.01, 8.29]
VAMPIRE	2	170	1	158	0.3%	1.86 [0.17, 20.30]
Yin 2011	2	73	4	91	0.6%	0.62 [0.12, 3.31]
Total (95% CI)		10433		10433	100.0%	0.89 [0.78, 1.01]
Total events	403		457			

Heterogeneity: Tau^2 = 0.00; Chi^2 = 11.21, df = 18 (P = 0.89); I^2 = 0%
Test for overall effect: Z = 1.78 (P = 0.08)

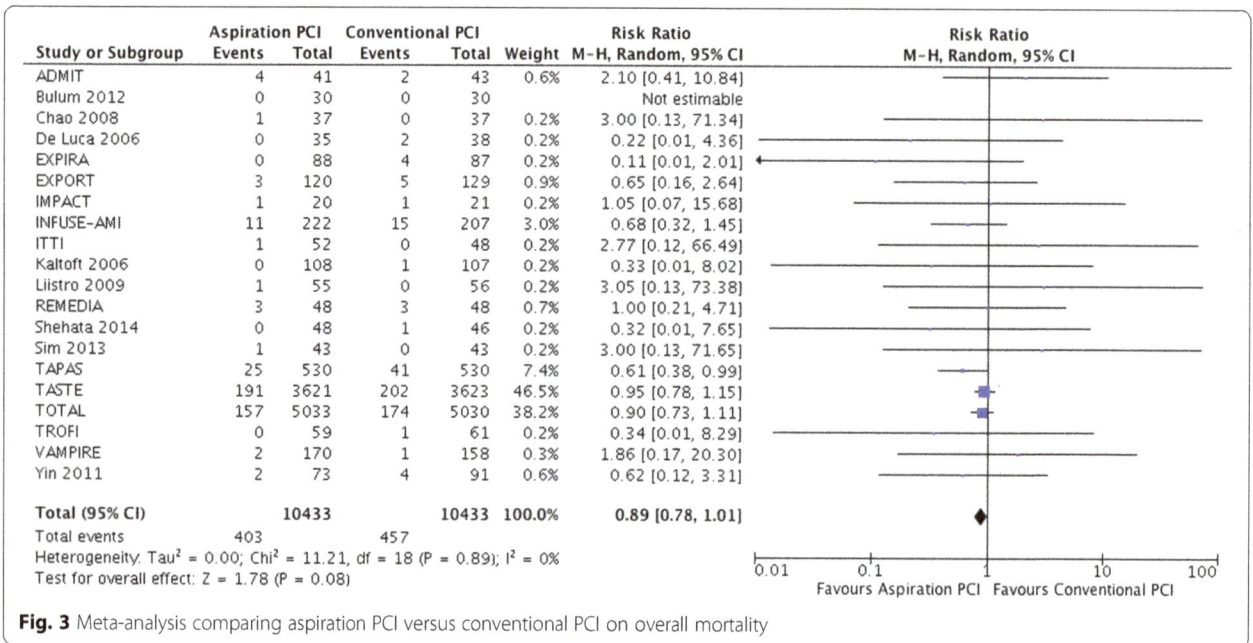

Fig. 3 Meta-analysis comparing aspiration PCI versus conventional PCI on overall mortality

More than 10 studies addressed overall mortality and recurrent MI; for both, funnel plots did not suggest publication bias (Appendix: Figures 1 and 2).

Meta-Regression analysis

Data from studies assessed in a meta-regression showed that the relationship between mortality rates decreased with increasing mean age; however was not significant (slope: −0.011; 95 % confidence interval: −.0980 to .0765; P = 0.784; Fig. 7). Similarly, the relationship between recurrent myocardial infarction rates decreased with increasing mean age; however was not significant (slope: −0.011; 95 % confidence interval: −.1175 to .0944; P = 0.811; Fig. 8).

Discussion
Main findings

Based on pooled data from 20 randomized trials with more than 20,000 patients, we found moderate quality evidence for a non-statistically significant reduction in overall mortality (4 fewer deaths/1000 treated over 6 months) (Table 4) and a small potential increase in stroke (3 additional strokes/1000 treated over 6 months) (Table 4) in patients treated with thrombectomy. Moderate quality evidence suggests no impact of thrombectomy on either recurrent MI or major bleeding (Table 4).

A number of factors decreased our certainty in the estimates for overall mortality. In particular, the confidence interval included both no reduction in deaths and a mortality reduction that although small (8 fewer deaths in 1,000 over six months), many would consider important. Similarly with stroke: the confidence interval includes no increase in stroke and an increase of 6 more strokes in 1,000 patients over 6 months with thrombectomy, which many would consider an important risk. Other issues decreasing confidence in our estimates included potential risk of bias imposed by lack of blinding of patients and health care providers in all studies, and lack of blinding of outcome adjudicators in some studies.

The meta-regression analyses showed that both mortality and recurrent myocardial infarction rates decreased with increasing mean age. However, there was a non-significant difference between these two variables and the mean age of participants in both studied groups. A study [49] evaluated through a meta-regression whether there is an association between age, gender, diabetes mellitus, previous myocardial infarction and ejection fraction, and the choice of revascularization, focusing on death, myocardial infarction, repeat revascularization and stroke. The authors found that the reduction in stroke was significantly higher in females, and that women and patients with diabetes mellitus were at increased risk of subsequent revascularization after PCI [49].

Strengths and limitations

Strengths of our review include a comprehensive search; assessment of eligibility, risk of bias, and data abstraction independently and in duplicate; use of the GRADE

Table 4 *GRADE evidence profile*: Aspiration thrombectomy (AT) prior to PCI in patients with STEMI

Quality assessment						Summary of findings					Certainty in estimates
						Study event rates		Relative risk (95 % CI)	Anticipated absolute effects over 6 months		
No of participants(studies) Range follow-up time	Risk of bias	Inconsistency	Indirectness	Imprecision	Publication bias	Without AT	With AT		Without AT	With AT	OR Quality of evidence
Overall mortality (Includes cardiovascular (CV) mortality for studies only reporting CV mortality)											
20866 (20) 6–12 mo	No serious limitations[1]	No serious limitations	No serious limitations[2]	Serious imprecision[1,3]	Undetected	457/ 10433	403/ 10433	0.89 (0.78–1.01)	35 per 1000[4]	4 fewer per 1000 (8 fewer to 0 more)	⊕⊕⊕⊖ MODERATE, due to imprecision
Recurrent myocardial infarction											
20662 (17) 6–12 mo	No serious limitations[1]	No serious limitations	No serious limitations	Serious imprecision[1,5]	Undetected	246/ 10331 (2.3 %)	229/10331 (2.2 %)	0.94 (0.79–1.12)	18 per 1000[4]	1 fewer per 1000 (4 fewer to 2 more)	⊕⊕⊕⊖ MODERATE, due to imprecision
Stroke											
18348 (8) 6–12 mo	No serious limitations[1]	No serious limitations	No serious limitations	Serious imprecision[1,6]	Undetected	48/ 9163 (0.5 %)	77/9185 (0.8 %)	1.56 (1.09–2.24)	5 per 1000[4]	3 more per 1000 (0 more to 6 more)	⊕⊕⊕⊖ MODERATE, due to imprecision
Major bleeding											
11655 (4) 6–12 mo	No serious limitations[1]	No serious limitations	No serious limitations	Serious imprecision[1,5]	Undetected	99/5823 (1.7 %)	101/5832 (1.7 %)	1.02 (0.78–1.35)	15 per 1000[4]	0 more per 1000 (3 fewer to 5 more)	⊕⊕⊕⊖ MODERATE, due to imprecision

[1] No studies were blinded to patient or caregiver. Some studies (minority of subjects enrolled) did not indicate blinded adjudication. While not specifically rating down for risk of bias, these additional concerns plus borderline clinically important imprecision led to downgrading of certainty in estimates for all outcomes

[2] Some studies only report cardiovascular and not all cause mortality. However cardiovascular mortality constituted significant proportion of overall mortality in studies reporting both types of mortality. Therefore we opted against rating down for indirectness

[3] 95% CI for absolute effects include clinically important benefit and no benefit

[4] Baseline risk estimates for mortality, recurrent MI, stroke, and major bleeds come from control arm of TOTAL study (largest and most recent randomized trial)

[5] 95% CI for absolute effects include benefit and harm

[6] 95% CI for absolute effects include clinically important harm and no harm

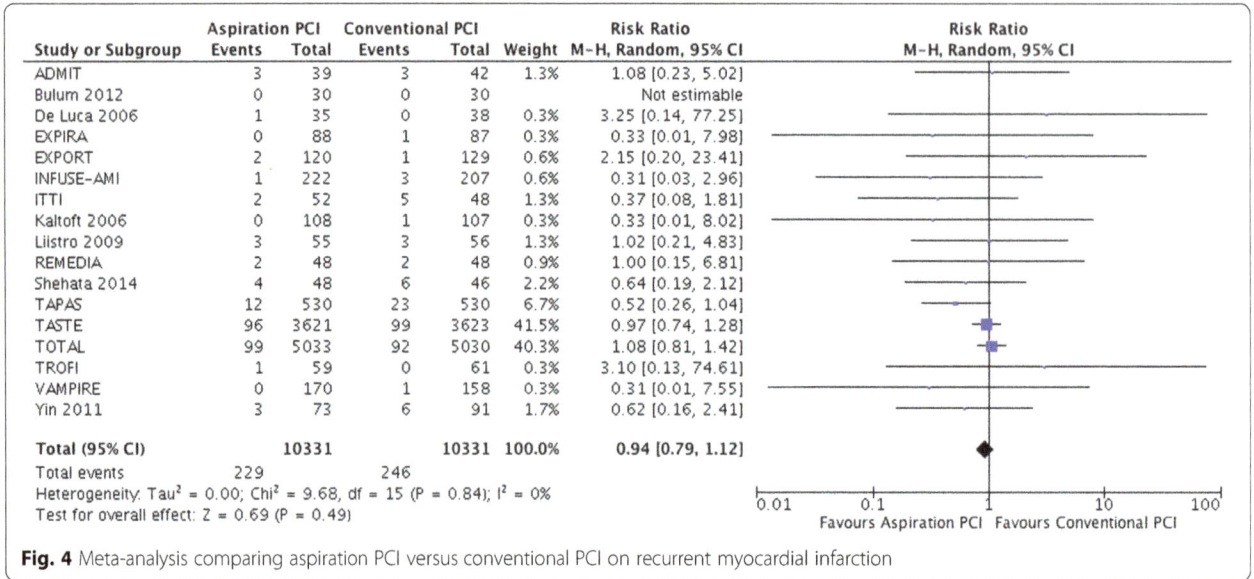

Fig. 4 Meta-analysis comparing aspiration PCI versus conventional PCI on recurrent myocardial infarction

approach in rating the quality of evidence for each outcome; and focus on absolute as well as relative effects of the intervention on patient-important outcomes. In this case, the small and more or less equivalent number of possible deaths prevented and strokes caused by thrombectomy, and the uncertainty consequent on the imprecision and risk of bias issues, are crucial in considering patient management (Table 4).

Potential limitations are related to the available data. Trials often suffered from incomplete outcome reporting, and lack of blinding consequent on the nature of the intervention, but for some studies also avoidable lack of blinding (outcome adjudication).

Relation to prior work

Recently published results from another meta-analysis [50] as well as data from a limited meta-analysis conducted as part of an evaluation of the outcome of stroke in the TOTAL study [12] are in general consistent with our findings. Results from all three analyses are in general consistent with our findings. Our systematic review and meta-analysis nevertheless adds important information as a result of our comprehensive assessment of risk of bias issues, our use of a complete case analysis that avoids assumptions regarding patients lost to follow-up, our use of the GRADE approach to rate quality of evidence, and our focus on absolute effects of thrombectomy required for optimal decision-making.

Furthermore, another review compared the effects of thrombectomy as an adjunct to PCI in the management of acute myocardial infarction in 20,853 patients [51]. The authors concluded that mortality; reinfarction and; stent thrombosis rates did not differ significantly between patients treated with or without AT; but stroke rates were increased with AT [51].

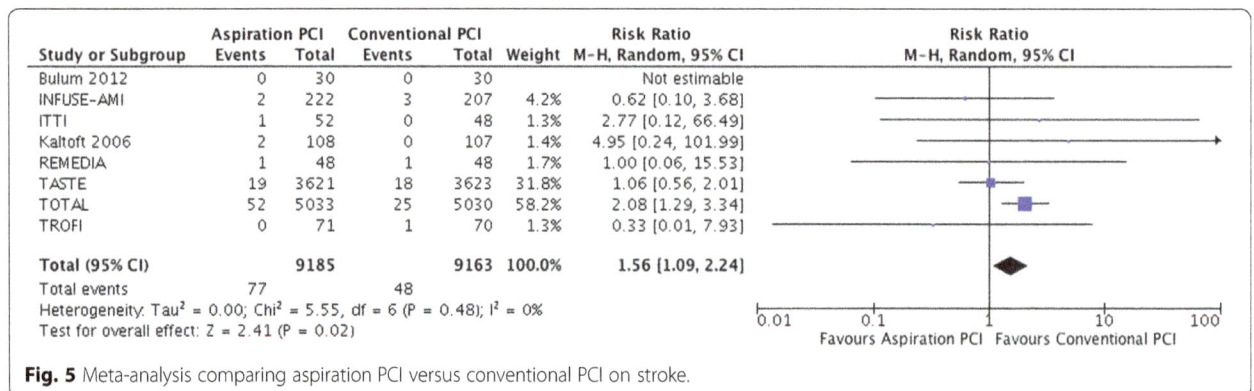

Fig. 5 Meta-analysis comparing aspiration PCI versus conventional PCI on stroke.

Study or Subgroup	Aspiration PCI Events	Total	Conventional PCI Events	Total	Weight	Risk Ratio M-H, Random, 95% CI
INFUSE-AMI	2	218	4	214	2.7%	0.49 [0.09, 2.65]
ITTI	0	52	0	48		Not estimable
TAPAS	20	529	18	531	19.3%	1.12 [0.60, 2.08]
TOTAL	79	5033	77	5030	78.0%	1.03 [0.75, 1.40]
Total (95% CI)		5832		5823	100.0%	1.02 [0.78, 1.35]
Total events	101		99			

Heterogeneity: Tau^2 = 0.00; Chi^2 = 0.80, df = 2 (P = 0.67); I^2 = 0%
Test for overall effect: Z = 0.15 (P = 0.88)

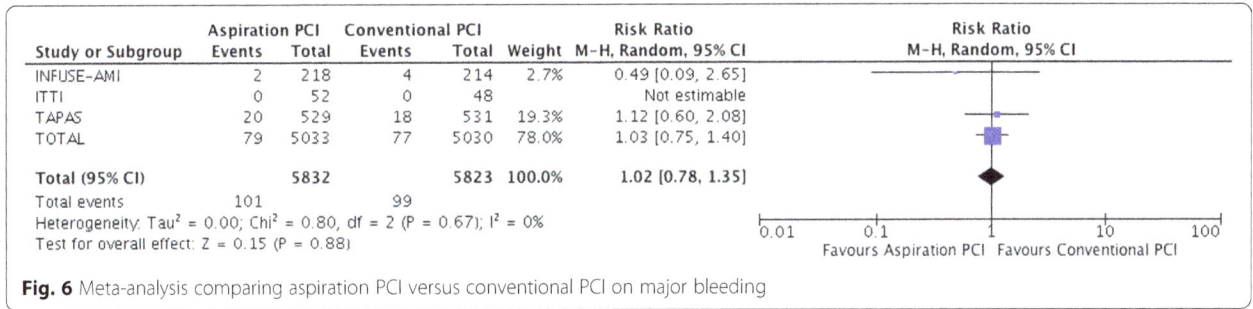

Fig. 6 Meta-analysis comparing aspiration PCI versus conventional PCI on major bleeding

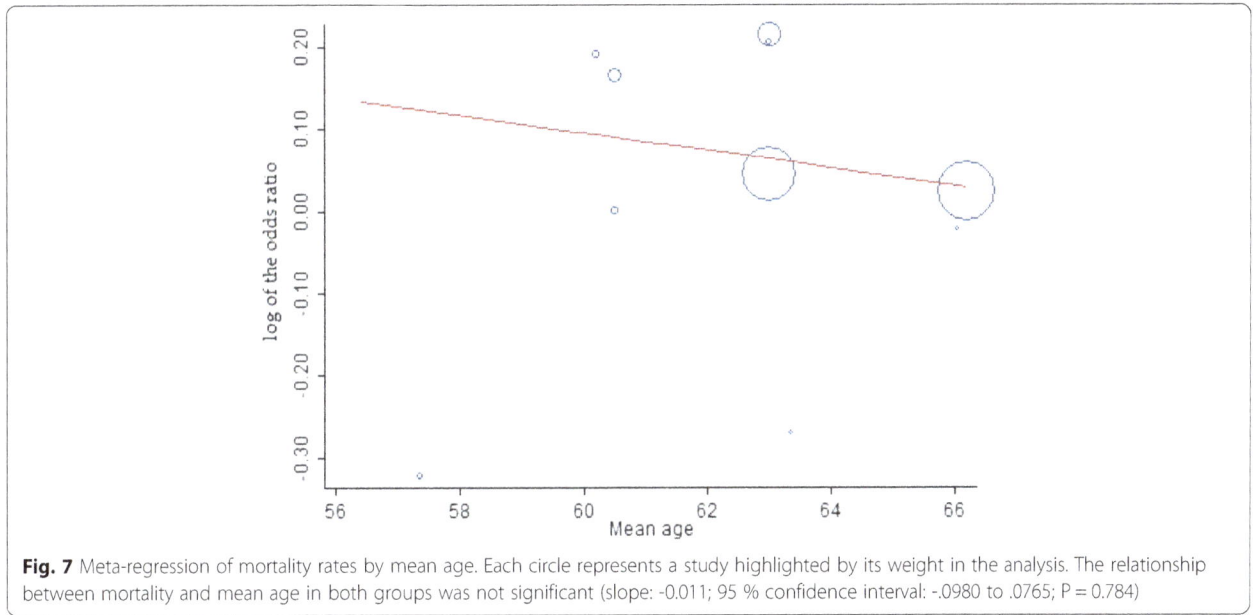

Fig. 7 Meta-regression of mortality rates by mean age. Each circle represents a study highlighted by its weight in the analysis. The relationship between mortality and mean age in both groups was not significant (slope: -0.011; 95 % confidence interval: -.0980 to .0765; P = 0.784)

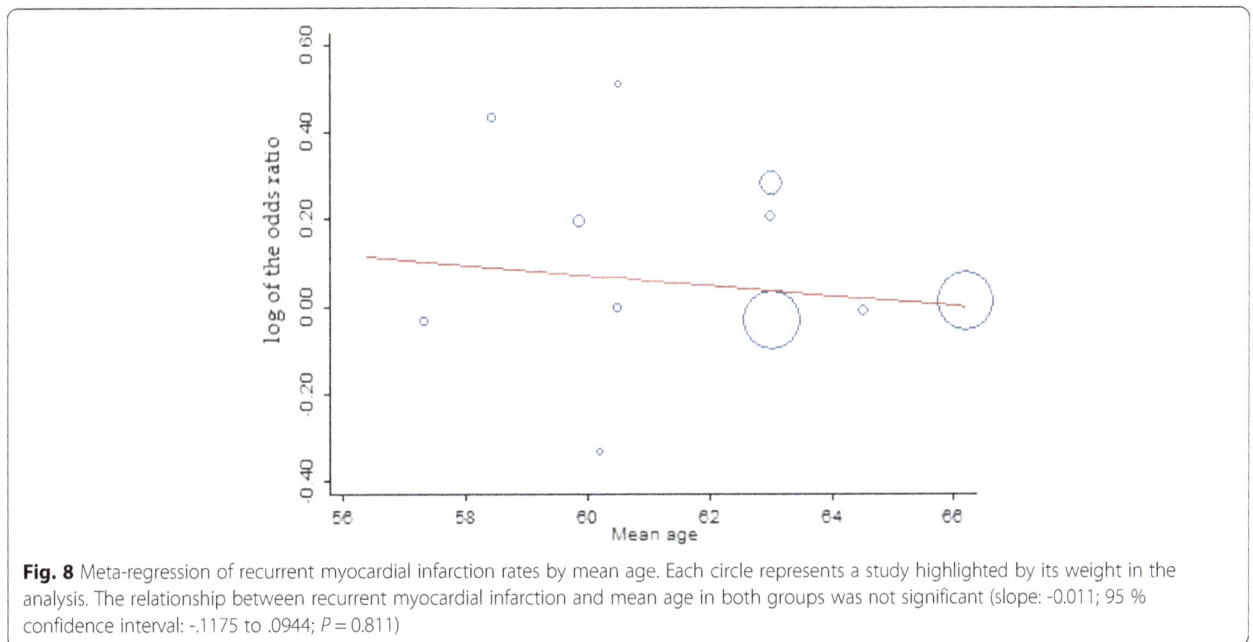

Fig. 8 Meta-regression of recurrent myocardial infarction rates by mean age. Each circle represents a study highlighted by its weight in the analysis. The relationship between recurrent myocardial infarction and mean age in both groups was not significant (slope: -0.011; 95 % confidence interval: -.1175 to .0944; *P* = 0.811)

Implications

The possible magnitude of benefit with respect to mortality and magnitude of harm with respect to stroke are small – some might say very small – and similar both with respect to magnitude and likelihood that the effects are real. With respect to mortality, the most likely mechanism of benefit would be a reduction in recurrent MI; the data, however, provide no support for an impact of thrombectomy on MI.

Similarly the mechanism of an increase in stroke is not immediately apparent. In a recent analysis of data from the TOTAL study, thrombectomy was associated with a small increase in procedure time as well as increased use of larger catheters (99.2 % vs. 97.5 % > 5 French) [12]. One could postulate this could lead to an increase in embolization of aortic atherosclerotic plaque leading to increased early ischemic events. More frequent development of subsequent atrial fibrillation would constitute another possible mechanism; no study reported this outcome.

Initial enthusiasm for thrombectomy was motivated by evidence of improvement in markers of myocardial tissue reperfusion. Our findings emphasize the need for caution with respect to surrogates, and the desirability of focus on outcomes important to patients. While it is not routinely justified there may be individual cases in which an operator may feel the potential benefit of the procedure outweighs potential risks.

The absolute effects of thrombectomy prior to primary PCI are very small and still associated with uncertainty. Given the best estimates of effect and associated quality of evidence, fully informed risk adverse patients - and particularly those who are highly stroke risk averse - would likely decline thrombectomy. Patients who place high value on an uncertain mortality reduction and have limited concern regarding a possible stroke increase would be more likely to choose to undergo the procedure. Given current concerns regarding overtreatment and efficient use of health care resources, a policy decision to not use thrombectomy in a particular catheterization laboratory is defensible.

Conclusions

Moderate certainty evidence suggests aspiration thrombectomy is associated with a possible small decrease in mortality (4 less deaths/1000 over 6 months) and a small increase in stroke (3 more strokes/1000 over 6 months). Because absolute effects are very small and closely balanced, thrombectomy prior to primary PCI should not be used as a routine strategy.

Appendix

Table 5 Search strategy

Ovid MEDLINE(R) 1946 to present with daily update	
Ovid MEDLINE(R) in-process & other non-indexed citations June 24, 2015	
1. myocardial infarction.ti,ab	194029
2 *Infarction/	4551
3 Myocardial Infarction/	145002
4 or/1-3	201604
5 thrombus aspiration.ti,ab.	400
6 thromboaspiration.ti,ab.	125
7 (aspiration adj5 mechanical).ti,ab.	214
8 Thrombectomy.ti,ab.	4995
9 (aspiration and catheter*).ti,ab.	2140
10 thrombosuction.ti,ab.	34
11 *Thrombectomy/	2028
12 or/5-11	7869
13 randomized controlled trial.pt.	398533
14 controlled clinical trial.pt.	89780
15 randomized.ab.	324620
16 placebo.ab.	163833
17 drug therapy.fs.	1786167
18 randomly.ab.	233298
19 trial.ab.	336144
20 groups.ab.	1465972
21 or/13-20	3564150
22 and/4,12,21	349
23 exp animals/ not humans.sh.	4063058
24 22 not 23	346
Embase 1974 to 2015 June 24	
1. Myocardial Infarction.ti,ab.	138908
2 heart infarction/ or acute heart infarction/ or infarction/ or ST segment elevation myocardial infarction/	298819
3 myocardial disease/	4499
4 or/1-3	335897
5 thrombus aspiration.ti,ab.	899
6 thromboaspiration.ti,ab.	227
7 (aspiration adj5 mechanical).ti,ab.	328
8 Thrombectomy.ti,ab.	7683
9 (aspiration and catheter*).ti,ab.	3379
10 thrombosuction.ti,ab.	59
11 *Thrombectomy/	1973
12 or/5-11	11913
13 random$.tw.	995701
14 factorial$.tw.	25787
15 (crossover$ or cross-over$).tw.	76738

Table 5 Search strategy *(Continued)*

16	placebo$.tw.	221322
17	(doubl$ adj blind$).tw.	158296
18	(singl$ adj blind$).tw.	16231
19	assign$.tw.	266556
20	allocat$.tw.	95221
21	volunteer$.tw.	195251
22	Crossover Procedure.sh.	43314
23	Double-blind Procedure.sh.	123817
24	Randomized Controlled Trial.sh.	377450
25	Single-blind Procedure.sh.	20454
26	or/13-25	1582267
27	animals/ not humans/	1258280
28	and/4,12,26	454
29	28 not 27	454

CENTRAL Issue 5 of 12, May 2015

#1	myocardial infarction:ti,ab,kw (Word variations have been searched)	17426
#2	MeSH descriptor: [Infarction] explode all trees	18
#3	MeSH descriptor: [Myocardial Infarction] explode all trees	8885
#4	#1 or #2 or #3	17525
#5	thrombus aspiration:ti,ab,kw (Word variations have been searched)	151
#6	thromboaspiration:ti,ab,kw (Word variations have been searched)	10
#7	aspiration mechanical:ti,ab,kw (Word variations have been searched)	251
#8	thrombectomy:ti,ab,kw (Word variations have been searched)	336
#9	aspiration catheter*:ti,ab,kw (Word variations have been searched)	293
#10	thrombosuction:ti,ab,kw (Word variations have been searched)	4
#11	MeSH descriptor: [Thrombectomy] explode all trees	144
#12	#5 or #6 or #7 or #8 or #9 or #10 or #11	860
#13	#4 and #12	216
	In Trials	195

Table 6 Mortality data

Acronym (author, year)	No. included in analysis (intervention/ control)	Follow-up time (month)*	Cardiac-specific mortality (intervention/ control)	Overall mortality (intervention/ control)
ADMIT [28]	41/43	6		4/41; 2/43
	47/47	1		3/47; 1/47
Bulum 2012 [29]	30/30	6		0/30; 0/30
Chao 2008 [30]	37/37	6	NA	1/37; 0/37
De Luca 2006 [31]	35/38	6		0/35; 2/38
EXPIRA[32, 33]	88/87	24	0/88; 6/87	0/88; 6/87
	88/87	9	0/88; 4/87	0/88; 4/87
EXPORT [34]	120/129	1	3/120; 5/129	3/120; 5/129
IMPACT[35]	20/21	6	1/20; 1/ 21	1/20; 1/ 21
INFUSE AMI [36, 37]	222/207	12	NA	11/222; 15/ 207
	218/214	1		0/218; 1/214
ITTI [38]	52/48	6		1/52; 0/48
Kaltoft 2006 [39]	108/107	1	NA	0/108 ; 1/107
Liistro 2009 [40]	55/56	6	1/55; 0/56	1/55; 0/56
REMEDIA[41]	48/48	1	NA	3/48; 3/48
Shehata 2014 [25]	48/46	8	0/48; 1/46	0/48; 1/46
Sim 2013 [42]	43/43	12	NA	1/43; 0/43
TAPAS [43, 44]	530/530	12	19/530; 36/530	25/530; 41/ 530
	529/531	1	NA	11/529; 21/ 531
TASTE [26, 27]	3621/3623	12		295/3621; 316/3623
	3621/3623	1-12		191/3621; 202/3623
TOTAL [6]	5033/5030	6	157/5033; 174/ 5030	157/5033; 174/5030
TROFI [45, 46]	59/61	12	0/59; 1/61	0/59; 1/61
VAMPIRE [47]	170/158	8		2/170; 1/158
Yin 2011 [48]	73/91	12	NA	2/73; 4/91

*Preference for 6-month mortality, then any defined period closest to 6 months, however abstract in-hospital mortality if that is the only one available was excluded from review

Table 7 Outcome data per study

Author, year	No. included in analysis (intervention/ control)	Follow-up time (Month)	No. (%) of major bleeding (intervention/ control)	No. (%) of non-fatal stroke (intervention/ control)	No. (%) of recurrent myocardial infarction (intervention/ control)
ADMIT [28]	39/42	6			3(7.7)/3(7)
	42/46	1			2(4.7)/0
	49/51	0			1(2)/0
Bulum 2012 [29]	30/30	6		0/0	0/0
Chao 2008 [30]	37/37				
De Luca 2006 [31]	35/38	6			1/0
EXPIRA [32, 33]	88/87	24			0/1(1.14)
EXPORT [34]	120/129	1			2(0.016)/1(0.77)
IMPACT [35]	20/21	6			
INFUSE AMI [36, 37]	222/207	12	NA	2(0.9)/3(1.4)	1(0.45)/3(1.4)
	218/214	1	2(0.9)/4(1.86)	0/1(0.46)	1(0.45)/2(0.93)
ITTI [38]	52/48	6	0/0	1(1.92)/0(0)	2(3.84)/5(10.41)
Kaltoft 2006 [39]	108/107	1		2(1.85)/0(0)	0/1(0.93)
Liistro 2009 [40]	55/56				3(5.4)/3(5.3)
REMEDIA [41]	48/48	1		1(2)/1(2)	2(4)/2(4)
Shehata 2014 [25]	48/46	8			4(8)/6(13)
Sim 2013 [42]	43/43	12			
TAPAS [43, 44]	529/531	1	20(3.78)/18(3)		4(0.75)/10(1.88)
	530/530	12			12(2.26)/23(4.3)
TASTE [26, 27]	3621/3623	12		19(0.52)/18(0.4)*	96(2.7)/99(2.7)
	3621/3623	1			19(0.52)/31(0.85)
TOTAL [6]	5033/5030	6	79(1.5)/77(1.5)	52(1)/25(0.5)	99(2)/92(1.8)
	5033/5030	1		33(0.65)/16(0.32)	
TROFI [45, 46]	59/61	12	NA	NA	1(1.7)/0
	71/70	0	NA	0/1(1.4)	0/0
VAMPIRE [47]	170/158	8			0/1(0.6)
	178/171	0			0/1(0.6)
Yin 2011 [48]	73/91	12			3(4)/6(6.6)

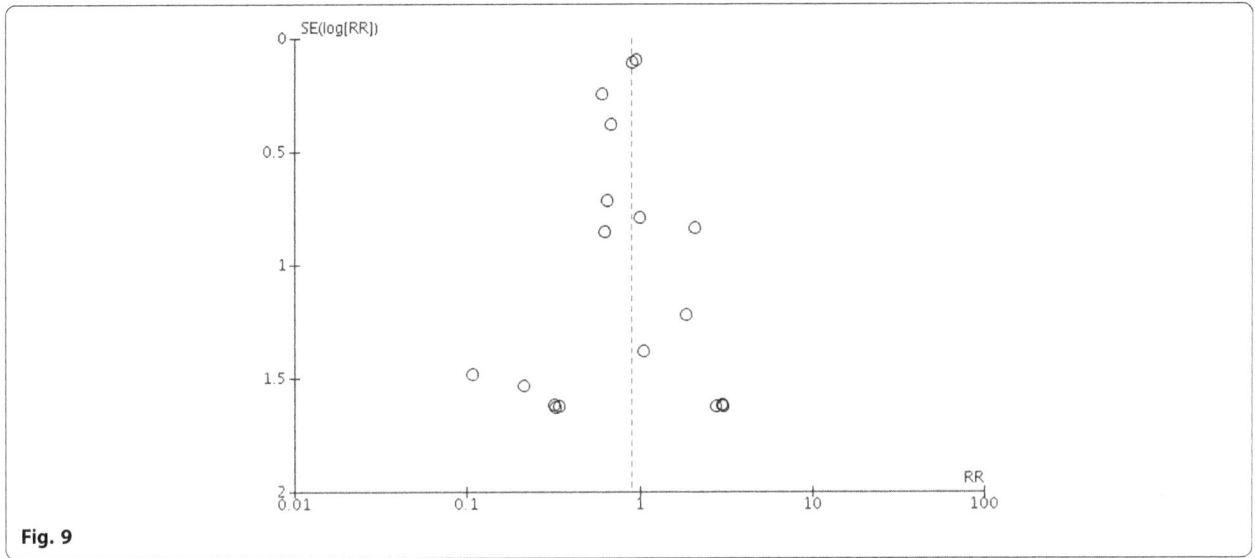

Fig. 9

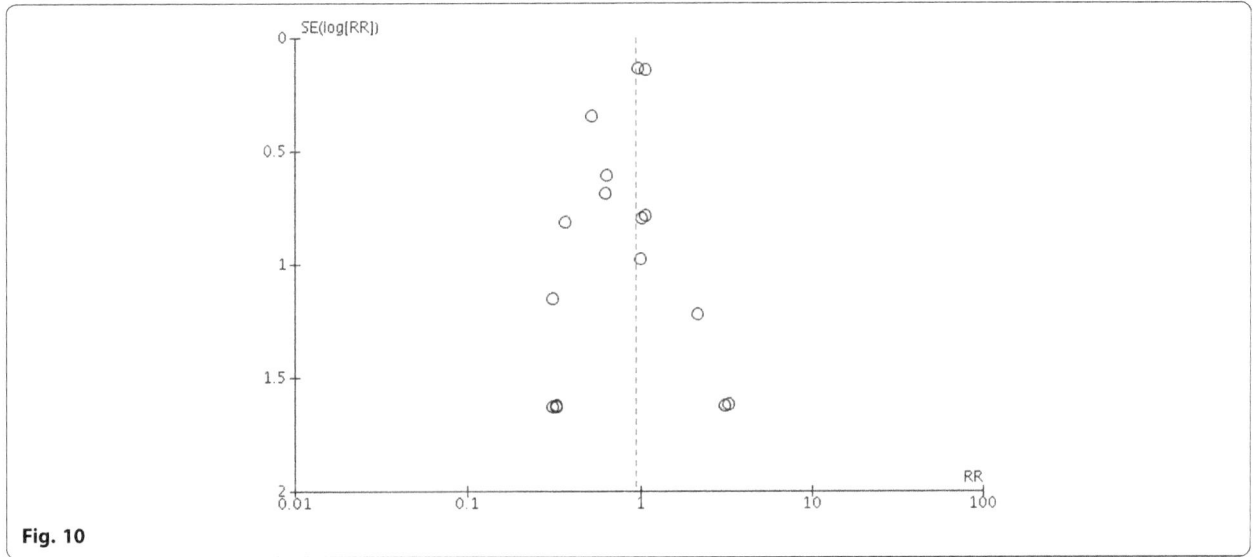

Fig. 10

Abbreviations

AT, aspiration thrombectomy; CV, cardiovascular; CENTRAL, cochrane controlled trials register; CIs, confidential intervals; GRADE, grading of recommendations assessment development and evaluation; MeSH, medical subject headings; MI, myocardial infarction; PRISMA, preferred reporting items for systematic reviews and meta-analyses statement; PCI, primary percutaneous intervention; RCTs, randomized controlled trials; RevMan, review manager; RRs, risk ratios; STEMI, ST-segment elevation MI; TOTAL, Trial of Routine Aspiration Thrombectomy with PCI versus PCI Alone in Patients with STEMI.

Funding

R El Dib received a Brazilian Research Council (CNPq) scholarship (CNPq 310953/2015-4).

Authors' contributions

Conceiving the review: GHG, FAS, POV and RED. Undertaking searches: JK. Screening search results: RED, EAS, HG, JK, POV. Organizing retrieval of papers: RED and EAS. Screening retrieved papers against inclusion criteria: RED, EAS, HG, JK and POV. Appraising quality of papers: RED, EAS, HG, JK and POV. Extracting data from papers: RED, EAS, HG, JK and POV. Writing to authors of papers for additional information: RED. Providing additional data about papers: RED. Obtaining and screening data on unpublished studies: RED and EAS. Managing data for the review: RED. Entering data into Review Manager (RevMan): RED. Analyzing RevMan statistical data: RED, FAS, GHG, POV. Interpreting data: RED, FAS, GHG, POV. Making statistical inferences: RED, FAS, GHG, POV. Writing the review: RED, FAS, GHG, POV. Taking responsibility for reading and checking the review before submission: RED, FAS, EAS, HG, JK, GHG, POV. All authors read and approved the final manuscript.

Competing interests

The authors declare that they have no competing interests.

Author details

[1]Department of Anaesthesiology, Botucatu Medical School, Unesp – Univ Estadual Paulista, São Paulo, Brazil. [2]McMaster Institute of Urology, McMaster University, Hamilton, Ontario, Canada. [3]Division of Cardiology, Department of Medicine, McMaster University, St. Joseph's Healthcare - 50 Charlton Avenue East, Hamilton, Ontario, Canada. [4]Research Institute - Hospital do Coração (HCor), São Paulo, Brazil. [5]Department of Pharmacy, Tanta Chest Hospital, Tanta, Egypt. [6]Division of Cardiology and Heart Education And Research Training (HEART) Centre, Department of Medicine and Therapeutics, Prince of Wales Hospital, and Institute of Vascular Medicine, The Chinese University of Hong Kong, Shatin, Hong Kong. [7]Department of Clinical Epidemiology and Biostatistics, McMaster University, Hamilton, Ontario, Canada. [8]Department of Medicine, McMaster University, Hamilton, Ontario, Canada. [9]Department of Medicine, Innlandet Hospital Trust-Division Gjøvik, Oppland, Norway. [10]Institute for Health and Society, Faculty of Medicine, University of Oslo, Oslo, Norway.

References

1. Keeley EC, Boura JA, Grines CL. Primary angioplasty versus intravenous thrombolytic therapy for acute myocardial infarction: a quantitative review of 23 randomised trials. Lancet. 2003;361(9351):13–20.

2. Stone GW, Peterson MA, Lansky AJ, Dangas G, Mehran R, Leon MB. Impact of normalized myocardial perfusion after successful angioplasty in acute myocardial infarction. J Am Coll Cardiol. 2002;39(4):591–7.

3. Kumbhani DJ, Bavry AA, Desai MY, Bangalore S, Bhatt DL. Role of aspiration and mechanical thrombectomy in patients with acute myocardial infarction undergoing primary angioplasty: an updated meta-analysis of randomized trials. J Am Coll Cardiol. 2013;62(16):1409–18.

4. Kumbhani DJ, Bavry AA, Desai MY, Bangalore S, Byrne RA, Jneid H, et al. Aspiration thrombectomy in patients undergoing primary angioplasty: totality of data to 2013. Catheter Cardiovasc Interv. 2014;84(6):973–7.

5. Spitzer E, Heg D, Stefanini GG, Stortecky S, Rutjes AW, Räber L, Blöchlinger S, Pilgrim T, Jüni P, Windecker S. Aspiration Thrombectomy for Treatment of ST-segment Elevation Myocardial Infarction: a Meta-analysis of 26 Randomized Trials in 11 943 Patients. Rev Esp Cardiol (Engl Ed). 2015;68(9):746–52.

6. Jolly SS, Cairns JA, Yusuf S, Meeks B, Pogue J, Rokoss MJ, Kedev S, Thabane L, Stankovic G, Moreno R, Gershlick A, Chowdhary S, Lavi S, Niemelä K, Steg PG, Bernat I, Xu Y, Cantor WJ, Overgaard CB, Naber CK, Cheema AN, Welsh RC, Bertrand OF, Avezum A, Bhindi R, Pancholy S, Rao SV, Natarajan MK, ten Berg JM, Shestakovska O, Gao P, Widimsky P, Džavík V. Randomized trial of primary PCI with or without routine manual thrombectomy. N Engl J Med. 2015;372(15):1389–98.

7. Ferreira-Gonzalez I, Busse JW, Heels-Ansdell D, Montori VM, Akl EA, Bryant DM, Alonso-Coello P, Alonso J, Worster A, Upadhye S, Jaeschke R, Schünemann HJ, Permanyer-Miralda G, Pacheco-Huergo V, Domingo-Salvany A, Mills EJ, Guyatt GH. Problems with use of composite end points in cardiovascular trials: systematic review of randomised controlled trials. BMJ. 2007;334(7597):786.

8. Lim E, Brown A, Helmy A, Mussa S, Altman DG. Composite outcomes in cardiovascular research: a survey of randomized trials. Ann Intern Med. 2008;149(9):612–7.

9. Moher D, Liberati A, Tetzlaff J, Altman DG. Preferred reporting items for systematic reviews and meta-analyses: The PRISMA statement. BMJ. 2009;339:b2535.

10. Moher D, Cook DJ, Eastwood S, Olkin I, Rennie D, Stroup DF. Improving the quality of reports of meta-analyses of randomised controlled trials: the QUOROM statement. Quality of Reporting of Meta-analyses. Lancet. 1999;354(9193):1896–900.

11. Higgins JPT, Green S (editors). Cochrane Handbook for Systematic Reviews of Interventions Version 5.1.0 [updated March 2011]. The Cochrane Collaboration, 2011. Available from www.cochrane-handbook.org

12. Jolly SS, Cairns JA, Yusuf S, Meeks B, Gao P, Hart RG, Kedev S, Stankovic G, Moreno R, Horak D, Kassam S, Rokoss MJ, Leung RC, El-Omar M, Romppanen HO, Alazzoni A, Alak A, Fung A, Alexopoulos D, Schwalm JD, Valettas N, Džavík V. Stroke in the TOTAL trial: a randomized trial of routine thrombectomy vs. percutaneous coronary intervention alone in ST elevation myocardial infarction. Eur Heart J. 2015;36(35):2364–72.

13. Higgins JP, Altman DG, Gøtzsche PC, Jüni P, Moher D, Oxman AD, Savovic J, Schulz KF, Weeks L, Sterne JA. The Cochrane Collaboration's tool for assessing risk of bias in randomised trials. BMJ. 2011;343:d5928.

14. Guyatt GH, Busse JW. Modification of Cochrane Tool to assess risk of bias in randomized trials. http://distillercer.com/resources/.

15. Guyatt GH, Oxman AD, Vist GE, Kunz R, Falck-Ytter Y, Alonso-Coello P, Schünemann HJ. GRADE: an emerging consensus on rating quality of evidence and strength of recommendations. BMJ. 2008;336:924–6.

16. Guyatt GH, Oxman AD, Vist G, Kunz R, Brozek J, Alonso-Coello P, Montori V, Akl EA, Djulbegovic B, Falck-Ytter Y, Norris SL, Williams JW Jr, Atkins D, Meerpohl J, Schünemann HJ. GRADE guidelines: 4. Rating the quality of evidence—study limitations (risk of bias). J Clin Epidemiol. 2011;64:407–15.

17. Guyatt GH, Oxman AD, Kunz R, Brozek J, Alonso-Coello P, Rind D, Devereaux PJ, Montori VM, Freyschuss B, Vist G, Jaeschke R, Williams JW Jr, Murad MH, Sinclair D, Falck-Ytter Y, Meerpohl J, Whittington C, Thorlund K, Andrews J, Schünemann HJ. GRADE guidelines 6. Rating the quality of evidence—imprecision. J Clin Epidemiol. 2011;64:1283–93.

18. Guyatt GH, Oxman AD, Kunz R, Woodcock J, Brozek J, Helfand M, Alonso-Coello P, Glasziou P, Jaeschke R, Akl EA, Norris S, Vist G, Dahm P, Shukla VK, Higgins J, Falck-Ytter Y, Schünemann HJ. GRADE guidelines: 7. Rating the quality of evidence—inconsistency. J Clin Epidemiol. 2011;64:1294–302.

19. Guyatt GH, Oxman AD, Kunz R, Woodcock J, Brozek J, Helfand M, Alonso-Coello P, Glasziou P, Jaeschke R, Akl EA, Norris S, Vist G, Dahm P, Shukla VK, Higgins J, Falck-Ytter Y, Schünemann HJ. GRADE guidelines: 8. Rating the quality of evidence—indirectness. J Clin Epidemiol. 2011;64:1303–10.

20. Guyatt GH, Oxman AD, Montori V, Vist G, Kunz R, Brozek J, Alonso-Coello P, Djulbegovic B, Atkins D, Falck-Ytter Y, Williams JW Jr, Meerpohl J, Norris SL, Akl EA, Schünemann HJ. GRADE guidelines: 5. Rating the quality of evidence—publication bias. J Clin Epidemiol. 2011;64:1277–82.

21. The Nordic Cochrane Centre. The Cochrane Collaboration. Review Manager (RevMan). 5.3. Copenhagen: The NordicCochrane Centre, The Cochrane Collaboration; 2011.

22. Orlic D, Ostojic M, Beleslin B, Borovic M, Tesic M, Milasinovic D, et al. The randomized physiologic assessment of thrombus aspiration in patients with ST-segment elevation acute myocardial infarction trial (PATA STEMI) [abstract]. Eur Heart J. 2014;35:Abstract Supplement, 45.

23. Woo SI, Park SD, Kim DH, Kwan J, Shin SH, Park KS, Kim SH, Ko KY, Hwang TH, Yoon GS, Choi WG, Kim SH. Thrombus aspiration during primary percutaneous coronary intervention for preserving the index of microcirculatory resistance: A randomised study. EuroIntervention. 2014;9(9):1057–62.

24. Shehata M. Impact of successful manual thrombus aspiration during primary PCI in diabetic patients: Angiographic and clinical follow-up [abstract]. Catheter Cardiovasc Interv. 2014;83:S3.

25. Shehata M. Angiographic and clinical impact of successful manual thrombus aspiration in diabetic patients undergoing primary PCI. Int J Vasc Med 2014b; 263926 doi:10.1155/2014/263926.

26. Lagerqvist B, Fröbert O, Olivecrona GK, Gudnason T, Maeng M, Alström P, Andersson J, Calais F, Carlsson J, Collste O, Götberg M, Hårdhammar P, Ioanes D, Kallryd A, Linder R, Lundin A, Odenstedt J, Omerovic E, Puskar V, Tödt T, Zelleroth E, Östlund O, James SK.. Outcomes 1 year after thrombus aspiration for myocardial infarction. N Engl J Med. 2014;371(12):1111–20.

27. Frobert O, Lagerqvist B, Olivecrona GK, Omerovic E, Gudnason T, Maeng M, Aasa M, Angerås O, Calais F, Danielewicz M, Erlinge D, Hellsten L, Jensen U, Johansson AC, Kåregren A, Nilsson J, Robertson L, Sandhall L, Sjögren I, Ostlund O, Harnek J, James SK. Thrombus aspiration during st-segment elevation myocardial infarction. N Engl J Med. 2013;369:1587–97.

28. Turgeman Y, Bushari LI, Antonelli D, Feldman A, Yahalom M, Bloch L, Suleiman K. Catheter Aspiration after Every Stage during Primary Percutaneous Angioplasty, ADMIT Trial. Intl J Angiol. 2014;23(1):29–40.

29. Bulum J, Ernst A, Strozzi M. The impact of successful manual thrombus aspiration on in-stent restenosis after primary PCI: Angiographic and clinical follow-up. Coron Artery Dis. 2012;23:487–91.

30. Chao CL, Hung CS, Lin YH, Lin MS, Lin LC, Ho YL, Liu CP, Chiang CH, Kao HL. Time-dependent benefit of initial thrombosuction on myocardial reperfusion in primary percutaneous coronary intervention. Int J Clin Pract. 2008;62:555–61.

31. De Luca L, Sardella G, Davidson CJ, De Persio G, Beraldi M, Tommasone T, Mancone M, Nguyen BL, Agati L, Gheorghiade M, Fedele F. Impact of intracoronary aspiration thrombectomy during primary angioplasty on left ventricular remodeling in patients with anterior ST elevation myocardial infarction. Heart. 2006;92:951–7.

32. Sardella G, Mancone M, Bucciarelli-Ducci C, Agati L, Scardala R, Carbone I, et al. Thrombus aspiration during primary percutaneous coronary intervention improves myocardial reperfusion and reduces infarct size: The EXPIRA (thrombectomy with export catheter in infarct-related artery during primary percutaneous coronary intervention) prospective, randomized trial. J Am Coll Cardiol. 2009;53:309–15.

33. Sardella G, Mancone M, Canali E, Di Roma A, Benedetti G, Stio R, Badagliacca R, Lucisano L, Agati L, Fedele F. Impact of thrombectomy with export catheter in infarct-related artery during primary percutaneous coronary intervention (EXPIRA trial) on cardiac death. Am J Cardiol. 2010;106:624–9.

34. Chevalier B, Gilard M, Lang I, Commeau P, Roosen J, Hanssen M, Lefevre T, Carrié D, Bartorelli A, Montalescot G, Parikh K. Systematic primary aspiration in acute myocardial percutaneous intervention: A multicentre randomised controlled trial of the Export aspiration catheter. EuroIntervention. 2008;4:222–8.

35. Hoole SP, Jaworski C, Brown AJ, McCormick LM, Agrawal B, Clarke SC, West NE. Serial assessment of the index of microcirculatory resistance during primary percutaneous coronary intervention comparing manual aspiration catheter thrombectomy with balloon angioplasty (IMPACT study): a randomised controlled pilot study. Open Heart. 2015;2(1):e000238.

36. Stone GW, Maehara A, Witzenbichler B, Godlewski J, Parise H, Dambrink JH, Ochala A, Carlton TW, Cristea E, Wolff SD, Brener SJ, Chowdhary S, El-Omar M, Neunteufl T, Metzger DC, Karwoski T, Dizon JM, Mehran R, Gibson CM. Intracoronary abciximab and aspiration thrombectomy in patients with large anterior myocardial infarction: The INFUSE-AMI randomized trial. JAMA. 2012;307:1817–26.

37. Stone GW, Witzenbichler B, Godlewski J, Dambrink JH, Ochala A, Chowdhary S, et al. Intralesional abciximab and thrombus aspiration in patients with large anterior myocardial infarction: One-year results from the INFUSE-AMI trial. Circ Cardiovasc Interv. 2013;6:527–34.

38. Liu CP, Lin MS, Chiu YW, Lee JK, Hsu CN, Hung CS, Kao HL. Additive benefit of glycoprotein IIb/IIIa inhibition and adjunctive thrombus aspiration during primary coronary intervention: results of the Initial Thrombosuction and Tirofiban Infusion (ITTI) trial. Int J Cardiol. 2012;156(2):174–9.

39. Kaltoft A, Bøttcher M, Nielsen SS, Hansen HH, Terkelsen C, Maeng M, Kristensen J, Thuesen L, Krusell LR, Kristensen SD, Andersen HR, Lassen JF, Rasmussen K, Rehling M, Nielsen TT, Bøtker HE. Routine thrombectomy in percutaneous coronary intervention for acute ST-segment-elevation myocardial infarction: A randomized, controlled trial. Circulation. 2006;114:40–7.

40. Liistro F, Grotti S, Angioli P, Falsini G, Ducci K, Baldassarre S, Sabini A, Brandini R, Capati E, Bolognese L. Impact of thrombus aspiration on myocardial tissue reperfusion and left ventricular functional recovery and remodeling after primary angioplasty. Circ Cardiovasc Interv. 2009;2:376–83.

41. Burzotta F, Trani C, Romagnoli E, Mazzari MA, Rebuzzi AG, De Vita M, Garramone B, Giannico F, Niccoli G, Biondi-Zoccai GG, Schiavoni G, Mongiardo R, Crea F. Manual thrombus-aspiration improves myocardial reperfusion: The randomized evaluation of the effect of mechanical reduction of distal embolization by thrombus-aspiration in primary and rescue angioplasty (REMEDIA) trial. J Am Coll Cardiol. 2005;46:371–6.

42. Sim DS, Ahn Y, Kim YH, Lee D, Seon HJ, Park KH, Yoon HJ, Yoon NS, Kim KH, Hong YJ, Park HW, Kim JH, Jeong MH, Cho JG, Park JC. Effect of manual thrombus aspiration during primary percutaneous coronary intervention on infarct size: Evaluation with cardiac computed tomography. Int J Cardio. 2013;168:4328–30.

43. Svilaas T, Vlaar PJ, van der Horst IC, Diercks GF, de Smet BJ, van den Heuvel AF, Anthonio RL, Jessurun GA, Tan ES, Suurmeijer AJ, Zijlstra F. Thrombus aspiration during primary percutaneous coronary intervention. N Engl J Med. 2008;358:557–67.

44. Vlaar PJ, Svilaas T, van der Horst IC, Diercks GF, Fokkema ML, de Smet BJ, van den Heuvel AF, Anthonio RL, Jessurun GA, Tan ES, Suurmeijer AJ, Zijlstra F. Cardiac death and reinfarction after 1 year in the thrombus aspiration during percutaneous coronary intervention in acute myocardial infarction study (tapas): A 1-year follow-up study. Lancet. 2008;371:1915–20.

45. Onuma Y, Thuesen L, van Geuns RJ, van der Ent M, Desch S, Fajadet J, Christiansen E, Smits P, Holm NR, Regar E, van Mieghem N, Borovicanin V, Paunovic D, Senshu K, van Es GA, Muramatsu T, Lee IS, Schuler G, Zijlstra F, Garcia-Garcia HM, Serruys PW. Randomized study to assess the effect of thrombus aspiration on flow area in patients with ST-elevation myocardial infarction: an optical frequency domain imaging study—TROFI trial. European Heart J. 2013;34:1050–60.

46. Garcia-Garcia HM, Muramatsu T, Nakatani S, Lee IS, Holm NR, Thuesen L, van Geuns RJ, van der Ent M, Borovicanin V, Paunovic D, Onuma Y, Serruys PW. Serial optical frequency domain imaging in STEMI patients: the follow-up report of TROFI study. European Heart J – Cardiovascular Imaging. 2014;15(9):987–95.

47. Ikari Y, Sakurada M, Kozuma K, Kawano S, Katsuki T, Kimura K, Suzuki T, Yamashita T, Takizawa A, Misumi K, Hashimoto H, Isshiki T. Upfront thrombus aspiration in primary coronary intervention for patients with ST-segment elevation acute myocardial infarction: Report of the VAMPIRE (vacuum aspiration thrombus removal) trial. JACC Cardiovasc Interv. 2008;1:424–31.

48. Yin D, Zhu H, Zhou X, Huang R, Wang J, Zheng Z. Thrombus aspiration before angiography during percutaneous coronary intervention in acute myocardial infarction. J Dalian Med Univ. 2011;33:235–9.

49. D'Ascenzo F, Barbero U, Moretti C, Palmerini T, Della Riva D, Mariani A, Omedè P, DiNicolantonio JJ, Biondi-Zoccai G, Gaita F. Percutaneous coronary intervention versus coronary artery bypass graft for stable angina: meta-regression of randomized trials. Contemp Clin Trials. 2014;38(1):51–8.

50. Elgendy IY, Huo T, Bhatt DL, Bavry AA. Is Aspiration Thrombectomy Beneficial in Patients Undergoing Primary Percutaneous Coronary Intervention? Meta-Analysis of Randomized Trials. Circ Cardiovasc Interv. 2015;8(7).

51. Barkagan M, Steinvil A, Berchenko Y, Finkelstein A, Keren G, Banai S, Halkin A. Impact of routine manual aspiration thrombectomy on outcomes of patients undergoing primary percutaneous coronary intervention for acute myocardial infarction: A meta-analysis. Int J Cardiol. 2016;204:189–95.

16

Risk factors and in-hospital outcome of acute ST segment elevation myocardial infarction in young Bangladeshi adults

Mohammad Azizul Karim[1], Abdullah Al Shafi Majumder[1], Khandaker Qamrul Islam[1], Muhammad Badrul Alam[2], Makhan Lal Paul[3], Mohammad Shafiqul Islam[4], Kamrun N. Chowdhury[5] and Sheikh Mohammed Shariful Islam[6,7,8*]

Abstract

Background: South Asians have a higher overall incidence rate and younger age of onset for acute myocardial infarction (AMI) compared to Western populations. However, limited information is available on the association of preventable risk factors and outcomes of AMI among young individuals in Bangladesh. The aim of this study was to determine the risk factors and in-hospital outcome of AMI among young (age ≤40 years) adults in Bangladesh.

Methods: We conducted a prospective observational study among consecutive 50 patients aged ≤40 years and 50 patients aged >40 years with acute ST Segment Elevation Myocardial Infarction (STEMI) and followed-up in-hospital at the National Institute of Cardiovascular Diseases (NICVD). Clinical characteristics, biochemical findings, diet, echocardiography and in-hospital outcomes were compared between the two groups. Multivariate logistic regression was performed to assess the association between risk factors and in-hospital outcome in young patients adjusting for other confounding variables.

Results: The mean age of the young and older patient groups was 36.5 ± 4.6 years and 57.0 ± 9.1 years respectively. Male sex (OR 3.4, 95 % CI 1.2 – 9.75), smoking (OR 2.4, 95 % CI 1.04 – 5,62), family history of MI (OR 2.4, 95 % CI 1.11 – 5,54), homocysteine (OR 1.2, 95 % CI 1.08 – 1.36), eating rice ≥2 times daily (OR 3.5, 95 % CI 1.15 – 10.6) and eating beef (OR 4.5, 95 % CI 1.83 – 11.3) were significantly associated with the risk of AMI in the young group compared to older group. In multivariate analysis, older patients had significantly greater chance of developing heart failure (OR 7.5, 95 % CI 1.51 to 37.31), re-infarction (OR 7.0, 95 % CI 1.08 – 45.72), arrhythmia (OR 15.3, 95 % CI 2.69 – 87.77) and cardiogenic shock (OR 69.0, 95 % CI 5.81 – 85.52) than the younger group.

Conclusion: Younger AMI patients have a different risk profile and better in-hospital outcomes compared to the older patients. Control of preventable risk factors such as smoking, unhealthy diet, obesity and dyslipidemia should be reinforced at an early age in Bangladesh.

Background

Cardiovascular disease (CVD) is a global health problem reaching epidemic proportions in both developed and developing countries and it is the leading cause of mortality and morbidity worldwide [1, 2]. The South Asian countries have among the highest incidences of CVD globally [3]. Estimates from the global burden of disease study suggests that by the year 2020 this part of the world will have more individuals with atherosclerotic CVD than any other region [3, 4].

South Asian populations have an increased risk and 5–10 years earlier onset for acute myocardial infarction (AMI) compared to Western populations. In recent years, the frequency of AMI in the younger population is increasing [3, 5, 6]. AMI in young individuals can cause death and disability in the prime of life and has serious consequences for the patients, their family and health systems of the nation, causing an increased economic burden. Previous studies have shown that young AMI patients (<40 years) had a high prevalence of smoking, family history and dyslipidemia and a

---

* Correspondence: shariful.islam@icddrb.org
[6]International Center for Diarrhoeal Disease Research, Bangladesh, Center for Control of Chronic Diseases, Dhaka, Bangladesh
[7]Center for International Health, University of Munich, Munich, Germany
Full list of author information is available at the end of the article

relatively high incidence of normal coronary arteries, non-obstructive stenosis or single-vessel disease [7–9]. Identifying the risk factors for AMI in this group of people is necessary for risk factor modification and developing cost-effective secondary prevention strategies as young AMI patients have different clinical characteristics and pathophysiology from that in older patients [10]. Several studies have documented the classical risk factors for ischemic heart disease (IHD). However, the role of these risk factors in the pathogenesis of IHD and whether they are equally important for the young patients in Bangladesh is still not yet convincingly established. Data on risk factors and in-hospital outcomes for young AMI patients are limited in Bangladesh. We therefore conducted this study to determine the risk factors and in-hospital outcome of AMI among young patients (≤40 years) compared to older (>40 years) patients in Dhaka, Bangladesh. Our hypothesis was that younger patients would have better outcomes and a different pattern of risk factors than older patients.

Methods

Study population and setting

We conducted a prospective observational study of 100 patients with AMI attending the Department of Cardiology, National Institute of Cardiovascular Diseases (NICVD), Dhaka between July 2010 and June 2011. We recruited 50 consecutive patients aged less than 40 years and 50 consecutive patients aged 40 years or older. The inclusion criteria were adult patients of both sexes presenting with first acute ST Segment Elevation Myocardial Infarction (STEMI) or AMI within 12 hours onset of chest pain and providing informed consent. The exclusion criteria were: patients with valvular heart disease, congenital heart disease and cardiomyopathy; patients with other major disorders such as severe renal impairment, cancers, systemic infection and those not willing to provide written informed consent. The diagnosis of AMI was established based on the following criteria: detection of rise and/or fall of cardiac biomarkers (preferably troponin) with at least one value above the 99th percentile of the upper reference limit (URL) together with evidence of myocardial ischemia with at least one of the following: symptoms of ischemia; ECG changes indicative of new ischemia (new ST-T changes or new left bundle branch block [LBBB]); development of pathological Q waves in the ECG; imaging evidence of new loss of viable myocardium or new regional wall motion abnormality [11].

Data collection

All participants presenting at the Emergency Room of NICVD with acute onset of chest pain during the last 12 hours were screened for eligibility by the attending physician. All eligible participants were referred to the study team by the attending physician and first interviewed by a member of the research team at the wards of Cardiology Department, NICVD after the patient's condition were stable. Blood for biochemical tests were collected from the wards by laboratory assistants experienced in blood collection and sent to NICVD laboratory for analysis. One of the investigator (MAK) performed bedside echocardiography tests in the wards. All participants were followed up during the hospitalization period.

Data were collected using a structured questionnaire and pretested clinical examination form (Supplementary File 1) through face-to-face interviews and clinical examination. The questionnaire contained the following information: demographic data , anthropometric measurements, risk factors (dietary pattern, current tobacco use, family history of premature CAD, history of angina). Dietary pattern was assessed by asking questions on specific food intake. Clinical and laboratory data included: blood pressure (BP), biochemical tests (random blood sugar (RBS), serum creatinine, serum electrolytes, fasting lipid profile, troponin-I, fasting blood sugar (FBS), 2 hours after fasting glucose, fasting plasma total homocysteine level, serum uric acid), electrocardiography (ECG), echocardiography and in-hospital outcomes (as defined below). Weight, height, waist circumference (WC), hip circumference (HC), waist-hip ratio (WHR) was measured using standard clinical guidelines [12]. Body mass index (BMI) was measured as weight in kilograms^2 divided by height in centimeters. Blood pressure was measured twice (at admission) and the average value was recorded. Echocardiography was done at least two times, first, within 24 hours of admission and last, on the day of discharge, or even more frequently if indicated. Echocardiographic variables included LVID (d), LVID (s), regional wall motion abnormality (RWMA) and left ventricular ejection fraction (LVEF).

Definition of variables

Hypertension was defined as > 140 mmHg systolic BP or >90 mmHg diastolic BP on at least two occasions or current use of any antihypertensive therapy [13]. Diabetes was diagnosed when patient had classical symptoms of diabetes plus random plasma glucose concentration ≥200 mg/dl (11.1 mmol/L) or FPG ≥126 mg/dl (7 mmol/L) or 2-hr post load glucose ≥ 200 mg/dl (11.1 mmol/L) during an OGTT or using anti-diabetic medications. Dyslipidemia was diagnosed according to ATP-III criteria: LDL cholesterol >100 mg/dl, Total cholesterol > 200 mg/dl, HDL cholesterol <40 mg/dl, triglycerides >150 mg/dl [14]. Family early history of ischemic heart disease (IHD) was considered when any direct blood relative (parents, siblings, children) had any of the following at age <55 years: angina, MI, sudden cardiac death without obvious cause [15]. Cardiogenic shock was defined as evidence of tissue hypo perfusion included by heart

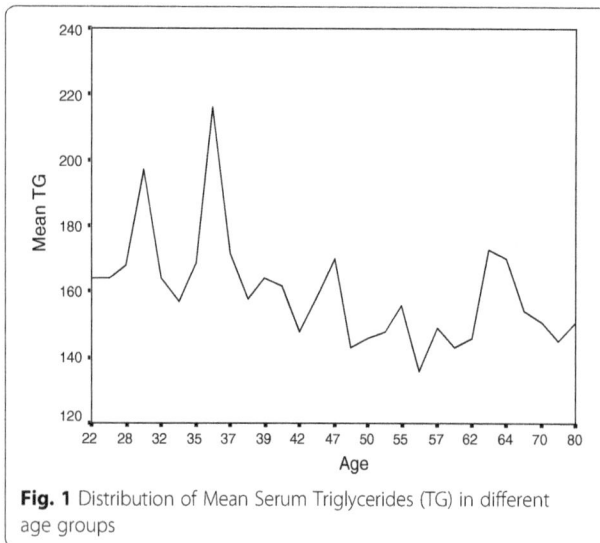

Fig. 1 Distribution of Mean Serum Triglycerides (TG) in different age groups

failure after correction of preload. Cardiogenic shock was usually characterized by: reduced BP (systolic BP <90 mmHg or a drop of mean arterial pressure >30 mmHg) and/or, low urine output (<0.5 ml/kg/h), pulse rate >60 bpm with or without evidence of organ congestion. For congestive cardiac failure we used Killip classification as follows: Class I: Absence of rales over the lung fields and absence of S3; Class II: Crackles/rales over 50 % or less of the lung fields ± presence of am S3 gallop; Class III: Crackles/rales over >50 % of the lung fields and S3 gallop. Class IV: Cardiogenic shock [15]. BMI was calculated as weight (kg)/height squared (m2) and classified as: underweight < 18.5, normal 18.5 – 24.9, overweight 25.0 – 29.9 and obesity ≥30 [16]. In-hospital outcomes: All patients were followed up during hospitalization and clinical outcome was recorded based

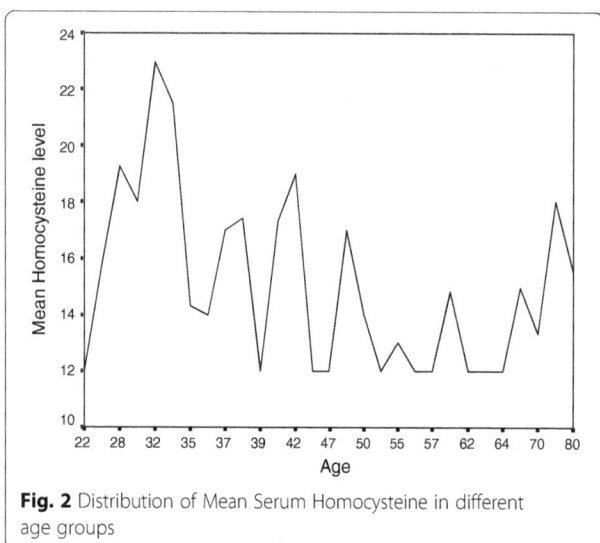

Fig. 2 Distribution of Mean Serum Homocysteine in different age groups

on standard criteria as: duration of hospital stay, heart failure, post-MI angina, re-infarction, mechanical complications, significant arrhythmia, cardiogenic shock (as defined below) and death.

Ethics
Written informed consent was taken from each patient before data collection. Confidentiality was strictly maintained and the patients were informed about the study and their rights to withdraw at any stage which would not hamper the rights to treatments. The study protocol was approved by the institutional review board of National Institute of Cardiovascular Diseases (NICVD), Dhaka.

Data analysis
Data were analyzed using SPSS version 17 (SPSS Corp. Texas, USA). Data are expressed in frequencies (n), percentage (%), and means ± standard deviation (Mean ± SD). The two study groups were compared using Student's t-test and Fisher's exact test for continuous variables and chi-square test for categorical variable, as applicable. Multivariate logistic regression analysis was performed to examine associated risk factors of AMI and in-hospital outcomes controlling for confounding variables (education and socioeconomic status). A p-value of less than 0.05 was considered to be statistically significant.

Results
Clinical characteristics and biochemical status
Table 1 shows the clinical characteristics and biochemical findings of the study participants. The mean ± SD age of the young and older groups was 36.5 ± 4.6 and 57.0 ± 9.1 years respectively. Majority of patients were male (young 88 % vs. old 68 %). The younger group had a significantly higher proportion of smoking (74 % vs 54 %), family history of IHD (56 % vs 34 %) and higher BMI. In contrast, hypertension (15 % vs 76 %), diabetes (22 % vs 46 %) and history of angina (12 % vs 48 %) were significantly higher among participants of the older group. Mean serum homocysteine and triglyceride were significantly higher in the younger group and mean HDL cholesterol was significantly higher in the older group. The mean C-reactive protein (CRP), uric acid, total cholesterol and LDL cholesterol levels were higher in the younger group, but the difference was not statistically significant. There was no significant difference in mean random blood sugar by age ($p = 0.37$) Figs. 1, 2 .

Food habits
The food habits of the study participants are presented in Table 2. The mean frequency of eating rice, beef, chicken and fish was significantly higher in the younger

Table 1 Clinical characteristics and biochemical status of study participants (n = 100)

Variables	Young group (age ≤ 40) (n = 50)	Older group (age > 40) (n = 50)	p-value
Clinical characteristics			
Age (Mean ± SD)	36.5 ± 4.6	57.0 ± 9.1	0.001[*]
Male sex	44 (88)	34 (68)	0.02
Smoking	37 (74)	27 (54)	0.04
Chewing tobacco	7 (14)	16 (32)	0.03
Dyslipidemia	26 (52)	20 (40)	0.22
Hypertension	7 (14)	38 (76)	0.001
Diabetes mellitus	11 (22)	23 (46)	0.01
Family history of IHD	28 (56)	17 (34)	0.02
BMI (mean ± SD)	25.21 ± 3.6	24.26 ± 3.61	0.19[a]
Normal (18.5 – 24.9)	23 (56)	28 (56)	0.32
Over weight (25 – 29.9)	16 (32)	14 (28)	0.66
Obese (≥30)	11 (22)	8 (16)	0.44
Waist hip ratio (mean ± SD)	0.96 ± 0.06	0.95 ± 0.05	0.42
Waist hip ratio (>1)	13 (26.0)	9 (18.0)	0.33
History of angina	6 (12)	17 (48)	0.02
Biochemical status			
Serum homocysteine	17.14 ± 5.12	13.84 ± 2.93	0.001
C-reactive protein (CRP)	14.66 ± 6.8	13.02 ± 2.53	0.11
Uric acid	6.7 ± 6.0	5.6 ± 0.6	0.21
Random blood sugar (RBS)	10.6 ± 6.2	11.7 ± 6.0	0.37
Total cholesterol	193.10 ± 21.95	186.58 ± 22.20	0.14
Triglyceride	165.26 ± 23.52	150.40 ± 16.88	0.01
LDL cholesterol	121.69 ± 22.36	113.80 ± 25.05	0.10
HDL cholesterol	38.36 ± 4.11	42.70 ± 4.83	0.01

Values are Mean ± SD or n(%) unless otherwise indicated
[*]p value reached from unpaired t-test
[a]chi-square test

Table 2 Distribution of study subjects by food consumption

Variables	Young group (age ≤ 40)	Older group (age > 40)	p-value
Rice	50 (100)	50 (100)	
Frequency (per day)	1.98 ± 0.42	1.78 ± 0.54	0.04
1 time	5 (10)	14 (28)	
≥2 times	45 (90)	36 (72)	
Bread	50 (100)	48 (96)	
Frequency (per day)	1.12 ± 0.32	1.28 ± 0.45	0.04
1 time	44 (88)	36 (72)	
2 times	6 (12)	14 (28)	
Beef	25 (50)	9 (18)	
Frequency (per week)	2.04 ± 0.84	1.33 ± 0.50	0.02
1 time	8 (32)	6 (66.7)	
≥2 times	17 (68)	3 (33.3)	
Mutton	4 (8)	2 (4)	
Frequency (per week)	1.50 ± 0.57	2 ± 0.5	0.31
Chicken	43 (86)	47 (94)	
Frequency (per week)	1.33 ± 0.52	1.13 ± 0.33	0.03
1 time	30 (69.8)	41 (87.2)	
≥2 times	13 (30.2)	6 (12.8)	
Fish	50 (100)	50 (100)	
Frequency (per week)	2.80 ± 0.90	1.13 ± 0.80	0.03
1 – 2 times	19 (38)	32 (64)	
≥3 times	31 (62)	18 (36)	
Egg	5 (10)	4 (8)	
Frequency (per week)	2.80 ± 2.3	1.00 ± 1.20	0.18
Milk	4 (8)	3 (6)	
Frequency (per week)	1.25 ± 0.50	1.33 ± 0.57	0.84
Fruits	50 (100)	49 (98)	
Frequency (per week)	1.74 ± 0.66	2.02 ± 0.24	0.02
1 time	19 (38)	1 (2)	
≥2 times	31 (62)	48 (98)	
Vegetables	50 (100)	50 (100)	
Frequency (per week)	3.40 ± 0.83	3.78 ± 0.58	0.01
2 times	9 (18)	4 (8)	
3 times	14 (28)	3 (6)	
>4 times	27 (54)	43 (86)	

values are n(%) and mean ± SD

group. The older group reported a significantly higher frequency of eating bread, fruits and vegetables. The younger group reported higher consumption of rice (≥2 times a day), beef ≥2 times per month, chicken ≥2 times per month and fish ≥3 times per month, while the older group reported higher proportion of fruit consumption (≥2 times) and vegetables ≥4 times per week.

Echocardiography findings
The frequency of anterior, inferior and anteroseptal MI was similar in both the groups (Table 3). The mean ± SD of left ventricular ejection fraction (LVEF) was significantly higher in the younger group (p = 0.004). The incidence of heart failure (according to Killip classification) and presence of any arrhythmia was not significantly different by age. The proportion of mechanical complications of MR was higher in the older group than younger group (p < 0.05).

In-hospital outcomes
Table 4 shows the in-hospital outcome of the study participants. The mean duration of hospitalization was almost double in the older group than in the younger

Table 3 Echocardiography findings of the study participants (N = 100)

Variables	Young group (age ≤ 40) n = 50 Number (%)	Older group (age > 40) n = 50 Number (%)	p-value
Wall involvement			
Anterior MI	23 (46)	22 (44)	NS
Inferior MI	16 (32)	18 (36)	NS
Antero-septal MI	11 (22)	10 (20)	NS
Left ventricular ejection fraction (LVEF)			
LVEF	54.4 ± 7.7	49.8 ± 7.8	0.004
<40	0 (0)	2 (4)	
40 – 49	10 (20)	22 (44)	0.01
≥50	40 (80)	26 (52)	0.003
Incidence of heart failure (Killip classification)			
Class I	2 (4)	5 (10)	0.23
Class II	2 (4)	3 (6)	0.64
Class III	0 (0)	2 (4)	
Class IV	1 (2)	3 (6)	0.30
Pattern of arrhythmia			
CHB	2 (4)	7 (14)	0.08
AF	1 (2)	3 (6)	0.30
VT/VF	2 (4)	3 (6)	0.60
Mechanical complications			
MR	1 (2)	6 (12)	0.05
VSR	0 (0)	1 (2)	

group ($p = 0.001$). The survival rates were higher in younger group but not statistically significant ($p = 0.05$). Older group had significantly worse clinical evolution in terms of higher rates of heart failure, significant arrhythmias and mechanical complications. Fatal outcome due to anterior

Table 4 Comparison of in-hospital outcome between two groups (N = 100)

Variables	Young group (age ≤ 40) (n = 50) Number (%)	Older group (age > 40) (n = 50) Number (%)	p-value
Duration of hospital stay (days) (Mean ± SD)	5.08 ± 1.8	10.7 ± 1.8	0.001
Heart failure	5 (10)	13 (26)	0.04
Post MI angina	3 (6)	8 (16)	0.11
Re-infarction	2 (4)	5 (10)	0.23
Significant arrhythmias	5 (10)	13 (26)	0.04
Cardiogenic shock	1 (2)	3 (6)	0.30
Mechanical complications	1 (2)	7 (14)	0.02
Death	1 (2)	6 (12)	0.05

and inferior MI was less frequent in the younger group (13.64 %) vs. older group (33.33 %) $p = 0.05$.

Table 5 presents the results of logistic regression analysis for risk factors and in-hospital outcomes in young patients. Male sex (OR 3.4, 95 % CI 1.2 to 9.75), smoking (OR 2.4, 95 % CI 1.04 to 5,62), family history of IHD (OR 2.4, 95 % CI 1.11 to 5,54), homocysteine level (OR 1.2, 95 % CI 1.08 to 1.36), taking rice ≥2 times daily (OR 3.5, 95 % CI 1.15 to 10.6) and taking beef (OR 4.5, 95 % CI 1.83 to 11.3) were significant risk factors for development of AMI in the younger group compared to the older group. Older patients had approximately 7.5 times more chance of developing heart failure (OR 7.5, 95 % CI 1.51 to 37.31), 7 times more chance of developing re-infraction (OR 7.0, 95 % CI 1.08 to 45.72), 15 times more chance of developing arrhythmia (OR 15.3, 95 % CI 2.69 to 87.77), 69 times more chance of developing cardiogenic shock (OR 69.0, 95 % CI 5.81 – 85.52) than the younger group, which was statistically significant.

Discussion

This study, to the best of knowledge, is the first in Bangladesh to demonstrate the risk factors and in-hospital outcomes of AMI in young people. The study shows that majority of young AMI patients were male and a family history of IHD, smoking, overweight, increased homocysteine and triglycerides were the most common risk factors among young patients. Young patients showed a different risk factor profile and better survival rates and in-hospital outcomes compared to the older group.

A majority of our participants were male, which is consistent with previous studies in Bangladesh by which the percentage of male patients were 85 – 92 % [17, 18]. A study by Khan and colleagues with young AMI patients reported smoking (84.4 %), hypertension (46.9 %), dyslipidemia (56.3 %), diabetes (12.5 %), family history (34.4 %) with higher triglyceride level and lower HDL [19]. These findings are consistent with previous studies [8, 19–21]. Another study in Bangladesh showed that AMI in young patients is most commonly seen in males and the most frequent risk factor was smoking [22]. In our study, males had 3.4 times significantly greater chances of developing AMI at younger age compared to females.

Almost half of our participants had higher BMI and one-quarter of young AMI patients had WHR < 1. Younger patients had higher BMI and WHR, but the difference was not statistically significant. Both BMI and WHR are predictors of CVD and mortality [23]. A study in Bangladesh showed an association between hypertension and dyslipidemia [24]. In our study young AMI patients had higher dyslipidemia and lower hypertension than older patients. Our findings support the emphasis on smoking cessation and life-style interventions to prevent

Table 5 Logistic regression for risk factors and in-hospital outcomes of AMI in young group

Independent variables	B	Wald	OR	95 % CI		p value
				Lower	Upper	
Male sex	1.239	5.454	3.451	1.220	9.759	0.02
Smoking	0.886	4.252	2.425	1.045	5.626	0.04
Family history of IHD	0.904	4.804	2.471	1.110	5.547	0.03
BMI (Overweight)	0.191	0.190	1.210	0.514	2.851	0.66
Homocysteine level	0.198	11.453	1.219	1.087	1.367	0.001
TG	0.036	10.633	1.037	1.014	1.059	0.001
LDL	0014	2.633	1.015	0.997	1.035	0.11
HDL	−0.356	17.316	0.70	0.592	0.826	0.001
Eating rice (≥2 times daily)	1.253	4.883	3.50	1.152	10.633	0.03
Eating beef (per week)	1.516	10.670	4.56	1.834	11.316	0.01
Vegetables (≥2 times) weekly	−1.655	11.105	0.191	0.072	0.506	0.001
Heart Failure	2.018	6.102	7.524	1.517	37.311	0.01
Re-infarction	1.952	4.179	7.040	1.084	45.727	0.04
Arrhythmia	2.733	9.464	15.385	2.696	87.776	0.002
Cardiogenic shock	4.234	11.246	69.00	5.809	85.519	0.001

CVD among young persons. Previous studies have suggested that in young AMI patients coronary artery spasm might lead to temporary occlusion of the vessel or thrombus or a combination as a result of smoking and dyslipidemia [7, 25]. Therefore, creating awareness for smoking cessation, healthy diet, early screening and interventions such as use of anti-platelet medications and distal protection might be more effective in this group of patients.

Results of our study showed that younger group had higher mean homocysteine, CRP, uric acid and TG and lower HDL cholesterol levels compared to the older group. A study in Bangladesh showed that elevated levels of CRP are significantly and inversely associated with angiographically visible coronary collateral development assessed by Rentrop classification [18]. The study also reported that young patients had significantly higher TG and lower HDL-C, which are known risk factors for AMI [18]. Therefore, our participants might have developed fewer coronary collaterals which might cause premature AMI in this younger group of patients. Previous studies showed significant increase in number of coronary artery involvement by atherosclerotic lesions with increasing levels of plasma homocysteine level [26], which is a strong predictor of mortality in patients with angiographically confirmed coronary artery disease [27]. A study in Bangladesh showed no vessel involvement was more common in young group than older group (21.9 % vs 12.5 %). The younger age group has less favorable lipid profile than older age group having raised total cholesterol, decreased HDL and raised LDL [19].

In this study the mean ejection fraction was significantly higher among young group, as was expected. In our younger and older group, anterior-MI, inferior-MI and antero-septal-MI was 46 % vs. 44 %, 32 % vs. 36 % and 22 % vs. 20 % between groups respectively. A study in Bangladesh among young patients with CVD showed 9.37 % non-Q MI, 28.12 % acute anterior MI, 14.06 % acute anteroseptal-MI, 26.56 % acute inferior-MI, 6.25 % acute infero-posterior-MI [28].

In this study, the younger group reported to consume significantly higher frequency of rice and beef and significantly lower frequency of fruits and vegetables compared to the older group. Previous studies have shown that unhealthy diet rich in carbohydrate and low in fruits and vegetables are a major risk factor for CVD [24, 29, 30]. Dietary results are difficult to compare due to differences in study design and variations of food habits in different countries. However, our result are consistent with other previous studies [31, 32].

AMI in young adults is not as well characterized as in older adults, and limited data suggest that prognosis may be better in this group [33]. Our results showed that AMI was associated with significantly higher mortality and cardiovascular events in the elderly compared with the young, which is similar to an Indian study. [34] In a study by Chowdhury & Marsh, the in-hospital mortality rate among young MI patients was approximately 1 – 6 % compared to 8 – 22 % in the older patients. [35] Another study showed that AMI in young patients presented with acute onset of symptoms, angiographically complex stenosis morphologic features, and less extensive CAD [36].

AMI in young patients causes significant morbidity, psychological effects, and financial constraints for the person and the family [37]. Screening for risk factors in the young population may help to improve prognosis and prevent AMI in young age [38].

Our result showing better clinical outcome among younger patient is in agreement with previous reports [10, 39]. However, studies in other countries have suggested that although in-hospital outcomes are better in young AMI patients due to less severe coronary vessel involvements, in the long run complications such as history of previous MI, peripheral vascular disease and low ejection fraction are high risks for mortality [40, 41].

Limitation of the study

Our study has features and limitations that should be kept in mind when using and interpreting its results. First, we conducted an observation study on limited number of patients in a single hospital. Therefore, the results might not be sufficient to change clinical practice or policy recommendations. Further multi-center longitudinal studies with adequate samples and power are recommended. Second, data were collected from one hospital and might not represent the overall AMI population. However, NICVD is the largest tertiary hospital for cardiovascular diseases in the country and patients are referred here for better management from all over Bangladesh. Third, dietary data were collected based on self-reports from patients and recall bias might be a problem. Forth, multiple comparisons were made with limited data and the probability for type I and type II errors can be ruled out as we could not adjust for multiple hypothesis testing. Finally, our patients were not evaluated angiographically and we did not collect the data on percutaneous revascularization and its outcome, which might provide better information.

Conclusion

This is the first study to present the risk factors and immediate in-hospital outcome of AMI in young patients in Bangladesh. Our results show that young patients with AMI commonly had different risk profile, less extensive MI and better in-hospital survival compared with older patients. Also, young AMI patients had higher prevalence of smoking, family history, unhealthy diet, overweight and dyslipidemia, which are preventable risk factors and should be considered for prevention of AMI in Bangladesh and other developing countries. Further large controlled studies with angiographic exploration and long-term follow up are needed to confirm the pathogenesis of AMI in young patients.

Competing interests

The authors declare that they have no competing interests.

Authors' contributions

MAK initiated the concept and conducted the data collection. AASM was the supervisor and KQI and MBA were co-supervisors for this study and contributed to study design, developing clinical guidelines, providing intellectual contribution. KNC and SMSI were involved in data analysis and manuscript writing. All authors have read the final version and agreed for publication.

Acknowledgements

The authors thank Professor Fabio Zicker, Senior Visiting Professor, International Health - Center for Technological Development in Health (CDTS) at Fiocruz Foundation, Rio de Janeiro, Brazil for editorial assistance. The authors are grateful to all the participants in the study for providing valuable data. We would also like to acknowledge the support of Faculty of NICVD at different stage of the study.

Author details

[1]National Institute of Cardiovascular Diseases (NICVD), Dhaka, Bangladesh. [2]Rangpur Medical College, Rangpur, Bangladesh. [3]Central Medical College, Comilla, Bangladesh. [4]Trishal Health Complex, Mymensingh, Bangladesh. [5]Department of Epidemiology, National Centre for Control of Rheumatic Fever and Heart Disease, Dhaka, Bangladesh. [6]International Center for Diarrhoeal Disease Research, Bangladesh, Center for Control of Chronic Diseases, Dhaka, Bangladesh. [7]Center for International Health, University of Munich, Munich, Germany. [8]Cardiovascular Division, The George Institute for Global Health, Sydney, Australia.

References

1. Murray CJ, Lopez AD. Measuring the global burden of disease. N Engl J Med. 2013;369(5):448–57.
2. Islam SMS, Purnat TD, Phuong NTA, Mwingira U, Schacht K, Fröschl G. Non-Communicable Diseases (NCDs) in developing countries: a symposium report. Global Health. 2014;10(1):81.
3. Joshi P, Islam S, Pais P, Reddy S, Dorairaj P, Kazmi K, et al. Risk factors for early myocardial infarction in South Asians compared with individuals in other countries. JAMA. 2007;297(3):286–94.
4. Yusuf S, Reddy S, Ôunpuu S, Anand S. Global burden of cardiovascular diseases part I: general considerations, the epidemiologic transition, risk factors, and impact of urbanization. Circulation. 2001;104(22):2746–53.
5. McKeigue P. Coronary heart disease in Indians, Pakistanis, and Bangladeshis: aetiology and possibilities for prevention. Br Heart J. 1992;67(5):341.
6. Sharma M, Ganguly NK. Premature coronary artery disease in Indians and its associated risk factors. Vasc Health Risk Manag. 2005;1(3):217.
7. Williams M, Restieaux N, Low C. Myocardial infarction in young people with normal coronary arteries. Heart. 1998;79(2):191–4.
8. Zimmerman FH, Cameron A, Fisher LD, Grace N. Myocardial infarction in young adults: angiographic characterization, risk factors and prognosis (Coronary Artery Surgery Study Registry). J Am Coll Cardiol. 1995;26(3):654–61.
9. Doughty M, Mehta R, Bruckman D, Das S, Karavite D, Tsai T, et al. Acute myocardial infarction in the young— The University of Michigan experience. Am Heart J. 2002;143(1):56–62.
10. Shiraishi J, Kohno Y, Yamaguchi S, Arihara M, Hadase M, Hyogo M, et al. Acute myocardial infarction in young Japanese adults. Circ J. 2005;69(12):1454–8.
11. Braunwald E, Antman EM, Beasley JW, Califf RM, Cheitlin MD, Hochman JS, et al. ACC/AHA 2002 guideline update for the management of patients with unstable angina and non–ST-segment elevation myocardial infarction—summary article: a report of the American College of Cardiology/American Heart Association task force on practice guidelines (Committee on the Management of Patients With Unstable Angina). J Am Coll Cardiol. 2002;40(7):1366–74.
12. Center for Disease Control (CDC). National Health and Nutrition Examination Survey (NHANES) Anthropometry Procedures. Centers for Disease Control and Prevention National Center for Health Statistics NHANES 1999-2000

Body Composition Procedures Manual (2000) Available at:http://www.cdc.gov/nchs/data/nhanes/bc.pdf. Accessed November 15, 2014.

13. Lenfant C, Chobanian AV, Jones DW, Roccella EJ. Seventh report of the joint national committee on the prevention, detection, evaluation, and treatment of high blood pressure (JNC 7) resetting the hypertension sails. Circulation. 2003;107(24):2993–4.

14. Lorenzo C, Williams K, Hunt KJ, Haffner SM. The National Cholesterol Education Program–Adult Treatment Panel III, International Diabetes Federation, and World Health Organization definitions of the metabolic syndrome as predictors of incident cardiovascular disease and diabetes. Diabetes Care. 2007;30(1):8–13.

15. Smith SC, Blair SN, Bonow RO, Brass LM, Cerqueira MD, Dracup K, et al. AHA/ACC guidelines for preventing heart attack and death in patients with atherosclerotic cardiovascular disease: 2001 update a statement for healthcare professionals from the American Heart Association and the American College of Cardiology. Circulation. 2001;104(13):1577–9.

16. WHO EC. Appropriate body-mass index for Asian populations and its implications for policy and intervention strategies. Lancet. 2004;363(9403):157.

17. Islam A, Faruque M, Chowdhury A, Khan H, Haque M, Ali M, et al. Risk factor analysis and angiographic profiles in first 228 cases undergone coronary angiography in cardiac Cath Lab of Dhaka medical college hospital. Cardiovasc J. 2011;3(2):122–5.

18. Majumder A, Karim M, Rahman M, Uddin M. Study of association of C-reactive protein with coronary collateral development. Cardiovasc J. 2010;3(1):26–32.

19. Khan A, Majumder A. Study of lipid profile and coronary angiographic pattern in young Bangladeshi patients with acute coronary syndrome. Cardiovasc J. 2009;1(2):183–8.

20. Islam M, Ali A, Khan N, Rahman A, Majumder A, Chowdhury W, et al. Comparative study of coronary collaterals in diabetic and nondiabetic patients by angiography. Mymensingh Med J. 2006;15(2):170–5.

21. Islam SMS, Alam DS, Wahiduzzaman M, Niessen LW, Froeschl G, Ferrari U, et al. Clinical characteristics and complications of patients with type 2 diabetes attending an urban hospital in Bangladesh. Diabetes Metab Syndr. 2014;9(1):7-13.

22. Patwary M, Reza A, Akanda M, Islam A, Majumder A, Mohibullah A, et al. Risk factors and pattern of coronary artery disease in young patients with acute myocardial infarction. Univ Heart J. 2008;4(1):20–3.

23. Myint PK, Kwok CS, Luben RN, Wareham NJ, Khaw K-T. Body fat percentage, body mass index and waist-to-hip ratio as predictors of mortality and cardiovascular disease. Heart. 2014; heartjnl-2014-305816.

24. Choudhury KN, Mainuddin A, Wahiduzzaman M, Islam SMS. Serum lipid profile and its association with hypertension in Bangladesh. Vasc Health Risk Manag. 2014;10:327.

25. Tun A, Khan IA. Myocardial infarction with normal coronary arteries: the pathologic and clinical perspectives. Angiology. 2001;52(5):299–304.

26. Kabir M, Majumder A, Bari M, Chowdhury A, Islam A. Coronary angiographic severity in patients with raised plasma homocysteine level. Cardiovasc J. 2009;1(2):169–73.

27. Nygård O, Nordrehaug JE, Refsum H, Ueland PM, Farstad M, Vollset SE. Plasma homocysteine levels and mortality in patients with coronary artery disease. N Eng J Med. 1997;337(4):230–7.

28. Haque A, Siddiqui A, Rahman S, Iqbal S, Fatema N, Khan Z. Acute coronary syndrome in the young-risk factors and angiographic pattern. Cardiovasc J. 2010;2(2):175–8.

29. Chen Y, McClintock TR, Segers S, Parvez F, Islam T, Ahmed A, et al. Prospective investigation of major dietary patterns and risk of cardiovascular mortality in Bangladesh. Int J Cardiol. 2013;167(4):1495–1.

30. Mirelman A, Koehlmoos TP, Niessen L. Risk-attributable burden of chronic diseases and cost of prevention in Bangladesh. Global Heart. 2012; 7(1):10.1016/j.gheart.2012.1001.1006.

31. Klein LW, Nathan S. Coronary artery disease in young adults*. J Am Coll Cardiol. 2003;41(4):529–31.

32. Malmberg K, Båvenholm P, Hamsten A. Clinical and biochemical factors associated with prognosis after myocardial infarction at a young age. J Am Coll Cardiol. 1994;24(3):592–9.

33. Rubin J, Borden W. Coronary heart disease in young adults. Curr Atheroscler Rep. 2012;14(2):140–9.

34. Mehta RH, Rathore SS, Radford MJ, Wang Y, Wang Y, Krumholz HM. Acute myocardial infarction in the elderly: differences by age. J Am Coll Cardiol. 2001;38(3):736–41.

35. Choudhury L, Marsh JD. Myocardial infarction in young patients. Am J Med. 1999;107(3):254–61.

36. Chen L, Chester M, Kaski JC. Clinical factors and angiographic features associated with premature coronary artery disease. CHEST J. 1995;108(2):364–9.

37. Egred M, Viswanathan G, Davis G. Myocardial infarction in young adults. Postgrad Med J. 2005;81(962):741–5.

38. Biswas T, Islam SMS, Islam A. Prevention of hypertension in Bangladesh: a review. Cardiovasc J. 2015;7(2):137–44.

39. Yeh RW, Sidney S, Chandra M, Sorel M, Selby JV, Go AS. Population trends in the incidence and outcomes of acute myocardial infarction. N Eng J Med. 2010;362(23):2155–65.

40. Mukherjee D, Hsu A, Moliterno DJ, Lincoff AM, Goormastic M, Topol EJ. Risk factors for premature coronary artery disease and determinants of adverse outcomes after revascularization in patients ≤ 40 years old. Am J Cardiol. 2003;92(12):1465–7.

41. Fournier JA, Cabezón S, Cayuela A, Ballesteros SM, Cortacero JA, Díaz De La Llera LS. Long-term prognosis of patients having acute myocardial infarction when ≤ 40 years of age. Am J Cardiol. 2004;94(8):989–92.

17

Socially disadvantaged city districts show a higher incidence of acute ST-elevation myocardial infarctions with elevated cardiovascular risk factors and worse prognosis

J. Schmucker[1]*[†] (iD), S. Seide[1†], H. Wienbergen[1], E. Fiehn[1], J. Stehmeier[1], K. Günther[2], W. Ahrens[2], R. Hambrecht[1], H. Pohlabeln[2] and A. Fach[1]

Abstract

Background: The importance of socioeconomic status (SES) for coronary heart disease (CHD)-morbidity is subject of ongoing scientific investigations. This study was to explore the association between SES in different city-districts of Bremen/Germany and incidence, severity, treatment modalities and prognosis for patients with ST-elevation myocardial infarctions (STEMI).

Methods: Since 2006 all STEMI-patients from the metropolitan area of Bremen are documented in the Bremen STEMI-registry. Utilizing postal codes of their home address they were assigned to four groups in accordance to the Bremen social deprivation-index (G1: high, G2: intermediate high, G3: intermediate low, G4: low socioeconomic status).

Results: Three thousand four hundred sixty-two consecutive patients with STEMI admitted between 2006 and 2015 entered analysis. City areas with low SES showed higher adjusted STEMI-incidence-rates (IR-ratio 1.56, G4 vs. G1). This elevation could be observed in both sexes (women IRR 1.63, men IRR 1.54) and was most prominent in inhabitants <50 yrs. of age (women IRR 2.18, men IRR 2.17). Smoking (OR 1.7, 95%CI 1.3–2.4) and obesity (1.6, 95%CI 1.1–2.2) was more prevalent in pts. from low SES city-areas. While treatment-modalities did not differ, low SES was associated with more extensive STEMIs (creatine kinase > 3000 U/l, OR 1.95, 95% CI 1.4–2.8) and severe impairment of LV-function post-STEMI (OR 2.0, 95% CI 1.2–3.4). Long term follow-up revealed that lower SES was associated with higher major adverse cardiac or cerebrovascular event (MACCE)-rates after 5 years: G1 30.8%, G2 35.7%, G3 36.0%, G4 41.1%, p (for trend) = 0.02. This worse prognosis could especially be shown for young STEMI-patients (<50 yrs. of age) 5-yr. mortality-rates(G4 vs. G1) 18.4 vs. 3.1%, p = 0.03 and 5-year-MACCE-rates (G4 vs. G1) 32 vs. 6.3%, p = 0.02.

Conclusions: This registry-data confirms the negative association of low socioeconomic status and STEMI-incidence, with higher rates of smoking and obesity, more extensive infarctions and worse prognosis for the socio-economically deprived.

* Correspondence: Johannes.Schmucker@klinikum-bremen-ldw.de
[†]Equal contributors
[1]The Bremer Institut für Herz- und Kreislaufforschung (BIHKF) am Klinikum Links der Weser, Bremen, Germany
Full list of author information is available at the end of the article

Background

The relationship between socioeconomic status (SES) and disease development in industrialized nations is well established [1–3]. The SES, usually measured by parameters like income, educational status and occupation, can be defined as individual level SES by assessing the social status of each study participant or area level SES, reflecting the subjects' living neighbourhood. Although distinctness of the results may differ, both, individual SES and area level SES, have shown to be valid predictors of morbidity and mortality [4, 5]. Other studies differentiate between contextual and compositional effects on health, the latter emphasizing the influence of individual characteristics'on disease, while the contextual approach focuses on the role of the patients' living environment. In previous studies an association of socioeconomic status and incidence as well as prognosis of cardiovascular disease (CVD) and myocardial infarctions has been observed [6–11]. For example Diez Roux et al. found an increased incidence of coronary heart disease associated with living in a disadvantaged neighbourhood with a hazard ratio (HR) of 3.1 among whites and 2.5 among blacks as compared to persons from most advantaged neighbourhoods [6]. In the Netherlands neighbourhood socioeconomic inequalities were observed in AMI incidence when comparing the most deprived with the most affluent neighbourhoods (RR for AMI was 1.34 in men (95% confidence interval (CI) 1.32 to 1.36) and 1.44 in women (95% CI 1.42 to 1.47) [10].

Recently a Canadian study group could show higher incidence of cardiovascular disease and rate of cardiovascular events (cardiovascular death, myocardial infarction, stroke and heart failure) in low-income countries compared to high- and middle-income countries [12]. In addition income ratios seem to have an influence on life expectancy. An actual investigation came to the result, that higher income was associated with greater longevity throughout the income distribution. Between the richest 1% and poorest 1% of individuals, life expectancy varied between 14.6 years (95% CI, 14.4 to 14.8 years) for men and 10.1 years (95% CI, 9.9 to 10.3 years) for women [13].

Several studies also described a negative impact of SES on treatment of patients with ST-elevation myocardial infarction (STEMI) [14–16], while others did not [17].

Since all incident cases of STEMI of residents of the city of Bremen are admitted to the Bremen heart center we are able to perform a comprehensive epidemiological analysis on a well defined clinical entity. We analysed the impact of socioeconomic status on incidence for STEMI-patients admitted between 2006 and 2015. Patients were assigned to SES-groups through the postal codes of their place of residence. Furthermore the influence of area level SES on the cardiovascular risk profile, infarction-severity and short- and long-term outcome after STEMI was analysed.

Methods

The Bremen STEMI-registry (BSR)

The BSR is a monocentric prospective registry of patients admitted with STEMI at the Bremen heart center. The Bremen heart center is exclusively responsible for 24-h-PCI-service in a large region in northwest Germany, serving a population of more than 800.000 residents from Bremen and in the northwestern part of Lower Saxony. Emergency services and regional hospitals are connected by telephone and fax for announcement of urgent coronary catheterization in case of STEMI. Since all STEMIs from the Bremen heart center are documented in the BSR it claims to give a complete statistical overview about the clinical course (short- and long-term) of STEMI-patients in the region of Bremen. The BSR was established in 2006 and is still running. Documentation is accomplished via data sheets completed by the responsible interventional cardiologist and/or through patient records after a physician has confirmed the exact diagnosis. Data about age, residence, sex, temporal delays of treatment, concomitant diseases, severity of STEMI and acute medical or interventional treatment are recorded. At discharge major adverse cardiac and cerebral events are documented. Follow-up examination is performed after 1 and 5 years by a telephone interview. Further details have been published previously [18].

Definition of STEMI and disease severity

STEMI was defined as persistent angina pectoris for ≥20 min in conjunction with a ST-segment elevation in two contigous leads of ≥0.25 mV in men below the age of 40 years, ≥0.2 mV in men over the age of 40 years, or ≥0.15 mV in women in leads V2-V3 and/or ≥0.1 mV in all other leads or new left bundle branch block [19].

Disease severity was evaluated using surrogate parameters, such as acute heart failure, pulmonary edema or cardiogenic shock at admission by the Killip-classification, multivessel disease with or without left-main-lesion and by measurement of the post-AMI ejection fraction. The peak creatine kinase (CK) was used to assess extension of myocardial infarction with laboratory controls routinely performed in STEMI-patients once to twice daily. To assess the quality of care, door-to-balloon time, interventional procedures and medication at hospital discharge were analysed.

The Bremen social deprivation index

The Bremen social deprivation index (SDI) was developed in 1993 to describe social inequalities in the city of Bremen in Germany. In its most recent update (2009) a ranking was established for 89 city districts, using census and public data on education, voting participation, unemployment, crime statistics and immigration flow. A positive composite index indicates a socially privileged, a negative composite index a socially disadvantaged city district with an overall mean SDI of 0 [20]. Since only postal codes were available in the BSR the SDIs of the 89 city districts were aggregated to 33 postal code regions of Bremen. Population data stem from municipial data of 2008.

Statistical analysis

Since a normal distribution of the social deprivation index across the postal code regions could be assumed (Kolgmorov-Smirnov-test of the 33 postal code regions: $p = 0.15$) distribution into groups was made according to the mean and standard deviation of the SDI: Within one standard deviation of the mean SDI postal codes were assigned to the groups G2 (social status: intermediate high) and G3 (social status: intermediate low). Postal codes with an SDI below −1 SD of the mean were assigned to G4 (social status: low), postal codes above +1 SD of the mean SDI were assigned to G1 (social status: high). Baseline characteristics of STEMI-patients were given as mean values ± standard deviation for continuous variables (age, left ventricular ejection fraction, door to balloon-time, number of coronary vessels affected) and in absolute numbers and percentages for categorical variables: (diabetes, obesity (body mass index > 30 kg/m^2), smoking, multivessel-disease, prehospital cardiopulmonal resuscitation (CPR), peak CK > 3000 U/l, acute heart failure, positive family history (FH) for CAD/CVD, primary PCI, CABG, LVEF ≤ 40%, medication at admission and at discharge) by using SAS/STAT (version 9.3., 2011). Statistical significance was tested using Chi-square for categorical and t-tests for continuous variables. For comparison of the groups ANOVA tests were used for continuous variables, Chi-square for trend-test (Cochrane-Armitage) for categorical variables. A p-value <0.05 was considered statistically significant. Sex-, age-, and SES-group-specific incidence rates (per 100.000 persons/year) were estimated as the sum of of STEMI-events during 2006–2015 divided by the sum of persons at risk in the strata of sex, age- and SES-group. Incidence rate ratios (IRRs) and 95% confidence intervals were estimated by log-linear Poisson regression of sex-, age- and SES-group-specific number of STEMI-events with logarithm of persons at risk as offset. Multivariate logistic regression analysis were performed with SES-groups, age, sex and prior CVD as the independent variable and age, sex, smoking, obesity, diabetes mellitus, CK > 3000 U/l, primary PCI, successful PCI

and LVEF < 40% as the dependent variable. Analysis of mortality and adverse-events-rates (major adverse cardiac and cerebrovascular events (MACCE): death, stroke, myocardial reinfarction) was performed after stratifying for age (<50 yrs., ≥50 yrs.).

Results
Study population

The total study population comprised the city of Bremen with approximately 550,000 inhabitants. Between January 1st 2006 and December 31th 2015 a total of 3462 residents of the city of Bremen a STEMI was newly diagnosed. They were assigned to groups (G1 to G4) according to the social deprivation index of their home address, with G1 representing the most affluent neighbourhoods and G4 representing the most deprived ones (Table 1).

Incidence of STEMI

The unadjusted incidence-rate (per 100.000 persons/year) of STEMI in the city of Bremen between 2006 and 2015 was 63 per 100,000 inhabitants/year or 74 per 100,000 inhabitants/year when excluding inhabitants <18 yrs. from the calculation model (Table 2). The hypothesis, that the number of STEMIs was equally distributed over time could not be rejected for any of the four SDI-Groups (p-values calculated by means of a chi-square goodness-of-fit test): G1 ($p = 0.45$), G2 ($p = 0.14$), G3 ($p = 0.14$), G4 ($p = 0.10$). A rising incidence of STEMI could be observed with declining SDI category. Adjusted relative risk (for age and sex) for STEMI showed a 56% increase of STEMI-incidence among pts. from low SES neighbourhoods as compared to the more affluent city regions. The association of rising STEMI incidence with increased social deprivation could be demonstrated in both sexes (Fig. 1a). The

Table 1 Sociodemographic baseline characteristics of SES-groups

	G1 (high SES)	G2 (intermediate high SES)	G3 (intermediate low SES)	G4 (low SES)
% of total population	19	24	43	14
Inhabitants <19 yrs. of age (%)	14	13	15	19
STEMIs 2006–2016 (n)	519	813	1554	576
SDI by definition	≥56	0 to 56	−56 to 0	≤ −56
SDI range	99 to 56	50 to 1	−3 to −50	−59 to −121
Mean SDI±SD	78 ± 16	26 ± 18	−31 ± 16	−86 ± 29

Table 2 Population ≥ 18 yrs. of age at risk and STEMI-events 2006–2015

		G1	G2	G3	G4
All STEMIs	Population at risk	87,783	114,107	200,548	64,087
	Events [a]	519	813	1554	576
	Incidence rate (IR/ 95%CI)	59 (54–65)	71 (66–76)	77 (74–81)	90 (83–98)
Men	Population at risk	41,345	58,548	102,460	32,357
	Events [a]	352	576	1097	407
	Incidence rate (IR/ 95%CI)	85 (77–95)	98 (91–107)	107 (101–114)	126 (114–139)
Women	Population at risk	46,438	55,559	98,088	31,730
	Events [a]	167	237	457	169
	Incidence rate (IR/ 95%CI)	36 (31–42)	43 (37–48)	47(42–51)	53 (46–62)
Age 18–49	Population at risk	42,972	61,834	104,873	33,326
	Events [a]	57	139	229	100
	Incidence rate (IR/ 95%CI)	13 (10–17)	22 (19–27)	22(19–25)	30 (24–36)
Age 50–64	Population at risk	19,873	26,569	44,815	14,861
	Events [a]	143	267	533	203
	Incidence rate (IR/ 95%CI)	72 (61–85)	100 (89–113)	119(109–130)	137 (118–157)
Age 65–79	Population at risk	18,171	18,524	37,191	11,863
	Events [a]	216	293	579	208
	Incidence rate (IR/ 95%CI)	118 (103–136)	158 (141–177)	156(143–168)	175 (154–202)
Age > 79	Population at risk	6767	7180	13,669	4037
	Events [a]	103	114	213	65
	Incidence rate (IR/ 95%CI)	152 (124–185)	159 (131–191)	156(137–178)	161 (124–205)

[a]STEMIs 2006–2015

socioeconomic gradient was most prominent in young patients (<50 years of age) showing a 2.18 fold elevation of STEMI-incidence when comparing G4 to G1 in women (Fig. 1b) and a 2.17 fold elevation in men (Fig. 1c). In the older ages groups this gradient consistently decreased until being no longer significant in pts. ≥ 80 years for men and women alike (Fig. 1b and c).

Baseline characteristics of STEMI-patients

The 3462 patients admitted with STEMI between 2006 and 2015 were on average 64.8+/–13 years old, 71% were male, 44% were active smokers, 21% had diabetes and 23% were obese (BMI > 30 kg/m^2). Patients from neighbourhoods with a lower SDI were on average younger at time of STEMI, more likely to smoke and more likely to be obese than those from more affluent city districts. In contrast the prevalence of a positive family history for CAD was significantly lower in patients from low-SES city districts. Gender distribution as well as prevalence of diabetes in STEMI patients did not differ substantially between SDI categories (Table 3). A multivariate analysis confirmed these results: higher degrees of social disadvantage was positively associated with higher likelihood of suffering the STEMI at young age, to smoke or to be obese at time of

STEMI. In contrast social deprivation and the prevalence of positive family history for CAD were inversely related while gender and diabetes mellitus did not show significant differences in prevalence between SDI-categories (Fig. 2).

Severity of STEMI

While the prevalence of multi-vessel-disease did not differ substantially between SES-classes, pts. from low-SES city districts showed greater extension of STEMI, measured by the peak creatine kinase (peak CK) and had on average lower left-ventricular-ejection-fraction (LVEF) post-STEMI (Table 4). The relation between social deprivation and infarct size and subsequent LV-EF-reduction post STEMI remained significant in a multivariate model (Fig. 3). Rates of prehospital resuscitation as well as the rate of cardiogenic shock in STEMI patients did not differ between SES-classes (Table 4).

Treatment modalities

The proportion of patients receiving a successful primary PCI was >89%, with no significant disparities when comparing the socioeconomic groups (Fig. 3). Moreover, comparable proportions of STEMI-patients had early

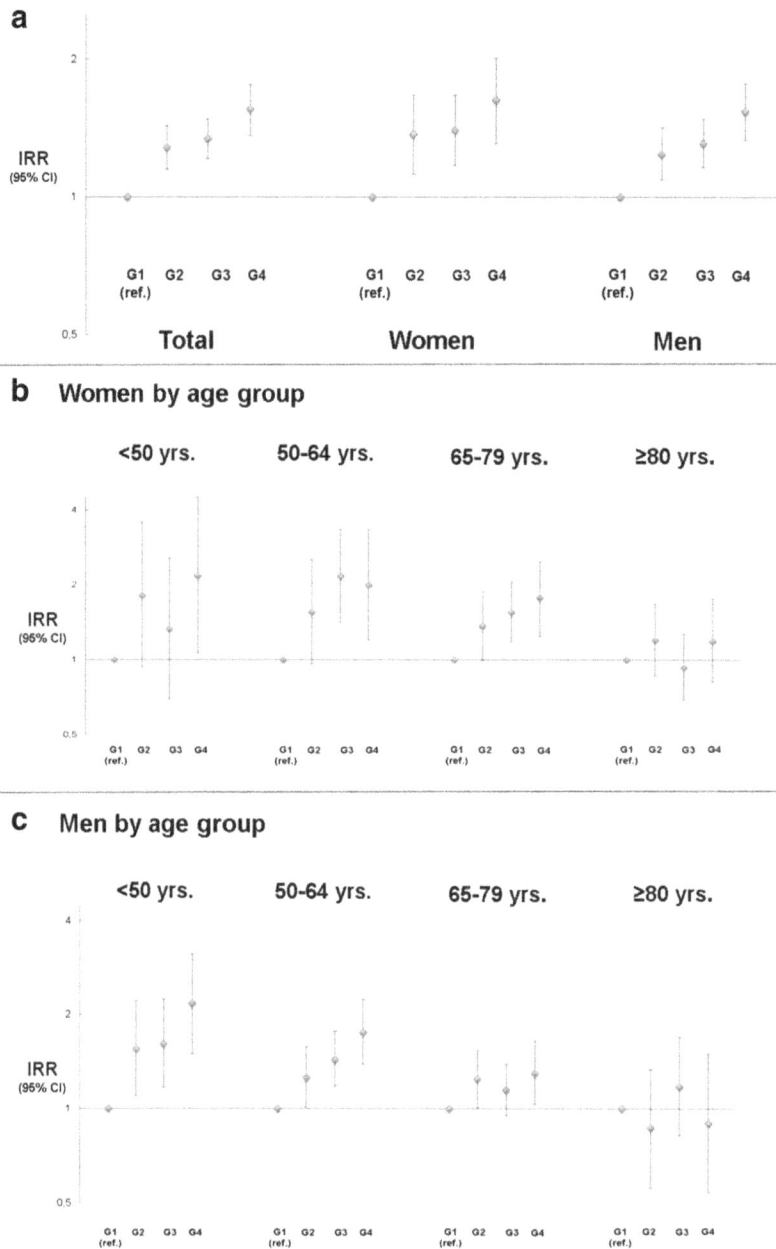

Fig. 1 Incidence rate ratios by SES. Adjusted incidence rate ratios (IRRs) with 95% CI, calculated for SES-class G2 to G4 with G1 as baseline (1). Calculation based on total numbers (**a**) or prestratified by age for women (**b**) and men (**c**)

surgical revascularisation procedures (CABG) or a conservative therapy regime. Prior to the coronary angiography pts. from all SES-groups showed similar average door-to-balloon-times. Patients from all quartiles received additional Gp2b3A-antagonist-medication (Tirofiban or Abciximab) at a similar frequency. At discharge from hospital there was no difference in standard medication (ASA, ADP-antagonists, beta blockers, statins, ACE/ATR-Inhibitors) between the groups (Table 4).

Impact of SES on prognosis

While SES had no significant impact on inhospital-mortality, 1-year-mortality, 1-year-MACCE-rates and 5-year-mortality-rates, lower SES was associated with a significant increase in MACCE-events within 5 years after STEMI, showing a 34% increase in event rates when comparing pts. from the most socially deprived city areas to those from the city areas with the highest SES (Table 4). When stratifying follow-up-data by age (<50 yrs. of age and ≥50 yrs. of age) a negative impact of

Table 3 Cardiovascular risk profile of STEMI-patients according to SES-group

	G1 ($n = 519$)	G2 ($n = 813$)	G3 ($n = 1554$)	G4 ($n = 576$)	p-value
Age (yrs) ± SD	67.6 ± 13	64.1 ± 13	63.1 ± 13	63.1 ± 13	<0.01
Female Gender (%)	31.8	29.1	29.4	29.3	0.08
Smoking (%)	33.3	44.2	45.9	49.1	<0.01
Mean BMI (kg/sqm) ± SD	26.7 ± 5	27.3 ± 5	27.6 ± 5	27.9 ± 5	<0.01
BMI > 30 kg/sqm (%)	17.0	21.4	25.2	26.8	<0.01
Diabetes mellitus (%)	18.8	21.9	20.5	20.4	0.3
Family history (FH) for CAD (%)	22.2	22.3	18.6	18.5	0.02
Known CV disease (%)	23.8	24.8	27.5	24.6	0.9

social deprivation on long-term-outcome could be shown for the young STEMI-cohort with elevated 1-year mortality-, 1-year-MACCE-rates as well as 5-year-mortality- and 5-year-MACCE-rates for the socially deprived (Fig. 4a). In contrast short-term- (<72 h) (G1: 1.3%, G2: 0.9%, G3 1.0%, G4:1.6%; p (for trend) = 0.8) and in-hospital mortality-rates (G1: 2.6% G2: 2.4%, G3: 3.9%, G4: 3.6%, p (for trend) = 0.1) were not significantly affected by SES-class. For pts. ≥ 50 yrs. SES did not show an impact on 1- and 5-year mortality-and MACCE-rates, while overall event-rates were generally higher due to the advanced patients' age (Fig. 4b).

Discussion

The present data of the Bremen STEMI registry show a significant association between socioeconomic status and incidence of STEMI. This negative association could be observed most strikingly for the young with a 2.2 fold higher risk for inhabitants younger than 50 years for suffering a STEMI when living in low SES city areas. Patients with STEMI from socially disadvantaged city districts were more likely to smoke and to be obese. Neither in-hospital treatment nor short-term mortality showed significant differences between the different SES-groups. However patients living in low-SES city-districts were more likely to suffer severe myocardial infarctions measured by peak-CK and showed higher rates of severe left-ventricular-impairment (EF < 40%) post-STEMI. Evaluation of long-term-prognosis showed higher 5-year-MACCE-rates for STEMI-patients from socially deprived city districts. The association of social deprivation and elevated mortality and MACCE-rates was most prominent for young-STEMI-populations showing a 3 fold elevation in 1-year-mortality, a 5.9 fold elevation in 5-year mortality and a 4.9 fold elevation in 5-year-MACCE-rates when comparing patients younger 50 yrs. from the city districts with the lowest SES to those from the most affluent ones.

Our findings are based on area-level-SES. Effects of socioeconomic inequity might therefore be attenuated and would be even more pronounced if individual-level socioeconomic data had been available. Whether the higher incidence and severity of STEMI as well as the poorer outcome of STEMI-pts. in the G4 group are attributable to contextual and/or compositional effects of the place of residence cannot be differentiated by our results but might be subject to latter investigation.

Association of socioeconomic status and prevalence of CAD /incidence of AMI

An association between socioeconomic deprivation and increased risk for suffering from CAD and AMI has been described by prior investigations [10, 21]. Besides the observation of an increased risk for coronary events in socioeconomic disadvantaged neighbourhoods in four US study sites by Diez Roux [21], a social down-gradient of STEMI incidence could be observed in both sex groups and most significantly in young inhabitants in a Dutch study (relative risk in women 1.44, in men 1.34, decreasing social gradient with increasing age) [10]. These results are in good accordance to our data.

Influence of SES on the cardiovascular risk profile for STEMI-patients

The elevated cardiovascular risk profile in patients with a low SES, in particular the higher rates of smokers and obese pts., might partly explain the elevated STEMI incidence. The association of active smoking and obesity with CAD and CAD-related mortality has been proven [22–25] and the influence of tobacco smoking in public areas on non-smokers` risk for AMI has been demonstrated by recent investigations [18]. Additionally there is some evidence, that beyond the classic risk factors for CAD the SES may have biological, behavioral and psychosocial components affecting the deprived [7, 26, 27]. Chetty et al. found that life expectancy more likely depends on health behaviors (i.e. smoking, obesity, exercise) rather than access to medical supplies or environmental factors (i.e. air pollution) [13]. In concern of CVD and MI disease determinants are varied. One aspect could be the neighbourhood in which people live, but social influences on health are complex and seem to

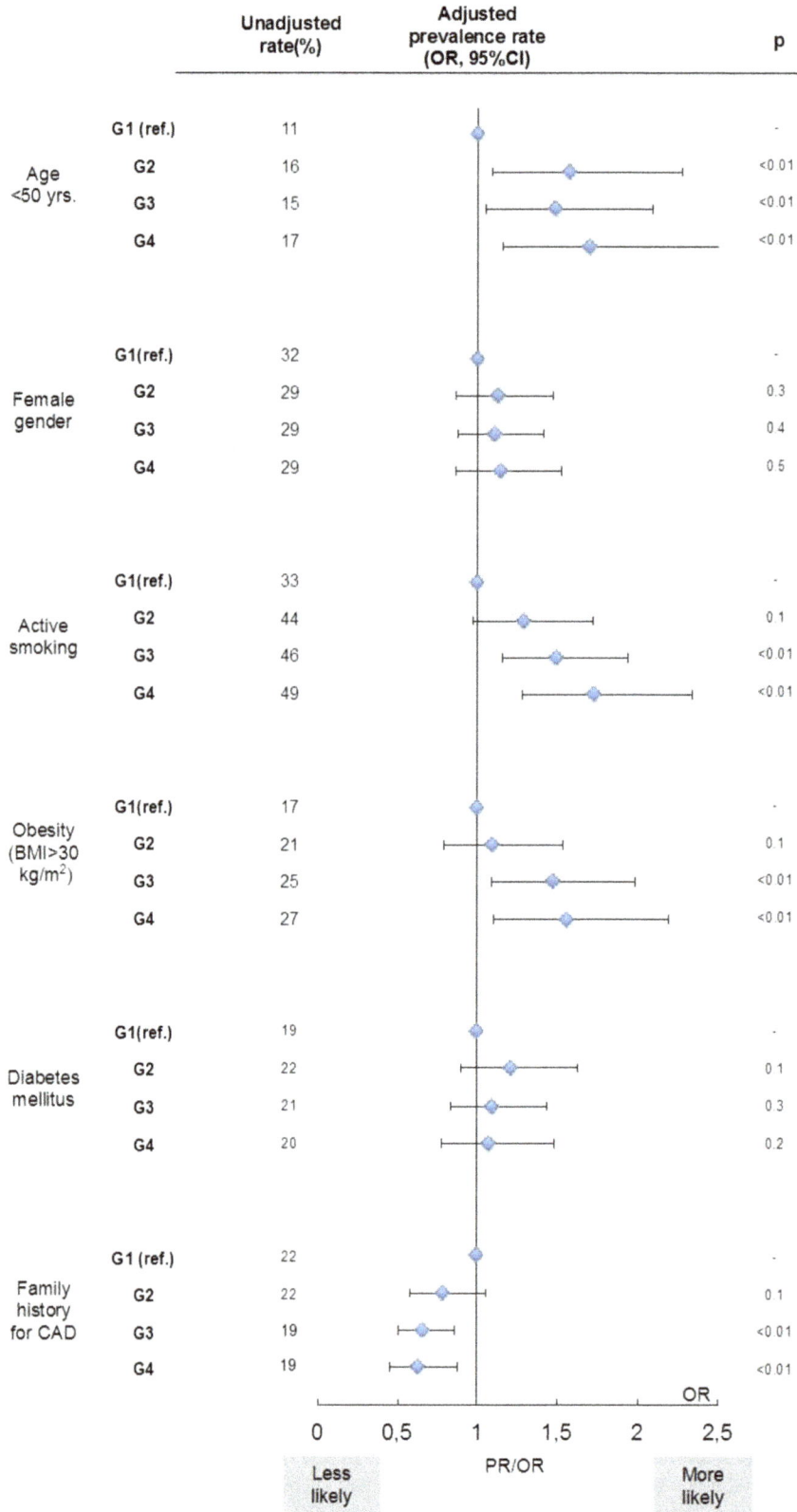

Fig. 2 Association of SES with age, gender and cardiovascular risk profile. Impact of SES-class (G2-G4, G1 = baseline) on prevalence of young age, female gender and cardiovascular risk factors in STEMI-patients. OR calculated with multivariate adjustment for age, gender and known cardiovascular disease

Table 4 Severity of CAD/ STEMI, treatment modalities and outcome according to SES-group

	G1 (n = 519)	G2 (n = 813)	G3 (n = 1554)	G4 (n = 576)	p-value
Severity of myocardial infarction					
Number of coronary vesssels affected ±SD	1.99 ± 0.8	1.94 ± 0.8	1.91 ± 0.8	1.84 ± 0.8	0.09
Cardiogenic shock (%)	12.1	13.1	12.0	12.4	0.8
Prehospital CPR (%)	10.9	11.3	10.8	10.3	0.5
Subacute MI(%) [a]	19.3	23.9	20.5	19.9	0.8
Mean peak CK (U/l) ± SD	1599 ± 1679	1838 ± 2019	1913 ± 2188	2025 ± 2167	<0.01
Peak CK > 3000 U/l (%)	13.7	20.5	20.9	23.3	<0.01
Post AMI LVEF in % ± SD	49.6 ± 9	48.9 ± 10	48.4 ± 11	47.5 ± 10	<0.01
LVEF <40% (%)	10.4	13.8	15.8	16.3	0.01
Treatment modalitites					
Primary PCI (%)	89.0	91.1	89.9	90.9	0.9
CABG (%)	6.1	3.9	4.8	3.4	0.14
Conservative therapy regimen (%)	4.8	4.9	5.2	5.7	0.8
Door to balloon time in min (median ± SD)	48 ± 32	43 ± 44.5	46 ± 40	44 ± 41	0.74
GP2b3a-Inhibitors (%)	70	67	66	70	0.7
ASA (at discharge) (%)	94	96	94	95	0.64
ADP-Antagon. (ad) (%)	90	90.5	90	94	0.23
Beta-blockers (ad) (%)	83	84	80	84	0.25
Statins (ad) (%)	86	87	87	86	0.9
ACE/ATR-Inhibitors (ad) (%)	77	80	79	79	0.9
Outcome					
Mortality <72 h (%)	3.9	3.6	3.9	4.2	0.71
Inhospital mortality (%)	8.8	7.6	7.9	8.1	0.71
1-year-mortality (%)	15.7	15.1	14.9	16.3	0.9
1-year-MACCE (%)	19.2	19.5	19.1	20.4	0.8
5-year-mortality (%)	23.9	27.7	25.7	28.3	0.46
5-year-MACCE (%)	30.8	35.7	36.0	41.1	0.02

[a] subacute MI was defined as onset of symptoms >12 h before admission to PCI- center and/or signs of subacute STEMI in initial ECG

operate through many different processes. Worldwide debate about to what extend contextual and/or compositional effects account for higher morbidity and mortality of the underprivileged is ongoing [28].

Impact of SES on quality of care and treatment modalities
With respect to quality of care (door-to-balloon-times, PCI rates and medication) as well as with respect to short-term outcome there were no significant differences between the four SES groups. These results are in contrast to findings from Finland and the US, where low-income pts. received fewer therapy with antiplatelets, beta-blockers, lipid-lowering medication [13, 29] and reperfusion therapy [13]. In addition obtaining similar invasive procedures in treatment of STEMI was unlikely for ethnic minority members in the US, where racial disparities led to lower rates of primary PCI and longer door-to-balloon times in Afro-Americans

[30, 31]. Alter et al. reported a negative association of SES and access to cardiac services, leading to elevated long -term mortality for patients from low SES areas even for Canada with its universal health care system [32]. Differences in findings about treatment strategies within different countries might still be attributed to altering health care systems. The fact, that there is no striking inequity in acute therapy and medication between the social groups in Bremen suggests, that the German health care system provides a guideline conform treatment for STEMI pts. independent of their social background.

Impact of SES on severity of myocardial infarction, post-AMI-cardiac performance and short-term-mortality
Data from the BSR showed that living in low SES areas was associated with more severe myocardial infarctions, measured by the peak creatine kinase (CK)

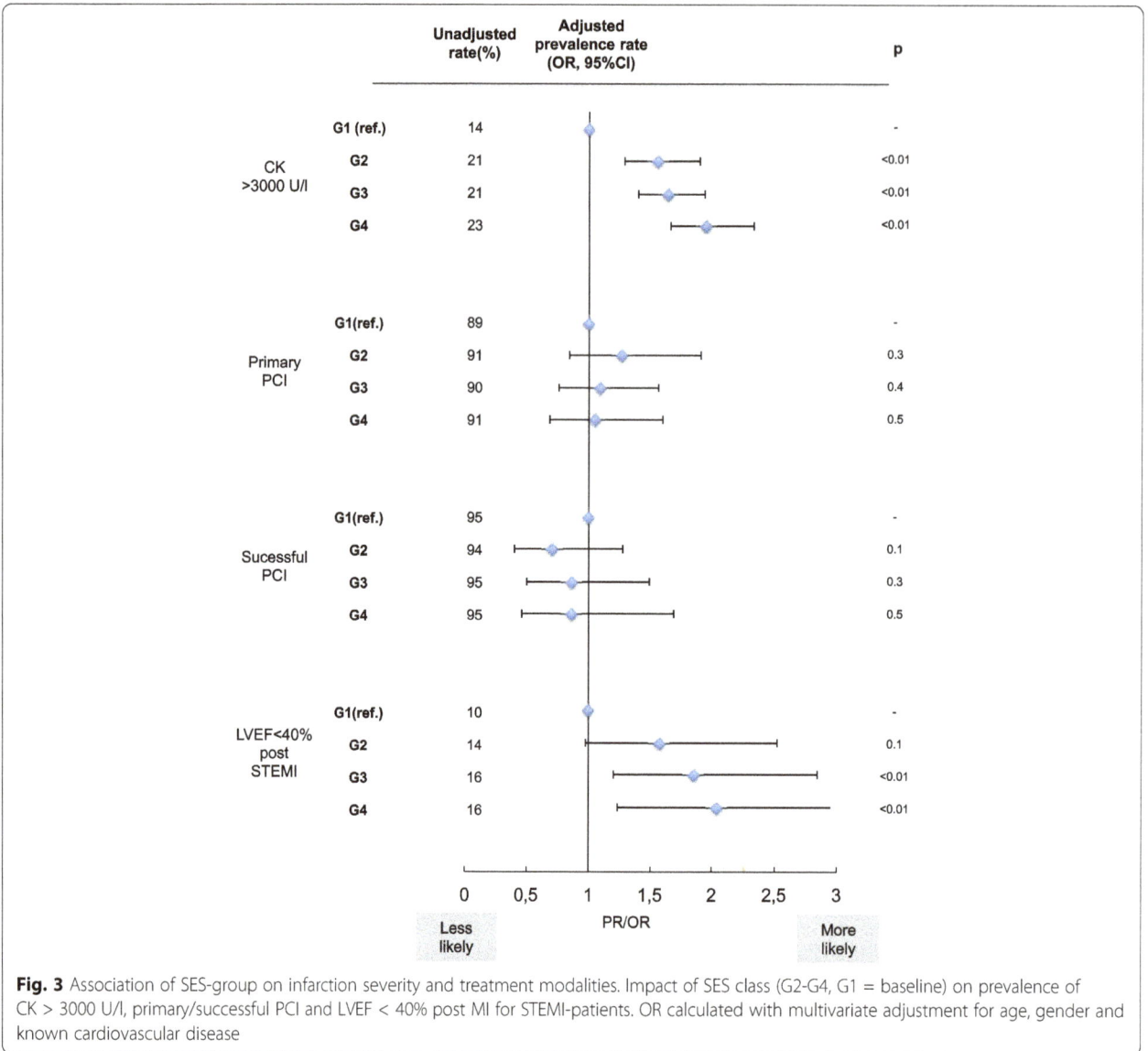

Fig. 3 Association of SES-group on infarction severity and treatment modalities. Impact of SES class (G2-G4, G1 = baseline) on prevalence of CK > 3000 U/l, primary/successful PCI and LVEF < 40% post MI for STEMI-patients. OR calculated with multivariate adjustment for age, gender and known cardiovascular disease

and higher rates of severe impairment of left ventricular ejection fraction post-STEMI. While Gerber et al. [33] showed higher rates of infarction-associated left-heart-failure for patients with low SES the impact of socioeconomic status on extent of MI has, to our knowledge, not been described before. However our data does not offer an explanation for the greater extent of MIs for the socially deprived since pre- as well as in-hospital-treatment modalities were similar across all SES-groups. While the rate of subacute MIs was similar in all SES-groups it however cannot be excluded, that the pain-to-alarm-interval, which is not coherently registered in this database, might have been longer for patients from socially deprived neighbourhoods.

Social deprivation and long-term outcome after STEMI

Although acute treatment strategies were comparable between the different SES groups in the BSR, 5-year-MACCE-rates were significantly higher for STEMI-patients from low SES city areas. Stratification for age revealed, that the worse prognosis after STEMI was evident for young-STEMI patients showing a steep elevation in 1-year-mortality and 5-year mortality and MACCE-rates. This disadvantage could no longer be shown for elder patients. Similar findings with increased long-term mortality after AMI in pts. with lower SES have been described by prior studies [9, 32–38]. Winkleby et al. [38] demonstrated that 1-year case fatality from CAD was 1.6 times higher for women and 1.7 times higher for men in high versus low deprivation

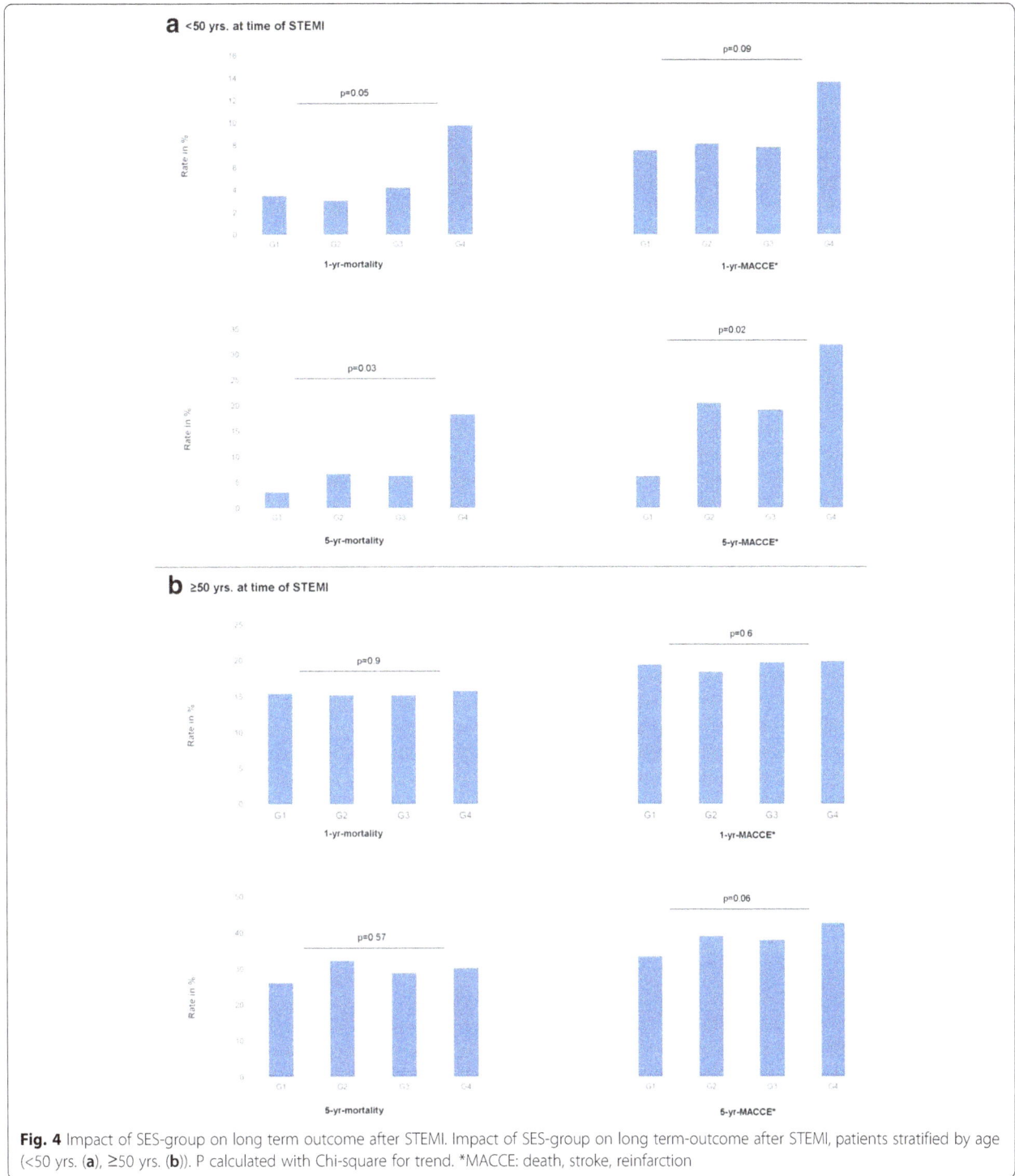

Fig. 4 Impact of SES-group on long term outcome after STEMI. Impact of SES-group on long term-outcome after STEMI, patients stratified by age (<50 yrs. (**a**), ≥50 yrs. (**b**)). P calculated with Chi-square for trend. *MACCE: death, stroke, reinfarction

neighbourhoods. In Israel low income was shown to be associated with an increase in mortality risk when accompanied by low education among STEMI pts. (HR 2.64, 95% CI: 1.92–3.63) [34]. This disadvantage for STEMI-patients from underprivileged city areas regarding long-term outcome may be the result of poor treatment compliance especially in young STEMI patients, as previously

low SES was found to be a predictor for non-adherence to post-discharge medication and lifestyle recommendations [39, 40]. Patients from low SES city areas were more likely to smoke at the index event. Since previous investigations have shown that the rate of smoking cessation after AMI is lower in the less educated [40], higher rates of remaining smokers even after STEMI should be assumed among the socially deprived patients contributing to their worse long-term-prognosis.

In total the elevated STEMI incidence and the higher long-term mortality in low SES city areas of Bremen may indicate a lack of efficacy of primary and secondary prevention strategies in those city districts. Consequently prevention programs should focus on socially disadvantaged neighbourhoods to further improve primary and secondary prevention strategies.

Study limitations

Limited data on long-term medical adherence and risk-factor-adjustment of pts. after STEMI was available in the BSR, so that further studies are required to complete knowledge about adherence to secondary prevention strategies.

Due to the catchment area of the Bremen heart center, we are limited to a relative small study population, but on the other hand for the same reason we can give a comprehensive view of the clinical care of STEMI in Bremen, which minimizes bias due to regional differences in treatment strategies. Although the Bremen heart center is the only regional provider for emergency PCI in case of STEMI, we cannot rule out that single cases of STEMI were treated elsewhere, were not presented to receive emergency-PCI or died before admission to the cath-lab. This might have generated a selection bias.

Our database did not provide individual level SES. The analysis therefore relied on area level SES. This and the pooling from city district-SES to postal-code district SES to ultimately 4 SES-groups probably weakened the effect of social inequalities. However both, area level SES and individual level SES are valid for investigating the impact of socioeconomic status, only that the effects of area level SES are supposed to be weaker. Despite this, our study demonstrates a clear effect of SES on incidence and long-term-outcome, which might have been even more prominent if data on individual level SES had been available.

Conclusions

In the present study a clear social gradient with an increased incidence of STEMI in socially deprived city districts could be observed. Patients with STEMI from socially disadvantaged city districts tend to be younger at time of infarction and are more likely to smoke and to be obese. The elevation in cardiovascular risk factors might partly explain the increased STEMI incidence. Patients from socially below average city districts furthermore showed larger myocardial infarctions and higher rates of severe impairment of cardiac function post STEMI.

While the social background does not seem to influence acute treatment modalities in STEMI nor short-term outcome, patients from low SES-city areas showed an elevation in 5-year-MACCE-rates. Which, besides pts.´ compliance and differences in infarction severity, may be the result of differences in secondary prevention strategies. The disadvantage in mortality and MACCE-rates however could especially be shown for STEMI-patients younger 50 years, where a 5.9 fold higher risk of death and a 4.9 fold elevation in MACCE-events within 5 years after STEMI could be observed.

Efforts and programs in primary and secondary prevention of CAD should therefore concentrate especially on city areas with a low socioeconomic profile.

Abbreviations

ADP: Adenosine diphosphate; AMI: Acute myocardial infarction; ASA: Acetylsalicylic acid; ATR: Angiotensin receptor; BSR: Bremen STEMI registry; CABG: Coronary artery bypass graft; CAD: Coronary artery disease; CHD: Coronary heart disease; CI: Confidence interval; CVD: Cardiovascular disease; LMCA: Left main coronary artery; LVEF: Left ventricular ejection fraction; MI: Myocardial infarction; PCI: Percutaneous coronary intervention; Pts: Patients; PY: Person years; SD: Standard deviation; SDI: Social deprivation index; SEM: Standard error of mean; SES: Socioeconomic status; STEMI: ST elevation myocardial infarction; US: United States; Yrs: Years

Acknowledgments

None.

Funding

No specific funding to declare.

Authors' contributions

JS study design, preparation of the manuscript. SS study design, preparation of the manuscript. HW writing and correction of manuscript. EF overseeing collection of data in the Bremen STEMI registry, revision of manuscript and results. JS revision of manuscript, data collection in the STEMI-registry. KG statistical models and analysis. WA statistical models and analysis, revision of manuscript. RH overseeing collection of data and statistical analysis, revision of manuscript. HP statistical analysis and revision of the manuscript. AF writing and revision of manuscript, data collection in the STEMI-registry. All authors read and approved the final manuscript.

Competing interests

The authors declare that they have no competing interests.

Author details

[1]The Bremer Institut für Herz- und Kreislaufforschung (BIHKF) am Klinikum Links der Weser, Bremen, Germany. [2]The Leibniz-Institut für Präventionsforschung und Epidemiologie Bremen – BIPS, Bremen, Germany.

References

1. Adler NE, Boyce T, et al. Socioeconomic status and health: the challenge of the gradient. Am Psychol. 1994;49:15–24.
2. Pickett KE, Pearl M. Multilevel analyses of neighbourhood socioeconomic context and health outcomes: a critical review. J Epidemiol Community Health. 2001;55:111–22.

3. Mackenbach JP, Stirbu I, Roskam A-JR, et al. Socioeconomic inequalities in health in 22 european countries. N Engl J Med. 2008;358(23):2468–81.
4. Winkleby MA, Cubbin C. Influence of individual and neighbourhood socioeconomic status on mortality among black, Mexican-American, and white women and men in the United States. J Epidemiol Community Health. 2003;57:444–52.
5. Janssen I, Boyce WF, Simpson K, et al. Influence of individual- and area-level measures of socioeconomic status on obesity, unhealthy eating, and physical inactivity in Canadian adolescents. Am J Clin Nutr. 2006;83:139–45.
6. Diez Roux AV, Merkin SS, Arnett D, Chambless L, Massing M, Nieto FJ, Sorlie P, Szklo M, Tyroler HA, Watson RL. Neighbourhood of residence and incidence of coronary heart disease. N Engl J Med. 2001;345:99–106.
7. Manderbacka K, Elovainio M. The complexity of the association between socioeconomic status and acute myocardial infarction. Rev Esp Cardiol. 2010;63:1015–8.
8. Clark AM, DesMeules M, Luo W, Duncan AS, Wielgosz A. Socioeconomic status and cardiovascular disease: risk and implications for care. Nat Rev Cardiol. 2009;6:712–22.
9. Morrison C, Woodward M, Leslie W, Tunstall-Pedoe H. Effect of socioeconomic group on incidence of, management of, and survival after myocardial infarction and coronary death: analysis of community coronary event register. BMJ. 1997;314:541–6.
10. Koopman C, van Oeffelen AA, Bots ML, Engelfriet PM, Verschuren WM, van Rossem L, van Dis I, Capewell S, Vaartjes I. Neighborhood socioeconomic inequalities in incidence of acute myocardial infarction: a cohort study quantifying age- and gender-specific differences in relative and absolute terms. BMC Public Health. 2012;12:3–11.
11. Stjärne MK, Fritzell J, De Leon AP, Hallqvist J, SHEEP Study Group. Neighborhood socioeconomic context, individual income and myocardial infarction. Epidemiology. 2006;17:14–23.
12. Yusuf S, Rangarajan S, Teo K, et al. Cardiovascular risk and events in 17 low-, middle-, and high-income countries. N Engl J Med. 2014;371(9):818–27.
13. Chetty R, Stepner M, et al. The association between income and life expectancy in the United States, 2001–2014. JAMA. 2016 April 26; 315(16):1750–66.
14. Foraker RE, Rose KM, Whitsel EA, Suchindran CM, Wood JL, Rosamond WD. Neighborhood socioeconomic status, Medicaid coverage and medical management of myocardial infarction: atherosclerosis risk in communities (ARIC) community surveillance. BMC Public Health. 2010;10:1–7.
15. Kitzmiller JP, Foraker RE, Rose KM. Lipid-lowering pharmacotherapy and socioeconomic status: atherosclerosis risk in communities (ARIC) surveillance study. BMC Public Health. 2013;13:1–3.
16. Rathore SS, Berger AK, Weinfurt KP, Feinleib M, Oetgen WJ, Gersh BJ, Schulman KA. Race, sex, poverty, and the medical treatment of acute myocardial infarction in the elderly. Circulation. 2000;102:642–8.
17. Hawkins NM, Scholes S, Bajekal M, Love H, O'Flaherty M, Raine R, Capewell S. Delivering equitable treatment across the spectrum of coronary disease. Circ Cardiovasc Qual Outcomes. 2013;6:208–16.
18. Schmucker J, Wienbergen H, Seide S, Fiehn E, Fach A, Würmann-Busch B, Gohlke H, Günther K, Ahrens W, Hambrecht R. Smoking ban in public areas is associated with a reduced incidence of hospital admissions due to ST-elevation myocardial infarctions in non-smokers: results from the Bremen STEMI registry. Eur J Prev Cardiol. 2014;21:1180–6.
19. Steg PG, James SK, Atar D, Badano LP, et al. ESC guidelines for the management of acute myocardial infarction in patients presenting with ST-segment elevation. Eur Heart J. 2012;33:2569–619.
20. Die Senatorin für Arbeit Frauen Gesundheit Jugend und Soziales. Sozialindikatoren. Aktualisierung der Sozialindikatoren 2010. Bremen: Sozialindikatoren; 2009.
21. Diez-Roux AV, Nieto FJ, Muntaner C, Tyroler HA, Comstock GW, Shahar E, Cooper LS, Watson RL, Szklo M. Neighborhood environments and coronary heart disease: a multilevel analysis. Am J Epidemiol. 1997;1(146):48–63.
22. Doyle JT, Dawber TR, Kannel WB, Heslin AS, Kahn HA. Cigarette smoking and coronary disease; combined experience of the Albany and Framingham studies. N Engl J Med. 1962;266:796–801.
23. Edwards R. The problem of tobacco smoking. BMJ. 2004;328:217–9.
24. Hubert HB, Feinleib M. Obesity as an independent risk factor for cardiovascular disease: a 26-year follow-up of participants in the Framingham hart study. Circulation. 1983;67:968–77.
25. Berrington de Gonzalez A, Hartge P, Cerhan JR, Flint AJ, Hannan L, RJ MI, Moore SC, Tobias GS, Anton-Culver H, Freeman LB, Beeson WL, Clipp SL, English DR, Folsom AR, Freedman DM, Giles G, Hakansson N, Henderson KD, Hoffman-Bolton J, Hoppin JA, Koenig KL, Lee IM, Linet MS, Park Y, Pocobelli G, Schatzkin A, Sesso HD, Weiderpass E, Willcox BJ, Wolk A, Zeleniuch-Jacquotte A, Willett WC, Thun MJ. Body-mass index and mortality among 1. 46 million white adults. N Engl J Med. 2010;363:2211–9.
26. Yusuf S, Hawken S, Ounpuu S, Dans T, Avezum A, Lanas F, McQueen M, Budaj A, Pais P, Varigos J, Lisheng L. Effect of potentially modifiable risk factors associated with myocardial infarction in 52 countries (the INTERHEART study): case-control study. Lancet. 2004;364:937–52.
27. Brunner E, Shipley MJ, Blane D, Smith GD, Marmot MG. When does cardiovascular risk start? Past and present socioeconomic circumstances and risk factors in adulthood. J Epidemiol Community Health. 1999;53:757–64.
28. Diez-Roux AV. Investigating neighborhood and area effects on health. Am J Public Health. 2001 November;91(11):1783–9.
29. Salomaa V, Miettinen H, Niemelä M, et al. Relation of socioeconomic position to the case fatality, prognosis and treatment of myocardial infarction events; the FINMONICA MI register study. J Epidemiol Community Health. 2001;55:475–82.
30. Mohamad T, Panaich SS, Alani A, Badheka A, Shenoy M, Mohamad B, Kanaan E, Ali O, Elder M, Schreiber TL. Racial disparities in left main stenting: insights from a real world inner city population. Journal Intervent Cardiol. 2013;26:43–8.
31. Bradley EH, Herrin J, Wang Y, McNamara RL, Webster TR, Magid DJ, Blaney M, Peterson ED, Canto JG, Pollack CV Jr, Krumholz HM. Racial and ethnic differences in time to acute reperfusion therapy for patients hospitalized with myocardial infarction. JAMA. 2004;292:1563–72.
32. Alter DA, Naylor CD, Austin P, Tu JV. Effects of socioeconomic status on access to invasive cardiac procedures and on mortality after acute myocardial infarction. N Engl J Med. 1999;341:1359–67.
33. Gerber Y, Benyamini Y, Goldbourt U, Drory Y. Israel study group on first acute myocardial infarction. Neighborhood socioeconomic context and long-term survival after myocardial infarction, Circulation. 2010;121:375–83.
34. Gerber Y, Goldbourt U, Drory Y. Interaction between income and education in predicting long-term survival after acute myocardial infarction. Eur J Prev Cardiol. 2008;15:526–32.
35. Smith GD, Hart C, Blane D, Gillis C, Hawthorne V. Lifetime socioeconomic position and mortality: prospective observational study. BMJ. 1997;314:547–52.
36. Lynch JW, Kaplan GA, Cohen RD, Tuomilehto J, Salonen JT. Do cardiovascular risk factors explain the relation between socioeconomic status, risk of all-cause mortality, cardiovascular mortality, and acute myocardial infarction? Am J Epidemiol. 1996;144:934–42.
37. Avendano M, Kunst AE, Huisman M, et al. Socioeconomic status and ischaemic heart disease mortality in 10 western European populations during the 1990s. Heart. 2006;92:461–7.
38. Winkleby M, Sundquist K, Cubbin C. Inequalities in CHD incidence and case fatality by neighborhood deprivation. Am J Prev Med. 2007;32:97–106.
39. Tofler GH, Muller JE, Stone PH, Davies G, Davis VG, Braunwald E. Comparison of long-term outcome after acute myocardial infarction in patients never graduated from high school with that in more educated patients. Milticenter investigation of the limitation of infarct size (MILIS). Am J Cardiol. 1993;71:1031–5.
40. Ho PM, Spertus JA, Masoudi FA, Reid KJ, Peterson ED, Magid DJ, Krumholz HM, Rumsfeld JS. Impact of medication therapy discontinuation on mortality after myocardial infarction. Arch Intern Med. 2006;166:1842–7.

18

Serum neutrophil gelatinase-associated lipocalin has an advantage over serum cystatin C and glomerular filtration rate in prediction of adverse cardiovascular outcome in patients with ST-segment elevation myocardial infarction

Olga L. Barbarash[1,2], Irina S. Bykova[1], Vasiliy V. Kashtalap[1,2], Mikhail V. Zykov[1], Oksana N. Hryachkova[1], Victoria V. Kalaeva[1], Kristina S. Shafranskaya[1], Victoria N. Karetnikova[1,2] and Anton G. Kutikhin[1*]

Abstract

Background: The aim of this study was to assess significance of serum neutrophil gelatinase-associated lipocalin (sNGAL) and cystatin C (sCC) in prediction of adverse cardiovascular outcome after ST-segment elevation myocardial infarction (STEMI).

Methods: We recruited 357 consecutive patients who were admitted to the hospital within 24 h after onset of STEMI. On the 1st and 12th-14th day after hospital admission, we measured levels of sNGAL and sCC. We also determined presence of renal dysfunction (RD), defined as glomerular filtration rate < 60 mL/min/1.73 m^2. After 3 years of follow-up, we performed a logistic regression and assessed the value of RD, sNGAL, and sCC in prediction of combined endpoint, defined as cardiovascular death or any cardiovascular complication.

Results: RD, sCC level ≥ 1.9 mg/L, and sNGAL level ≥ 1.25 ng/mL on the 12th-14th day of hospitalization were associated with a 1.6-fold, 1.9-fold, and 2.9-fold higher risk of adverse cardiovascular outcome, respectively. Area under the ROC curve was the highest for the model based on sNGAL level compared to the models based on sCC level or RD presence.

Conclusions: Measurement of sNGAL level in patients with STEMI on the 12th-14th day after hospital admission may improve prediction of adverse cardiovascular outcome.

Keywords: ST-segment elevation myocardial infarction, Renal dysfunction, Glomerular filtration rate, Cystatin C, Neutrophil gelatinase-associated lipocalin

* Correspondence: antonkutikhin@gmail.com
[1]Research Institute for Complex Issues of Cardiovascular Diseases, Sosnovy Boulevard 6, 650002 Kemerovo, Russian Federation
Full list of author information is available at the end of the article

Background

According to the World Health Organization statistics, coronary artery disease (CAD) is a leading cause of death worldwide [1]. An estimated 7.4 million people died from CAD in 2012, representing 11.2% of all global deaths [1]. In the Russian Federation alone, there were 597,921 deaths from CAD, which is the highest number amongst all countries included into analysis [1].

A number of investigations revealed a significant association of renal dysfunction [RD, defined as glomerular filtration rate (GFR) < 60 mL/min/1.73 m^2] with a high risk of cardiovascular death or acute cardiovascular events [2–4]. Moreover, RD is significantly associated with an adverse cardiovascular outcome in patients with CAD [5]. A critical decrease in GFR and albuminuria commonly occur at the late stage of chronic kidney disease (CKD) when > 30% of nephrons are affected [6]. However, there is a crucial need in novel, highly sensitive and specific markers of RD at the early stages of CKD. Recently, serum cystatin C (sCC) and serum neutrophil gelatinase-associated lipocalin (sNGAL) were suggested as the promising candidates [7, 8].

It is known that CC arises in all nucleated cells and is one of the most important endogenous inhibitors of cysteine proteinases whilst NGAL is produced by tubular epithelial cells and neutrophils in response to inflammation or ischemia, inhibiting bacterial growth and inducing epithelial cell proliferation [9]. The diagnostic value of sCC and sNGAL was shown for acute kidney injury, progression of CKD, and acute cardiorenal syndrome [10, 11]. Moreover, there is growing evidence of sCC and sNGAL importance in atherosclerosis and myocardial remodeling [12, 13]. In addition, sCC and sNGAL are associated with the risk factors of atherosclerosis [14, 15].

We carried out this study with the aim to investigate the value of sCC and sNGAL in prediction of an adverse cardiovascular outcome after ST-segment elevation myocardial infarction (STEMI).

Methods

We recruited 357 patients who were admitted within 24 h of STEMI onset to Research Institute for Complex Issues of Cardiovascular Diseases (Kemerovo, Russian Federation) in 2012–2013. The study was performed in accordance with the principles of Good Clinical Practice and the Declaration of Helsinki. The local ethical committee approved the study and all the participants provided written informed consent after a full explanation of the study was given to them.

The criteria of inclusion into the study were 1) age > 18 years; 2) diagnosis of STEMI according to the European Society of Cardiology (ESC) Guidelines [16]; 3) written informed consent to participate in the study. Criteria of

Table 1 Clinicopathological features of the patients, n = 357

Feature	Value
Female gender, n (%)	99 (27.7)
Mean age, years (95% confidence interval)	61.3 (59.9–62.6)
Stable angina, n (%)	176 (49.3)
Congestive heart failure, n (%)	75 (21.0)
Arterial hypertension, n (%)	301 (84.3)
Hypercholesterolemia, n (%)	87 (24.4)
Diabetes mellitus, n (%)	60 (16.8)
Smoking, n (%)	180 (50.4)
Body mass index > 25 kg/m^2, n (%)	265 (74.2)
Past medical history of myocardial infarction, n (%)	65 (18.2)
Past medical history of stroke, n (%)	31 (8.7)
Family history of coronary artery disease, n (%)	91 (25.5)

exclusion were 1) age < 18 years; 2) past medical history of cancer, concomitant autoimmune and/or mental disorders; 3) recurrent MI after percutaneous coronary intervention (PCI) or coronary artery bypass graft (CABG) surgery.

Stable angina, congestive heart failure, arterial hypertension, hypercholesterolemia, and diabetes mellitus were diagnosed according to ESC guidelines on the management of stable CAD [17], ESC guidelines for the diagnosis and treatment of acute and chronic heart failure [18], ESH/ESC Guidelines for the management of arterial hypertension [19], ESC/EAS Guidelines for the management of dyslipidemias [20], and ESC/EASD Guidelines on diabetes, pre-diabetes, and cardiovascular diseases [21], respectively. Smoking, body mass index, past medical history of MI or stroke, and family history of CAD were defined using the medical records. Clinicopathological features of the patients are represented in Table 1.

Selective coronary angiography was performed within the first hours after hospital admission using GE Healthcare Innova 3100 Cardiac Angiography System (General Electric Healthcare). Colour duplex screening of the extracranial arteries (ECA) and lower extremity arteries (LEA) was performed on the 5th-7th day after hospital admission in all patients using the cardiovascular ultrasound system Vivid 7 Dimension (General Electric Healthcare) with a 5.7 MHz linear array transducer (for ECA), a 2.5–3 MHz curved array transducer, and a

Table 2 In-hospital non-lethal cardiovascular complications, n = 357

Complication	Value
Early postinfarction angina, n (%)	50 (14.0)
Recurrent myocardial infarction, n (%)	18 (5.0)
Stroke, n (%)	2 (0.6)
Arrhythmia or heart block, n (%)	96 (26.9)
Any non-lethal cardiovascular complications, n (%)	166 (46.5)

Table 3 Study endpoints after 3 years of follow-up, n = 281

Study endpoint	Value
Cardiovascular death, n (%)	43 (15.3)
Recurrent myocardial infarction, n (%)	40 (14.2)
Stroke, n (%)	12 (4.3)
Hospital admission due to unstable angina, n (%)	81 (28.8)
Acute decompensated heart failure, n (%)	23 (8.2)
Combined endpoint, n (%)	199 (70.8)

5 MHz linear array transducer (for LEA). An extent of arterial stenosis was assessed in B regimen and by dopplerography (visualizing the local haemodynamics in the stenosis zone). Common and internal carotid arteries, vertebral, and subclavian arteries were visualized from both sides during the ECA screening; common and deep femoral arteries, popliteal, anterior and posterior tibial arteries were visualized from both sides during the LEA screening. The intima-media thickness (IMT) of common carotid artery was measured in the automatic mode (the value < 1 mm was considered normal). Polyvascular disease was defined as an increase in IMT ≥ 1 mm or ECA and/or LEA stenosis.

The preferable methods of myocardial reperfusion were defined in the shortest terms and included PCI or systemic thrombolytic therapy (TLT). Myocardial revascularization was not conducted when technical problems occurred or in patients with complex coronary anatomy or those with contraindications to TLT or PCI. All patients received the standard therapy of unfractionated heparin, aspirin, clopidogrel, angiotensin-converting enzyme inhibitors, beta-blockers, and statins. Long-acting nitrates, calcium channel blockers, diuretics, inotropic and antiarrhythmic drugs were prescribed if needed.

Serum creatinine level was measured at hospital admission and before hospital discharge with the further calculation of GFR by Modification of Diet in Renal Disease (MDRD) formula. In the case of in-hospital death, the final level of serum creatinine was taken into account. RD was defined as GFR < 60 mL/min/1.73 m^2. The levels of sCC and sNGAL were measured on the 1st and 12th-14th day after hospital admission by enzyme-linked immunosorbent assay using the respective kits of

R&D Systems according to the manufacturer's protocols. Reference values for sCC were 0.52–0.90 mg/L and 0.56–0.98 mg/L for females and males, respectively. Reference values for sNGAL were 0.037–0.106 ng/mL.

In-hospital case fatality rate was 10.4% (37/357 patients). The prevalence of in-hospital non-lethal cardiovascular complications is represented in Table 2. After 3 years of follow-up, we collected data from 87.8% (281/320) discharged patients. Follow-up was conducted by a telephone-based interview. Cardiovascular death, recurrent MI, stroke, hospital admission due to unstable angina, and acute decompensated heart failure were considered as an adverse cardiovascular outcome, or the study endpoints. The prevalence of the study endpoints is represented in Table 3.

Statistical analysis was performed using MedCalc (MedCalc Software) and SPSS (IBM). A sampling distribution was assessed by D'Agostino-Pearson test. Descriptive data were represented by median, interquartile range (25th and 75th percentiles), mean, and standard deviation of the mean. Two independent groups were compared by Mann-Whitney U-test. An adjustment for multiple comparisons was performed using false discovery rate (FDR). P-values, or q-values if FDR was applied (q-values are the name given to the adjusted p-values found using an optimized FDR approach), ≤ 0.05 were regarded as statistically significant. For multivariate analysis, we performed a stepwise linear logistic regression using forward Wald method with the plotting of the receiver operating characteristic (ROC) curve and further calculation of the area under the curve (AUC). Cut-off levels for sCC and sNGAL were defined according to the linear logistic regression to determine the optimal predictive values but were not linked to GFR.

Results

At hospital admission, all the patients were divided into two groups, with (n = 104, 29.1%) and without (n = 253, 70.9%) RD. The same stratification was carried out before hospital discharge [n = 86 (24.1%) and n = 271 (75.9%) patients with and without RD, respectively].

Medians of sCC and sNGAL levels on the 1st day after hospital admission were 1.21 (0.89–1.63) mg/L and 1.33

Table 4 Concentrations of serum cystatin C and neutrophil gelatinase-associated lipocalin in patients with and without renal dysfunction at hospital admission, n = 357

Feature	Renal dysfunction at hospital admission, n = 104	No renal dysfunction at hospital admission, n = 253	P value
Serum cystatin C on the 1st day after hospital admission, mg/L	1.76 (1.06–1.96)	1.16 (0.86–1.34)	0.037
Serum cystatin C on the 12th-14th day after hospital admission, mg/L	1.75 (1.15–2.16)	1.31 (0.95–1.66)	0.001
Serum neutrophil gelatinase-associated lipocalin on the 1st day after hospital admission, ng/mL	1.41 (1.01–1.82)	1.36 (1.08–1.64)	0.95
Serum neutrophil gelatinase-associated lipocalin on the 12th-14th day after hospital admission, ng/mL	1.78 (1.43–2.12)	1.85 (1.65–2.06)	0.68

Table 5 Concentrations of serum cystatin C and neutrophil gelatinase-associated lipocalin in patients with and without renal dysfunction before hospital discharge, $n = 357$

Feature	Renal dysfunction before hospital discharge, $n = 86$	No renal dysfunction before hospital discharge, $n = 271$	P value
Serum cystatin C on the 1st day after hospital admission, mg/L	1.27 (1.04–1.69)	1.12 (0.95–1.4)	0.14
Serum cystatin C on the 12th-14th day after hospital admission, mg/L	1.74 (1.29–2.17)	1.41 (0.96–1.7)	0.024
Serum neutrophil gelatinase-associated lipocalin on the 1st day after hospital admission, ng/mL	1.42 (1.05–2.28)	1.23 (0.2–1.76)	0.06
Serum neutrophil gelatinase-associated lipocalin on the 12th-14th day after hospital admission, ng/mL	1.93 (1.55–2.52)	1.53 (1.18–2.62)	0.031

(0.36–1.91) ng/mL, respectively. Medians of sCC and sNGAL levels on the 12th-14th day after hospital admission were 1.50 (1.02–1.90) mg/L and 1.63 (1.25–2.62) ng/mL, respectively.

Patients with RD at hospital admission had significantly higher levels of sCC on the 1st and 12th-14th day after hospital admission [1.76 (1.06–1.96) and 1.75 (1.15–2.16) mg/L, respectively) compared to those without RD [1.16 (0.86–1.34) and 1.31 (0.95–1.66) mg/L], $p = 0.037$ and 0.001, respectively (Table 4). Patients with RD at hospital discharge had significantly higher levels of sCC [1.74 (1.29–2.17) mg/L] and sNGAL [1.93 (1.55–2.52) ng/mL] on the 12th-14th day after hospital admission in comparison with those without RD [1.41 (0.96–1.7) mg/L and 1.53 (1.18–2.62) ng/mL], $p = 0.024$ and 0.031, respectively (Table 5). Regarding all other comparisons, we did not find any significant differences.

An increased level of sNGAL on the 1st day after admission was significantly associated with in-hospital non-lethal cardiovascular complications [1.42 (1.17–2.27) and 1.20 (0.20–1.86) ng/mL in patients with and without them, respectively, $p = 0.019$]. Moreover, a higher level of sNGAL on the 12th-14th day after hospital admission was significantly associated with a cardiovascular death after 3 years of follow-up (Fig. 1). In addition, elevated concentrations of sCC and sNGAL on the 12th-14th day after hospital admission were significantly associated with a combined endpoint (Figs. 1 and 2). Notably, 132 patients

had a level of sNGAL ≥ 1.25 ng/mL at hospital discharge that could possibly point on an infection [9]; however, none of them had signs or symptoms of any infectious disease both at hospital admission and hospital discharge. Nevertheless, we did not perform a specialized screening for latent infections.

For the determination of the independent factors of an adverse cardiovascular outcome, we performed a stepwise linear logistic regression. Factors included into regression were age, gender, past medical history of MI or stroke, diabetes mellitus, arterial hypertension, smoking, Killip class of acute heart failure at hospital admission, left ventricular ejection fraction (LVEF), localization of MI, number of affected coronary arteries, polyvascular disease, myocardial revascularization, sCC or sNGAL level on the 12th-14th day after hospital admission, and RD before hospital discharge. We identified anterior MI, LVEF < 40%, 3 affected coronary arteries, past medical history of stroke, level of sCC ≥ 1.9 mg/L on the 12th-14th day after hospital admission, level of sNGAL ≥ 1.25 ng/mL on the 12th-14th day after hospital admission, and RD before hospital discharge as the factors significantly associated with an adverse cardiovascular outcome after 3 years of follow-up (Table 6). Performance of PCI was associated with a significant decrease in risk of an adverse cardiovascular outcome (Table 6).

Finally, we compared AUC of the models based on RD before hospital discharge, level of sCC ≥ 1.9 mg/L, and level of sNGAL ≥ 1.25 ng/mL on the 12th-14th day after

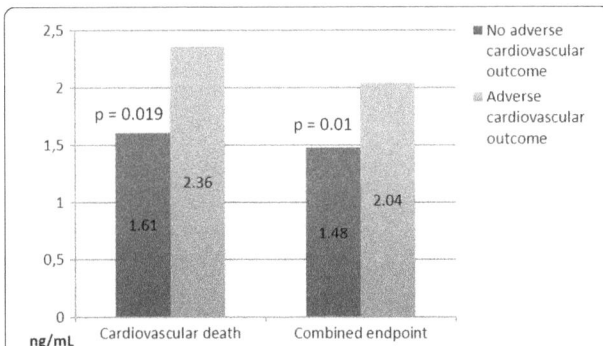

Fig. 1 Medians of sNGAL levels on the 12th-14th day after hospital admission depending on cardiovascular outcome after 3 years of follow-up

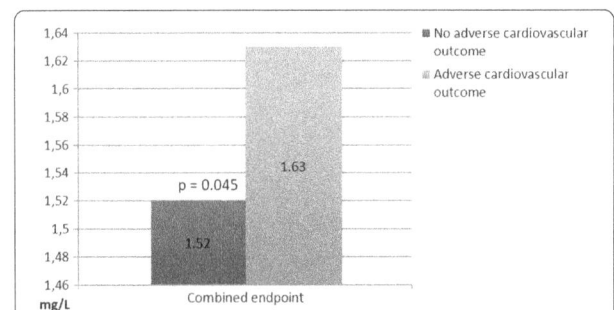

Fig. 2 Medians of sCC levels on the 12th-14th day after hospital admission depending on cardiovascular outcome after 3 years of follow-up; the Y axis is cut from 0 to 1.46 for the better visualization of the results

Table 6 Independent predictors of an adverse cardiovascular outcome after 3 years of follow-up

Predictor	P value	Odds ratio	95% confidence interval	
			Lower bound	Upper bound
Anterior localization of myocardial infarction	0.009	2.3	1.2	4.1
Left ventricular ejection fraction < 40%	0.001	3.6	1.7	7.6
Three affected coronary arteries	0.022	2.0	1.1	3.7
Past medical history of stroke	0.001	1.6	1.2	2.2
Level of serum cystatin C on the 12th-14th day after hospital admission ≥ 1.9 mg/L	0.004	1.9	1.2	2.9
Level of serum neutrophil gelatinase-associated lipocalin on the 12th-14th day after hospital admission ≥ 1.25 ng/mL	0.003	2.9	1.4	6.0
Renal dysfunction before hospital discharge	0.001	1.6	1.2	2.2
Percutaneous coronary intervention	0.001	0.4	0.3	0.7

hospital admission. The latter model had the highest predictive value (AUC = 0.78) whilst two other models had equally lower predictive value (AUC = 0.70, Fig. 3).

Discussion

In this study, we assessed the value of sCC and sNGAL level in prediction of an adverse cardiovascular outcome after STEMI. While sCC is a well-established marker of GFR [22, 23], sNGAL is mainly a neutrophil biomarker related to the bacterial infections; however, a number of studies also demonstrated an increase in sNGAL as a response to renal tubular damage [24–26]. Despite sNGAL is not well-recognized GFR marker compared to sCr and sCC and is not used for the calculation of GFR, sCr, sCC, and sNGAL all being the markers of renal tubular damage can be compared directly to each other for estimating efficiency in prediction of adverse outcome.

We previously demonstrated that sCC measured 1 day before and 7 days after CABG surgery is an appropriate predictor of in-hospital adverse cardiovascular and renal outcomes [27]. Here we showed that sCC and sNGAL can be potential markers of RD in patients with STEMI if measured on the 12th-14th day after hospital admission. Moreover, the level of sCC ≥ 1.9 mg/L and level of sNGAL ≥ 1.25 ng/mL on the 12th-14th day after hospital admission were associated with an adverse cardiovascular outcome in these patients after 3 years of follow-up. Out of three predictive models based on GFR < 60 mL/min/1.73 m², level of sCC ≥ 1.9 mg/L, and level of sNGAL ≥ 1.25 ng/mL on the 12th-14th day after hospital admission, the latter had the highest predictive value.

This corresponds to the results of Akerblom et al. who identified high level of sCC as an independent predictor of cardiovascular death or MI in patients with acute coronary syndrome (ACS) after 1 year of follow-up [28]. In

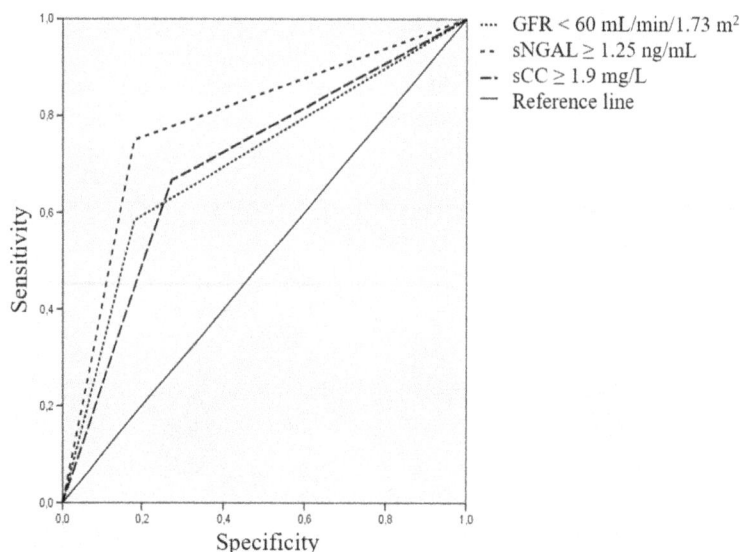

Fig. 3 Comparison of the predictive value of the models based on different markers of renal dysfunction regarding adverse cardiovascular outcome

addition, our results are in accordance with the data of Lindberg et al. who detected that high level of sNGAL is an independent predictor of an adverse cardiovascular outcome after 2 years of follow-up in patients with STEMI who underwent PCI [29]. Noteworthy, one of the recent studies demonstrated that a multimarker approach using sCC and a number of other biomarkers added prognostic information to the GRACE risk score in patients with ACS and high risk defined by GRACE, with increasing 6-month mortality in patients with a higher number of elevated biomarkers at hospital admission [30].

In our study, 39 patients were lost to follow-up; however, all of them were alive at that moment. Out of them, 17 (43.6%) patients had major cardiovascular risk factors, i.e., diabetes mellitus, CKD, or arterial hypertension; 15 (38.5%) and 24 (61.5%) respectively had cardiovascular complications and a decrease in GFR during the hospital stay. All these variables were comparable to the general sample; hence, exclusion of the patients lost to follow-up from the statistical analysis was unlikely to affect the results. However, this still can be considered as a study limitation along with a single-center design.

Therefore, both sCC and sNGAL have high predictive value for the stratification of cardiovascular risk in patients with STEMI; however, sNGAL has an advantage over sCC.

Conclusion

Patients with STEMI and in-hospital RD have higher levels of sCC and sNGAL compared to those without in-hospital RD. Elevated concentrations of sCC and sNGAL on the 12th-14th day after hospital admission can be suggested as the significant predictors of an adverse cardiovascular outcome in these patients after 3 years of follow-up. The model based on increased level of sNGAL has higher predictive value compared to those based on elevated concentration of sCC and decreased GFR.

Abbreviations

ACS: Acute coronary syndrome; AUC: Area under the ROC curve; CABG: Coronary artery bypass graft; CAD: Coronary artery disease; CKD: Chronic kidney disease; ECA: Extracranial arteries; ESC: European Society of Cardiology; FDR: False discovery rate; GFR: Glomerular filtration rate; IMT: Intima-media thickness; LEA: Lower extremity arteries; LVEF: Left ventricular ejection fraction; MDRD: Modification of diet in renal disease; PCI: Percutaneous coronary intervention; RD: Renal dysfunction; ROC: Receiver operating characteristic; sCC: serum cystatin C; sNGAL: serum neutrophil gelatinase-associated lipocalin; STEMI: ST-segment elevation myocardial infarction; TLT: Thrombolytic therapy

Acknowledgements

Not applicable.

Funding

This study was funded by Russian Foundation for Basic Research (№13-04-021620-a).

Authors' contributions

All authors fulfill the criteria for authorship. OLB and VaVK conceived and designed the study. ISB, MVZ, ViVK, KSS, and VNK collected the patient data and performed the statistical analysis. ONH performed the laboratory measurements. AGK wrote the manuscript. All authors read and approved the final version of the manuscript. All authors have agreed to authorship and order of authorship for this manuscript.

Competing interests

The authors declare that they have no competing interests.

Author details

[1]Research Institute for Complex Issues of Cardiovascular Diseases, Sosnovy Boulevard 6, 650002 Kemerovo, Russian Federation. [2]Kemerovo State Medical University, Voroshilova Street 22a, 650029 Kemerovo, Russian Federation.

References

1. Nowbar AN, Howard JP, Finegold JA, Asaria P, Francis DP. 2014 global geographic analysis of mortality from ischaemic heart disease by country, age and income: statistics from World Health Organisation and United Nations. Int J Cardiol. 2014;174:293–8.
2. Lin WY, Lin YJ, Chung FP, Chao TF, Liao JN, Chang SL, et al. Impact of renal dysfunction on clinical outcome in patients with low risk of atrial fibrillation. Circ J. 2014;78:853–8.
3. Choi JS, Kim CS, Park JW, Bae EH, Ma SK, Jeong MH, et al. Renal dysfunction as a risk factor for painless myocardial infarction: results from Korea Acute Myocardial Infarction Registry. Clin Res Cardiol. 2012;101:795–803.
4. Guo Y, Wang H, Zhao X, Zhang Y, Zhang D, Ma J, et al. Sequential changes in renal function and the risk of stroke and death in patients with atrial fibrillation. Int J Cardiol. 2013;168:4678–84.
5. Moukarbel GV, Yu ZF, Dickstein K, Hou YR, Wittes JT, McMurray JJ, et al. The impact of kidney function on outcomes following high risk myocardial infarction: findings from 27 610 patients. Eur J Heart Fail. 2014;16:289–99.
6. Stevens PE, Levin A. Kidney Disease: Improving Global Outcomes Chronic Kidney Disease Guideline Development Work Group Members. Evaluation and management of chronic kidney disease: synopsis of the kidney disease: improving global outcomes 2012 clinical practice guideline. Ann Intern Med. 2013;158:825–30.
7. Shlipak MG, Matsushita K, Ärnlöv J, Inker LA, Katz R, Polkinghorne KR, et al. Cystatin C versus creatinine in determining risk based on kidney function. N Engl J Med. 2013;369:932–43.
8. Zhou F, Luo Q, Wang L, Han L. Diagnostic value of neutrophil gelatinase-associated lipocalin for early diagnosis of cardiac surgery-associated acute kidney injury: a meta-analysis. Eur J Cardiothorac Surg. 2016;49:746–55.
9. Charlton JR, Portilla D, Okusa MD. A basic science view of acute kidney injury biomarkers. Nephrol Dial Transplant. 2014;29:1301–11.
10. Wasung ME, Chawla LS, Madero M. Biomarkers of renal function, which and when? Clin Chim Acta. 2015;438:350–7.
11. Bouquegneau A, Krzesinski JM, Delanaye P, Cavalier E. Biomarkers and physiopathology in the cardiorenal syndrome. Clin Chim Acta. 2015;443:100–7.
12. Angelidis C, Deftereos S, Giannopoulos G, Anatoliotakis N, Bouras G, Hatzis G, et al. Cystatin C: an emerging biomarker in cardiovascular disease. Curr Top Med Chem. 2013;13:164–79.
13. Iqbal N, Choudhary R, Chan J, Wentworth B, Higginbotham E, Maisel AS. Neutrophil gelatinase-associated lipocalin as diagnostic and prognostic tool for cardiovascular disease and heart failure. Expert Opin Med Diagn. 2013;7:209–20.
14. Wang J, Sim AS, Wang XL, Salonikas C, Moriatis M, Naidoo D, et al. Relations between markers of renal function, coronary risk factors and the occurrence and severity of coronary artery disease. Atherosclerosis. 2008;197:853–9.
15. Lindberg S, Jensen JS, Mogelvang R, Pedersen SH, Galatius S, Flyvbjerg A, et al. Plasma neutrophil gelatinase-associated lipocalin in the general population: association with inflammation and prognosis. Arterioscler Thromb Vasc Biol. 2014;34:2135–42.
16. Task Force on the management of ST-segment elevation acute myocardial infarction of the European Society of Cardiology (ESC), Steg PG, James SK, Atar D, Badano LP, Blömstrom-Lundqvist C, et al. ESC Guidelines for the management of acute myocardial infarction in patients presenting with ST-segment elevation. Eur Heart J. 2012;33:2569–619.

17. Task Force Members, Montalescot G, Sechtem U, Achenbach S, Andreotti F, Arden C, et al. 2013 ESC guidelines on the management of stable coronary artery disease: the Task Force on the management of stable coronary artery disease of the European Society of Cardiology. Eur Heart J. 2013;34:2949–3003.

18. McMurray JJ, Adamopoulos S, Anker SD, Auricchio A, Böhm M, Dickstein K, et al. ESC guidelines for the diagnosis and treatment of acute and chronic heart failure 2012: The Task Force for the Diagnosis and Treatment of Acute and Chronic Heart Failure 2012 of the European Society of Cardiology. Developed in collaboration with the Heart Failure Association (HFA) of the ESC. Eur J Heart Fail. 2012;14:803–69.

19. Mancia G, Fagard R, Narkiewicz K, Redon J, Zanchetti A, Böhm M, et al. 2013 ESH/ESC guidelines for the management of arterial hypertension: the Task Force for the Management of Arterial Hypertension of the European Society of Hypertension (ESH) and of the European Society of Cardiology (ESC). Eur Heart J. 2013;34:2159–219.

20. European Association for Cardiovascular Prevention & Rehabilitation, Reiner Z, Catapano AL, De Backer G, Graham I, Taskinen MR, et al. ESC/EAS Guidelines for the management of dyslipidaemias: the Task Force for the management of dyslipidaemias of the European Society of Cardiology (ESC) and the European Atherosclerosis Society (EAS). Eur Heart J. 2011;32:1769–818.

21. Authors/Task Force Members, Rydén L, Grant PJ, Anker SD, Berne C, Cosentino F, et al. ESC Guidelines on diabetes, pre-diabetes, and cardiovascular diseases developed in collaboration with the EASD: the Task Force on diabetes, pre-diabetes, and cardiovascular diseases of the European Society of Cardiology (ESC) and developed in collaboration with the European Association for the Study of Diabetes (EASD). Eur Heart J. 2013;34:3035–87.

22. Pottel H, Delanaye P, Schaeffner E, Dubourg L, Eriksen BO, Melsom T, et al. Estimating glomerular filtration rate for the full age spectrum from serum creatinine and cystatin C. Nephrol Dial Transplant. 2017. doi:10.1093/ndt/gfw425 . [Epub ahead of print]

23. Ye X, Liu X, Song D, Zhang X, Zhu B, Wei L, et al. Estimating glomerular filtration rate by serum creatinine or/and cystatin C equations: an analysis of multi-centre Chinese subjects. Nephrology (Carlton). 2016;21:372–8.

24. Quintavalle C, Anselmi CV, De Micco F, Roscigno G, Visconti G, Golia B, et al. Neutrophil gelatinase-associated lipocalin and contrast-induced acute kidney injury. Circ Cardiovasc Interv. 2015;8:e002673. doi:10.1161/CIRCINTERVENTIONS.115.002673.

25. Yavuz S, Anarat A, Acartürk S, Dalay AC, Kesiktaş E, Yavuz M, et al. Neutrophil gelatinase associated lipocalin as an indicator of acute kidney injury and inflammation in burned children. Burns. 2014;40:648–54.

26. Urbschat A, Gauer S, Paulus P, Reissig M, Weipert C, Ramos-Lopez E, et al. Serum and urinary NGAL but not KIM-1 raises in human postrenal AKI. Eur J Clin Invest. 2014;44:652–9.

27. Shafranskaya KS, Kashtalap VV, Gruzdeva OV, Kutikhin AG, Barbarash OL, Barbarash LS. The role of cystatin C in the prognosis of adverse outcomes after the coronary artery bypass graft surgery during hospitalisation. Heart Lung Circ. 2015;24:193–9.

28. Akerblom Å, Wallentin L, Siegbahn A, Becker RC, Budaj A, Buck K, et al. Cystatin C and estimated glomerular filtration rate as predictors for adverse outcome in patients with ST-elevation and non-ST-elevation acute coronary syndromes: results from the Platelet Inhibition and Patient Outcomes study. Clin Chem. 2012;58:190–9.

29. Lindberg S, Pedersen SH, Mogelvang R, Jensen JS, Flyvbjerg A, Galatius S, et al. Prognostic utility of neutrophil gelatinase-associated lipocalin in predicting mortality and cardiovascular events in patients with ST-segment elevation myocardial infarction treated with primary percutaneous coronary intervention. J Am Coll Cardiol. 2012;60:339–45.

30. Vieira C, Nabais S, Ramos V, Braga C, Gaspar A, Azevedo P, et al. Multimarker approach with cystatin C, N-terminal pro-brain natriuretic peptide, C-reactive protein and red blood cell distribution width in risk stratification of patients with acute coronary syndromes. Rev Port Cardiol. 2014;33:127–36.

19

A case of successful reperfusion through a combination of intracoronary thrombolysis and aspiration thrombectomy in ST-segment elevation myocardial infarction associated with an ectatic coronary artery

Yonggu Lee[1], Eunjin Kim[1], Bae Keun Kim[2] and Jeong-Hun Shin[1*]

Abstract

Background: Large thrombus burdens in ectatic coronary arteries that remain after aspiration thrombectomy can negatively impact outcomes following percutaneous coronary interventions in patients with acute myocardial infarction.

Case presentation: A 53-year-old man presented with ST-segment elevation myocardial infarction (STEMI). Coronary angiography revealed an ectatic right coronary artery (RCA) that was completely occluded in the mid portion by a large amount of thrombus. Catheter-directed intracoronary thrombolysis with alteplase led to recovery of coronary blood flow, which multiple attempts of aspiration thrombectomy had failed to achieve. Coronary angiography 9 days later showed good blood flow and insignificant stenosis remaining in the RCA; this had completely resolved in 6 months' follow-up coronary angiography.

Conclusion: Catheter-directed intracoronary thrombolysis can be performed effectively and safely when repeat aspiration thrombectomy fails to produce satisfactory coronary reperfusion in STEMI patients with large thrombus burdens in ectatic coronary arteries.

Keywords: Myocardial infarction, Aspiration thrombectomy, Intracoronary thrombolysis, Coronary ectasia, Case report

Background

Intracoronary thrombosis in patients with ST-segment elevation myocardial infarction (STEMI) can cause distal embolization, no-reflow phenomena and stent thrombosis, and increase the risk of adverse cardiac events and death following primary percutaneous coronary interventions (PCIs) [1, 2]. Although the beneficial effect of manual aspiration thrombectomy (MAT) during primary PCIs is still open to debate, it is frequently employed as a first-line therapy to reduce these adverse events [3]. However, there are no other effective options when MAT delivers insufficient coronary blood flow, especially in patients with large thrombus burdens. Here we report a case of successful coronary reperfusion through a combination of catheter-directed intracoronary thrombolysis and MAT in STEMI caused by thrombotic occlusion of an ectatic coronary artery.

Case presentation

A 53-year-old man presented in the emergency department with sudden chest pain lasting for 30 min. He was a 40-pack-year current smoker with high blood pressure on no medication. Blood pressure was 160/110 mmHg and pulse rate 60 beats/min. Electrocardiography showed ST-segment elevations in leads II, III, and aVF (Fig. 1a). Serum creatinine was 0.8 mg/dl and serum

* Correspondence: cardio.hyapex@gmail.com
[1]Division of Cardiology, Department of Internal Medicine, Hanyang University Guri Hospital, 153, Gyeongchun-ro, Guri-si, Gyeonggi-do 11923, South Korea
Full list of author information is available at the end of the article

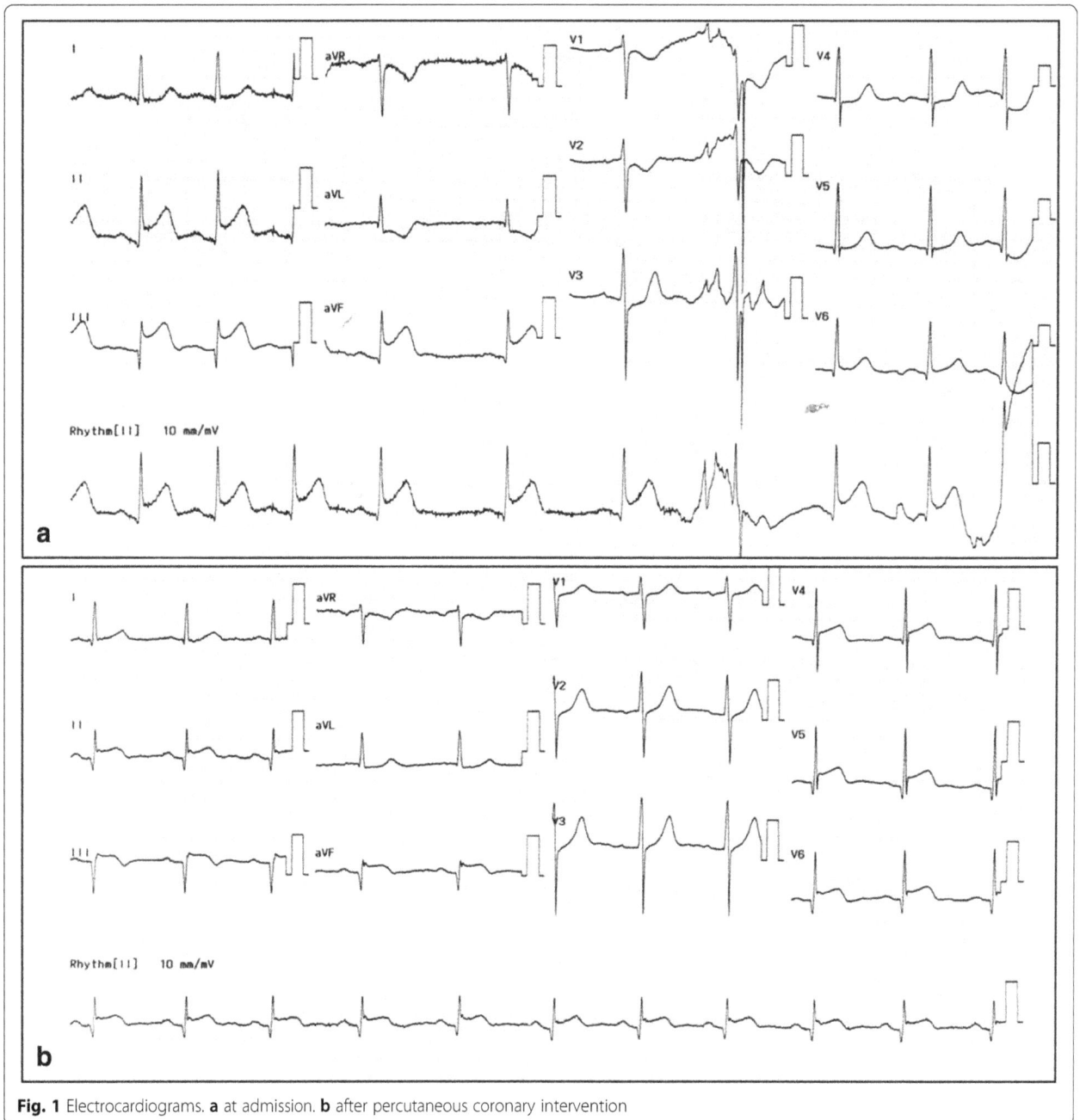

Fig. 1 Electrocardiograms. **a** at admission. **b** after percutaneous coronary intervention

troponin I 0.01 ng/ml. Killip classification was class I. Aspirin 300 mg and ticagrelor 180 mg were administered, and coronary angiography (CAG) was performed immediately under temporary ventricular pacing. CAG revealed an ectatic right coronary artery (RCA) completely occluded by a large amount of thrombus in the mid-portion (Fig. 2a). A bolus of unfractionated heparin (8000 IU) and glycoprotein IIb/IIIa antagonist (abciximab, 0.25 mg/kg) was administered intravenously and MAT was performed three times using a 6-Fr aspiration catheter (Rebirth, Goodman Co. Ltd., Nagoya, Japan). After red thrombi were aspirated, thrombolysis in

myocardial infarction (TIMI) grade 2 flow was achieved but a large filling defect persisted in the mid portion of the RCA, with distal embolization in the posterior descending artery (PDA) (Fig. 2b). Intravascular ultrasound (IVUS) (Atlantis, Boston Scientific, Natick, MA) revealed a ruptured plaque containing a large necrotic core and a large amount of thrombus remaining in the lesion. The external elastic membrane (EEM) diameter and the luminal diameter of the normal adjacent proximal segment of the occlusion were 7.5 mm and 6.5 mm, respectively (Fig. 3a). The culprit lesion was 7.7 mm in EEM diameter and 4.8 mm^2 in minimal luminal area

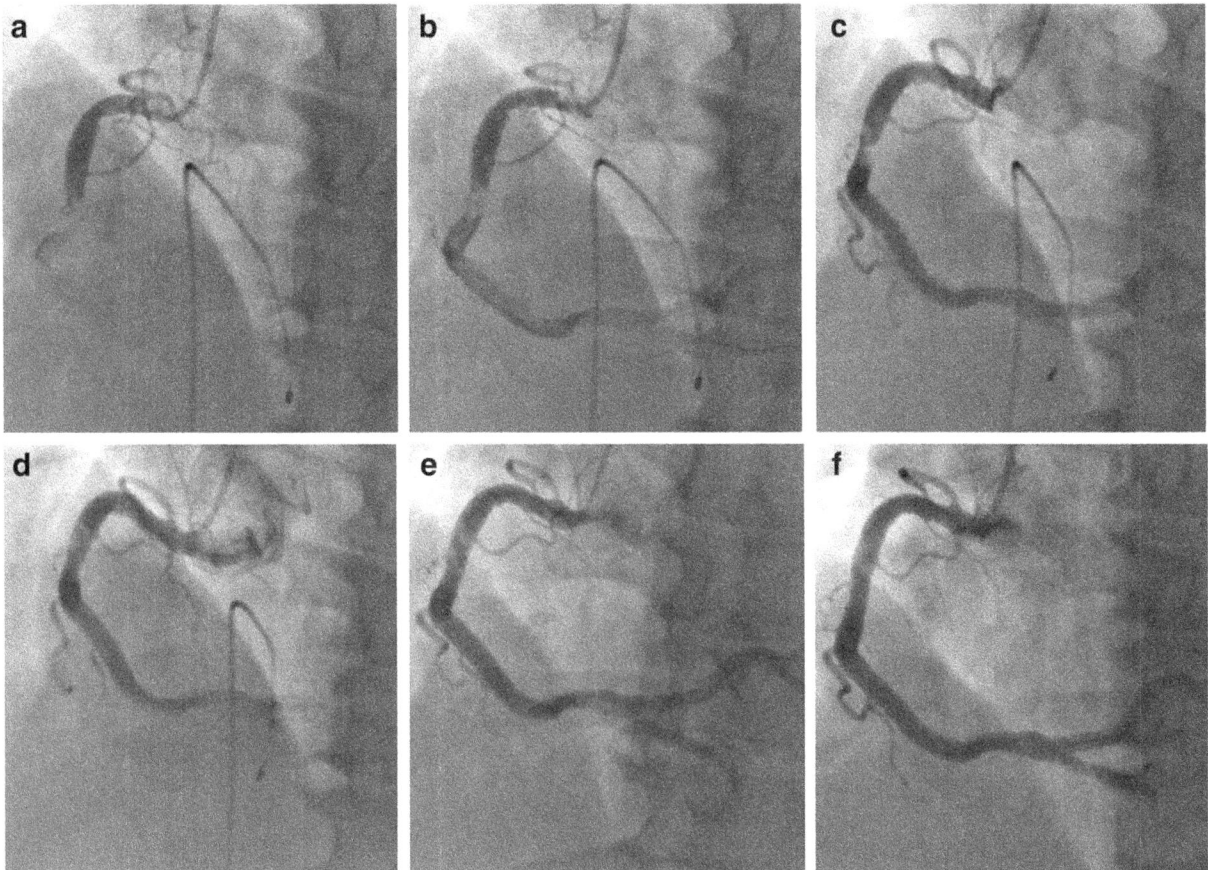

Fig. 2 Coronary angiography. **a** Thrombotic total occlusion of the mid portion of the right coronary artery (RCA) with TIMI grade 0 flow. **b** After thrombus aspiration, a large filling defect remained due to extensive thrombus in the mid portion of the RCA with distal embolization in the posterior descending artery (PDA). **c** After initial intracoronary thrombolysis and repeated thrombus aspiration, improvement of TIMI flow, distal embolization, and residual thrombus at the mid portion of the RCA were noted. **d** After balloon angioplasty and second intracoronary thrombolysis, the culprit stenotic lesion was dilated, but TIMI flow worsened with distal embolization. **e** On the ninth day after the primary percutaneous intervention, TIMI flow was restored, but focal eccentric intermediate stenosis with some residual thrombus remained at the mid portion of the RCA. **f** Six months after discharge, marked dissolution of the thrombus and only minimal stenosis at the mid portion of the RCA was noted

(MLA) (Fig. 3b). Because stent apposition might be difficult in such a large vessel, we decided to perform catheter-directed intracoronary thrombolysis using alteplase. The tip of a 2.7 Fr microcatheter (Progreat®, Terumo, Somerset, NJ, USA) was placed on the culprit lesion, and 5 mg of alteplase (Actilyse, Boehringer Ingelheim, Germany) in 5 mL normal saline was slowly administered over five minutes through the microcatheter. After 10 min, CAG showed improved coronary blood flow from the TIMI grade 2 to 3 in the mid portion of the RCA and from the TIMI grade 0 to 1 in the PDA, with remaining thrombi in the mid portion (Fig. 2c). Because significant stenosis persisted, a 4.5 × 8 mm noncompliant balloon (Quantum, Boston Scientific, Natick, MA) was inflated up to 16 atm in the mid portion of the RCA to disrupt the partially lysed thrombi. The lesion was dilated after the balloon angioplasty; however TIMI

flow of the RCA appeared to be worsened (Fig. 2d). Intracoronary thrombolysis was repeated in the same manner. Blood flow improved to TIMI grade 3 and IVUS showed increased MLA with remaining thrombi (Fig. 3c). The chest pain was completely relieved and the ST-segment elevation was resolved (Fig. 1b).

Intravenous infusion of the glycoprotein IIb/IIIa inhibitor was maintained for 12 h after PCI. Oral administration of aspirin (100 mg/day), ticagrelor (180 mg/day), rosuvastatin (20 mg/day), bisoprolol (1.25 mg/day), and candesartan (8 mg/day) was continued. Low molecular weight heparin (dalteparin 100 IU/kg every 12 h; Fragmin®, Pfizer Inc., New York, NY) was administered subcutaneously after the femoral sheath was removed. No significant bleeding complications occurred after PCI. CAG repeated 9 days after the PCI revealed TIMI grade 3 blood flow in the RCA and PDA, and insignificant

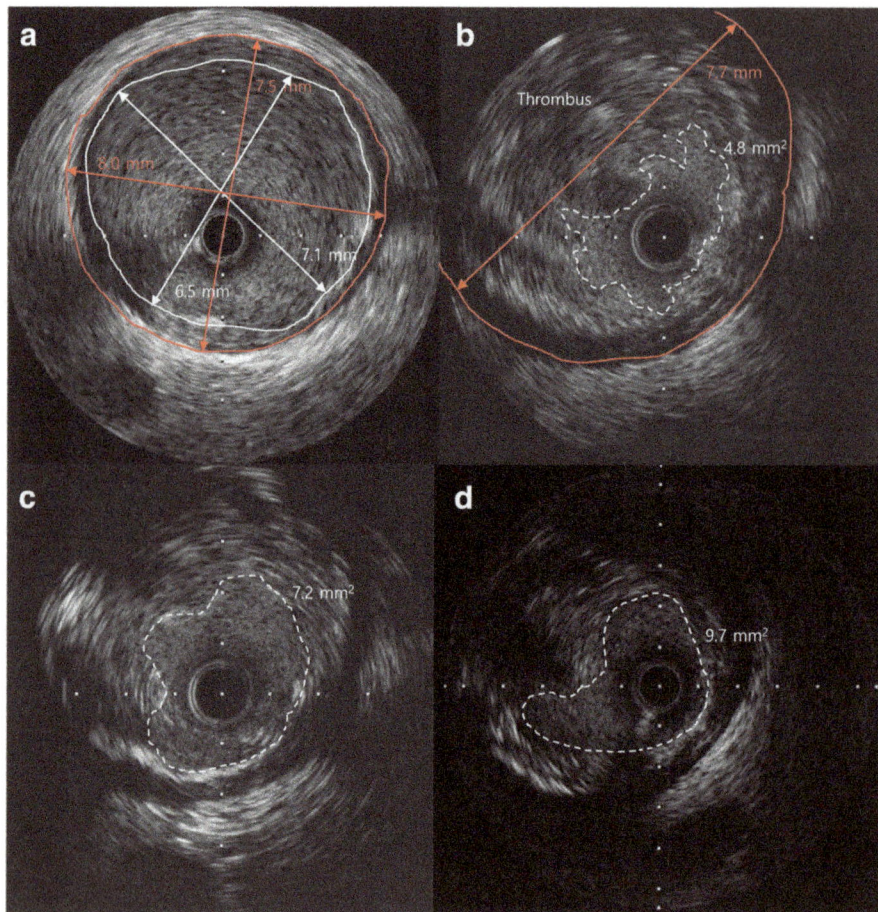

Fig. 3 Intravascular ultrasound (IVUS) findings. **a** Adjacent normal segment proximal to the occlusion site. The shortest EEM and luminal diameter were 7.5 mm and 6.5 mm, respectively. **b** A ruptured plaque containing many necrotic components and a large amount of thrombus. The diameter of the external elastic membrane was 7.7 mm. **c** After thrombus aspiration and intracoronary thrombolysis, intermediate stenosis with remnant thrombi was noted. **d** On the ninth day after the primary percutaneous intervention, a minimal lumen area of about 9.73 mm² with plaque was noted

focal stenosis with a small amount of remaining thrombus in the lesion (Fig. 2e). IVUS showed that the MLA was 9.7 mm² in the lesion (Fig. 3d) and the fractional flow reserve measured under maximal hyperemia was 0.98. Based on these assessments, we decided not to perform any additional intervention. The patient was discharged 12 days after PCI. CAG repeated 6 months after PCI showed complete dissolution of the thrombi and minimal remaining stenosis in the lesion with TIMI 3 blood flow in the RCA (Fig. 2f).

Discussion and conclusions

Massive intracoronary thrombi are associated with unsuccessful angiographic reperfusion and unfavorable clinical outcomes [1, 4]. Unresolved intracoronary thrombi can cause microvascular obstruction, known as the no-reflow phenomenon, and result in reduced myocardial perfusion at the microvascular level, increased infarct size and higher mortality [5]. Although

there have been improvements in antiplatelet and anti-coagulant regimens and technical advances in PCIs, intracoronary thrombus remains one of the most dreaded enemies of interventional cardiologists. MAT is one of the most frequently used thrombectomy methods in primary PCIs, because the procedure is simple and the risk of vascular injury and distal embolism is low. Clinical guidelines also suggest that MAT is a reasonable approach when intracoronary thrombi are encountered [3]. However, studies have yielded inconsistent results in terms of its benefits in primary PCI [6–8]. The TASTE trial showed no benefits of MAT for mortality, re-hospitalization and stent thrombosis [8]. More recently, Jolly et al. [7] also reported that MAT did not reduce cardiovascular events, whereas it increased stroke rate. This result may partly be related to insufficient thrombus removal and inadequate coronary blood flow recovery in cases with massive intracoronary thrombosis. Safe and feasible alternative strategies are needed when MAT fails during primary PCI.

Before coronary stents were much used, intracoronary thrombolysis was used in patients with all types of coronary artery disease [9, 10]. However, because studies gave discouraging results [11] and primary PCI with stent implantation became routine, intracoronary thrombolysis was rarely used in clinical practice. In recent years, intracoronary thrombolysis has regained popularity as an adjuvant therapy for primary PCI, as studies using different thrombolytic agents and improved antiplatelet regimens showed it to be safe and effective. Kelly et al. [12] reported that intracoronary infusion of tenecteplase was safe and effective for coronary flow recovery in patients with myocardial infarction. More recently, Boscarelli et al. [13] found that adjuvant intracoronary infusion of low dose tenecteplase and alteplase in STEMI significantly reduced the thrombi remaining after MAT and improved coronary blood flow. Several case reports of massive intracoronary thrombosis also described successful recovery of coronary blood flow after intracoronary thrombolysis using alteplase [14] and tenecteplase [15].

We used the glycoprotein IIb/IIIa inhibitor after intracoronary thrombolysis, which may significantly increase the risk of major bleeding events. However, the thrombolytic agent doses used through intracoronary routes are usually much lower than those used through intravenous routes. Kelly et al. [12] also reported that only 1 case of major bleeding (2.9%) among 34 patients after intracoronary thrombolysis using tenectaplase, which is similar to the major bleeding rates reported regularly in acute coronary syndrome [16]. Moreover, the majority of the patients (76%) in their study received glycoprotein IIb/IIIa inhibitors simultaneously with intracoronary thrombolysis.

In our case, a massive thrombotic occlusion occurred in the ectatic RCA. Coronary ectasia is defined as a diffuse dilation of a coronary artery to a diameter at least 1.5 times larger than normal coronary artery diameter [17]. It is present in 1–5% of patients undergoing CAG [18]. Various reperfusion strategies including MAT alone, simple balloon angioplasty, pulse-spray thrombolysis, intracoronary thrombolysis and mesh-covered stent implantation have been proposed in STEMI in ectatic coronary arteries [19–21]. Several randomized controlled trials have reported that rheolytic thrombectomy was more effective than MAT in thrombus removal and myocardial reperfusion in patients with STEMI, although there were no differences in infarct sizes and adverse cardiac events following PCI between rheolytic thrombolysis and MAT [22, 23]. Simple balloon angioplasty might increase the risk of distal embolization after intracoronary thrombus is incompletely removed. Prolonged intravenous heparin infusion is a viable option for the remaining thrombus after MAT

in ectatic coronary arteries [24]. However, for ectatic coronary arteries, because the sheer amount of thrombus is massive and blood flow is slow, no single strategy would be sufficient. In fact, we employed multiple strategies namely MAT, balloon angioplasty and intracoronary thrombolysis during the PCI to achieve a good immediate result. We think that the additional anatomical and physiological information obtained by IVUS and by measuring the fractional flow reserve helped us avoid stent implantation, which could have led to incomplete stent apposition. Self-expendable stents have been introduced for patients with complex coronary anatomy including aneurysmal dilation, which may also be an alternative strategy to avoid difficulty in stent apposition, as shown in our case [25].

In conclusion, catheter-directed intracoronary thrombolysis may be a safe and effective alternative reperfusion strategy that may be selected when MAT alone fails to achieve sufficient coronary blood flow in the culprit vessel in STEMI associated with massive thrombosis in ectatic coronary arteries.

Abbreviations

CAG: Coronary angiography; IVUS: Intravascular ultrasound; MLA: Minimal lumen area; PCI: Primary percutaneous coronary intervention; PDA: Posterior descending artery; RCA: Right coronary artery; STEMI: ST-elevation myocardial infarction; TIMI: Thrombolysis in myocardial infarction

Acknowledgements

No acknowledgements.

Funding

There was no funding pertaining to the manuscript.

Authors' contributions

JHS drafted the manuscript and performed the angioplasty. EK drafted the manuscript and edited the figures. BKK and YL critically revised the manuscript for important intellectual content. All authors read and approved the final manuscript.

Competing interests

The authors declare that they have no competing interests.

Author details

[1]Division of Cardiology, Department of Internal Medicine, Hanyang University Guri Hospital, 153, Gyeongchun-ro, Guri-si, Gyeonggi-do 11923, South Korea. [2]Department of Cardiology, Sungae Hospital, Seoul, Republic of Korea.

References

1. Ndrepepa G, Tiroch K, Fusaro M, Keta D, Seyfarth M, Byrne RA, Pache J, Alger P, Mehilli J, Schomig A, et al. 5-year prognostic value of no-reflow phenomenon after percutaneous coronary intervention in patients with acute myocardial infarction. J Am Coll Cardiol. 2010;55(21):2383–9.
2. Sianos G, Papafaklis MI, Daemen J, Vaina S, van Mieghem CA, van Domburg RT, Michalis LK, Serruys PW. Angiographic stent thrombosis after routine use

of drug-eluting stents in ST-segment elevation myocardial infarction: the importance of thrombus burden. J Am Coll Cardiol. 2007;50(7):573–83.

3. Kushner FG, Hand M, Smith Jr SC, King 3rd SB, Anderson JL, Antman EM, Bailey SR, Bates ER, Blankenship JC, Casey Jr DE, et al. 2009 focused updates: ACC/AHA guidelines for the management of patients with ST-elevation myocardial infarction (updating the 2004 guideline and 2007 focused update) and ACC/AHA/SCAI guidelines on percutaneous coronary intervention (updating the 2005 guideline and 2007 focused update) a report of the American College of Cardiology Foundation/American Heart Association task force on practice guidelines. J Am Coll Cardiol. 2009;54(23): 2205–41.

4. Napodano M, Dariol G, Al Mamary AH, Marra MP, Tarantini G, D'Amico G, Frigo AC, Buja P, Razzolini R, Iliceto S. Thrombus burden and myocardial damage during primary percutaneous coronary intervention. Am J Cardiol. 2014;113(9):1449–56.

5. Jaffe R, Dick A, Strauss BH: Prevention and treatment of microvascular obstruction-related myocardial injury and coronary no-reflow following percutaneous coronary intervention: a systematic approach. JACC Cardiovasc Interv 2010, 3(7):695-704.

6. Vlaar PJ, Svilaas T, van der Horst IC, Diercks GF, Fokkema ML, de Smet BJ, van den Heuvel AF, Anthonio RL, Jessurun GA, Tan ES, et al. Cardiac death and reinfarction after 1 year in the thrombus aspiration during Percutaneous coronary intervention in acute myocardial infarction study (TAPAS): a 1-year follow-up study. Lancet. 2008;371(9628):1915–20.

7. Jolly SS, Cairns JA, Yusuf S, Meeks B, Pogue J, Rokoss MJ, Kedev S, Thabane L, Stankovic G, Moreno R, et al. Randomized trial of primary PCI with or without routine manual thrombectomy. N Engl J Med. 2015;372(15):1389–98.

8. Frobert O, Lagerqvist B, Gudnason T, Thuesen L, Svensson R, Olivecrona GK, James SK. Thrombus aspiration in ST-elevation myocardial infarction in Scandinavia (TASTE trial). A multicenter, prospective, randomized, controlled clinical registry trial based on the Swedish angiography and angioplasty registry (SCAAR) platform. Study design and rationale. Am Heart J. 2010; 160(6):1042–8.

9. Zhu J, Liu XM, Du CJ, Zhang ZW, Qiu YQ, Gong Y, Liu JR, Hong YR, Luo ZY, Zhang Y. Diagnostic value of lesion-directed prostate biopsy under TRUS in early detection of prostate cancer. Zhonghua nan ke xue. 2009;15(5):437–40.

10. Goudreau E, DiSciascio G, Vetrovec GW, Chami Y, Kohli R, Warner M, Sabri N, Cowley MJ. Intracoronary urokinase as an adjunct to percutaneous transluminal coronary angioplasty in patients with complex coronary narrowings or angioplasty-induced complications. Am J Cardiol. 1992;69(1):57–62.

11. Simoons ML, Wijns W, Balakumaran K, Serruys PW, van den Brand M, Fioretti P, Reiber JH, Lie P, Hugenholtz PG. The effect of intracoronary thrombolysis with streptokinase on myocardial thallium distribution and left ventricular function assessed by blood-pool scintigraphy. Eur Heart J. 1982;3(5):433–40.

12. Kelly RV, Crouch E, Krumnacher H, Cohen MG, Stouffer GA. Safety of adjunctive intracoronary thrombolytic therapy during complex percutaneous coronary intervention: initial experience with intracoronary tenecteplase. Catheter Cardiovasc Interv. 2005;66(3):327–32.

13. Boscarelli D, Vaquerizo B, Miranda-Guardiola F, Arzamendi D, Tizon H, Sierra G, Delgado G, Fantuzzi A, Estrada D, Garcia-Picart J, et al. Intracoronary thrombolysis in patients with ST-segment elevation myocardial infarction presenting with massive intraluminal thrombus and failed aspiration. Eur Heart J Acute Cardiovasc care. 2014;3(3):229–36.

14. Kim JS, Kim JH, Jang HH, Lee YW, Song SG, Park JH, Chun KJ. Successful revascularization of coronary artery occluded by massive intracoronary thrombi with alteplase and percutaneous coronary intervention. J Atheroscler Thromb. 2010;17(7):768–70.

15. Gallagher S, Jain AK, Archbold RA. Intracoronary thrombolytic therapy: a treatment option for failed mechanical thrombectomy. Catheter Cardiovasc Interv. 2012;80(5):835–7.

16. Moscucci M, Fox KA, Cannon CP, Klein W, Lopez-Sendon J, Montalescot G, White K, Goldberg RJ. Predictors of major bleeding in acute coronary syndromes: the global registry of acute coronary events (GRACE). Eur Heart J. 2003;24(20):1815–23.

17. Swanton RH, Thomas ML, Coltart DJ, Jenkins BS, Webb-Peploe MM, Williams BT. Coronary artery ectasia–a variant of occlusive coronary arteriosclerosis. Br Heart J. 1978;40(4):393–400.

18. Swaye PS, Fisher LD, Litwin P, Vignola PA, Judkins MP, Kemp HG, Mudd JG, Gosselin AJ. Aneurysmal coronary artery disease. Circulation. 1983;67(1):134–8.

19. Yokokawa T, Ujiie Y, Kaneko H, Seino Y, Kijima M, Takeishi Y. Lone aspiration thrombectomy without stenting for a patient with ST-segment elevation

myocardial infarction associated with coronary ectasia. Cardiovasc Interv Ther. 2014;29(4):339–43.

20. Tanabe Y, Itoh E, Nakagawa I, Suzuki K. Pulse-spray thrombolysis in acute myocardial infarction caused by thrombotic occlusion of an ectatic coronary artery. Circ J. 2002;66(2):207–10.

21. Linares Vicente JA, Lukic A, Ruiz Arroyo JR, Revilla Marti P, Simo Sanchez B. Combined intracoronary thrombolysis, thrombus aspiration and mesh-covered stent implantation for organized massive thrombus burden in ectatic coronary. Cardiovasc Interv Ther. 2014;29(1):55–9.

22. Carrabba N, Parodi G, Maehara A, Pradella S, Migliorini A, Valenti R, Comito V, Marrani M, Rega L, Colagrande S, et al. Rheolityc thrombectomy in acute myocardial infarction: effect on microvascular obstruction, infarct size, and left ventricular remodeling. Catheter Cardiovasc Interv. 2016;87(1):E1–8.

23. Vergara R, Valenti R, Migliorini A, Parodi G, Giurlani L, Marrani M, Cantini G, Antoniucci D: Rheolytic Thrombectomy for acute myocardial infarction complicated by Cardiogenic shock. J Invasive Cardiol. 2016;28(12):E193–7.

24. Ielasi A, Anzuini A. Successful management of a huge thrombus in coronary aneurysmatic dilatation after failed mechanical thrombectomy during acute myocardial infarction. J Cardiovasc Med (Hagerstown). 2014;15(1):80–1.

25. La Manna A, Geraci S, Tamburino C. A self-expandable coronary stent system to treat complex coronary stenosis complicated by poststenotic aneurysm: an optical coherence tomographic evidence-based case report. J Invasive Cardiol. 2011;23(12):E277–80.

20

Influence of apelin-12 on troponin levels and the rate of MACE in STEMI patients

Xhevdet Krasniqi[2*] ⓘ, Blerim Berisha[2], Masar Gashi[2], Dardan Koçinaj[2], Fisnik Jashari[2] and Josip Vincelj[1]

Abstract

Background: During acute myocardial infarction, phosphorylated TnI levels, Ca^{2+} sensitivity and ATPase activity are decreased in the myocardium, and the subsequent elevation in Ca^{2+} levels activates protease I (caplain I), leading to the proteolytic degradation of troponins. Concurrently, the levels of apelin and APJ expression are increased by limiting myocardial injury.

Methods: In this prospective observational study, 100 consecutive patients with ST-elevation acute myocardial infarction were included. Patients meeting the following criteria were included in our study: (1) continuous chest pain lasting for >30 min, (2) observation of ST-segment elevation of more than 2 mm in two adjacent leads by electrocardiography (ECG), (3) increased cardiac troponin I levels, and (4) patients who underwent reperfusion therapy. We evaluated the levels of apelin-12 and troponin I on the first and seventh days after reperfusion therapy in all patients.

Results: Apelin-12 was inversely correlated with troponin I levels (Spearman's correlation = −0.40) with a p value <0.001. There was variability in the apelin values on the seventh day (Kruskal-Wallis test) based on major adverse cardiac events (MACE) (p = 0.012). Using ROC curve analyses, a cut-off value of >2.2 for the association of apelin with MACE was determined, and the AUC was 0.71 (95% CI, 0.58–0.84). Survival analysis using the Kaplan-Meier method showed a lower rate of MACE among patients with apelin levels >2.2 (p = 0.002), and the ROC curve analysis showed a statistically significant difference in the area under the curve (p = 0.004).

Conclusion: The influence of apelin levels on troponin levels in the acute phase of STEMI is inversely correlated, whereas in the non-acute phase, low apelin values were associated with a high rate of MACE.

Keywords: Apelin, Myocardial infarction, Major adverse cardiac events

Background

After acute myocardial infarction, the left ventricle undergoes a series of changes in shape, size, and thickness, which is referred to as ventricular remodelling; it precedes the development of clinically evident MACE by months to years. The apelin-APJ axis may be up-regulated with good left ventricular remodelling or down-regulated with cardiac troponin degradation and the release of cardiac natriuretic hormones that inhibit the pathophysiological mechanisms responsible for ventricular remodelling [1–3]. The role of hypoxia in the release of apelin, ischaemia reperfusion injury, and the action of apelin in cardiac contractility remains unclear.

Apelin and the cardiovascular system

The gene for the APJ receptor is located on chromosome 11 and encodes a G-protein coupled receptor that is recognized only by apelin [4, 5]. APJ receptor expression is particularly high in the heart, lung, kidney, cerebellum and vascular endothelium. In the heart, this receptor is expressed on a number of cell types, including the endothelium, smooth muscle and myocytes. The apelin gene is located on the human X chromosome, which, in response to hypoxia, encodes a 77-amino-acid preprotein that is cleaved by endopeptidases into a biologically active peptide such as apelin-12 [6]. The positive effects of apelin on the cardiovascular system include the regulation of vascular tone, cardiac contractile function and fluid balance [7–10]. Apelin plays a role in diuresis, pituitary hormone release, cardiomyocyte apoptosis and inflammation [11–14].

* Correspondence: xhevdeti_16@hotmail.com
[2]University Clinical Center of Kosova, Mother Theresa n.n, 10000 Prishtina, Republic of Kosovo
Full list of author information is available at the end of the article

In acute myocardial infarction, the levels of troponins are predictors of MACE [15–17]. The use of a sensitive troponin I assay improves early diagnosis [18], and these patients are more likely to undergo angiography [19, 20].

Relationship between apelin and troponin

After the binding of apelin with its receptor, phospholipase C (PLC) is activated and generates inositol trisphosphate (IP3) and diacylglycerol (DAG) from phosphatidyl inositol bisphosphate (PIP2). Diacylglycerol activates protein kinase C (PKC), increasing the activity of the sarco-lemmal Na^+/H^+ exchanger (NHE). This leads to an elevation in pH, which indirectly increases the intracellu-lar Ca^{2+} concentration through the reverse Na^+/Ca^{2+} ex-changer (NCX). On the other hand, apelin increases intracellular Ca^{2+} concentration via the calcium release channels associated with ryanodine receptors (RyRs) and via the activation of protein kinase C, which decreases the phosphorylation of phospholamban (PLB), reducing the function of the SR Ca^{2+} ATPase (SERCA) [21, 22].

Through protein kinase C, apelin activates its sites on troponin I, thereby regulating Ca^{2+} sensitivity and ATPase activity in the myocardium (Fig. 1) [23, 24].

During ischaemia/infarction, phosphorylated TnI levels, Ca^{2+} sensitivity and ATPase activity are decreased in the myocardium, and subsequently, the elevated Ca^{2+} levels activate protease I (caplain I), which may lead to the pro-teolytic degradation of troponins [25–28]. Concurrently, the levels of apelin and APJ expression are increased by limiting myocardial injury [1].

The aims of this study were to evaluate the influence of apelin on troponin levels and the rate of major adverse cardiac events (MACE) in STEMI patients.

Methods

Study population

In this dual-centre, prospective observational study, one hundred consecutive patients with ST-elevation acute myocardial infarction who presented or were referred to the coronary care unit of our institutions were included. Patients meeting the following criteria were included in our study: (1) continuous chest pain lasting >30 min, (2) the observation of ST-segment elevation of more than 2 mm in two adjacent leads by electrocardiography (ECG), (3) increased cardiac troponin I levels, and (4) patients who underwent reperfusion therapy [29]. We evaluated the levels of apelin-12 and troponin I on the first and seventh days after reperfusion therapy in all pa-tients. The study was approved by the institutional ethics committee of Dubrava University Hospital-Zagreb and the University Clinical Center of Kosova-Pristina. Written informed consent was obtained from all patients before inclusion in the study.

Patient characterization

Demographic data and clinical history were obtained during hospitalization using a standardized question-naire. Based on coronarography, the number of diseased vessels, culprit lesions and stenoses was determined. The culprit lesion was defined as the lesion with the highest degree of stenosis or with angiographic signs of endo-luminal thrombi and/or plaque rupture. Stenoses ≥50% of the lumen of the left main artery (LMA) or ≥70% of

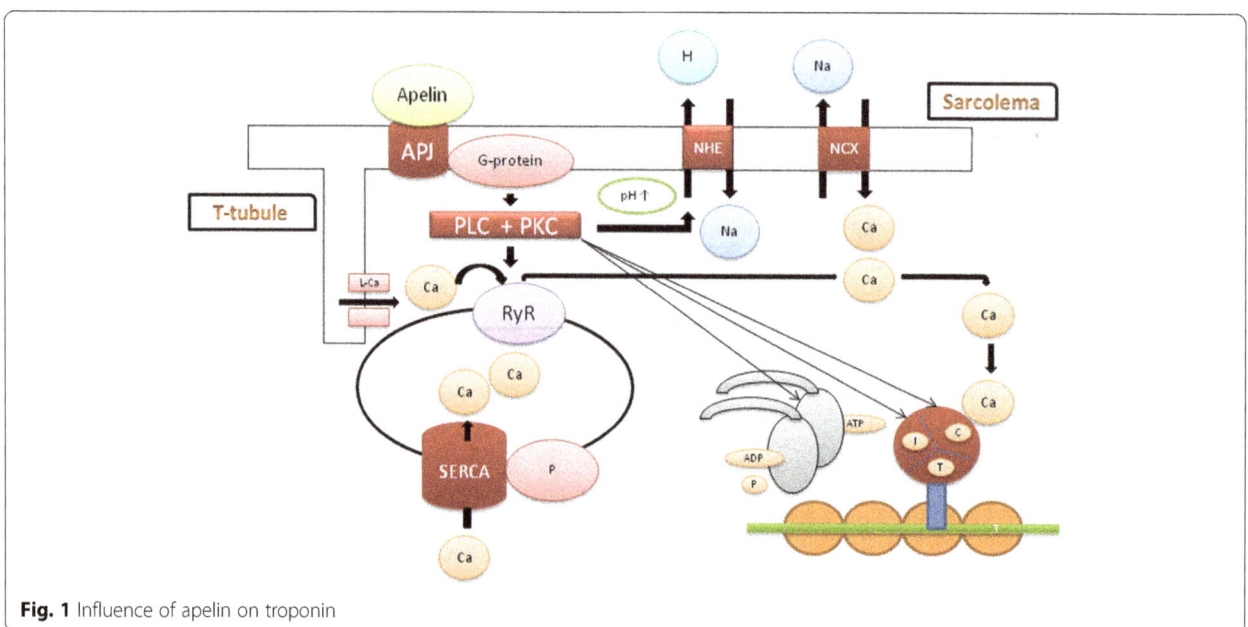

Fig. 1 Influence of apelin on troponin

the lumen of major epicardial vessels were considered significant. For the assessment of LV ejection fraction, transthoracic echocardiography was performed in all patients during their hospitalization.

Laboratory data

Blood samples for the measurement of routine laboratory parameters were collected at admission. On the first and seventh day after reperfusion therapy, blood samples were collected into lavender Vacutainer tubes (Catalogue No. VT-6450) that contain EDTA and can collect up to 7 ml of blood/tube. The blood was transferred from the lavender vacutainer tubes to centrifuge tubes containing aprotinin (0.6TIU/ml of blood) and then centrifuged at 1600 x g for 15 min at 4 °C. The serum was aliquoted and stored at –80 degrees Celsius to prevent degradation. Circulating apelin-12 and troponin I concentrations were analysed using a commercially available enzyme-linked immunosorbent assay (ELISA) kit (Phoenix Pharmaceuticals, Inc) according to the manufacturer's instructions.

Statistical analysis

The primary endpoint of the study was the influence of apelin-12 on troponin levels and its association with major adverse cardiac events in STEMI patients. Continuous variables are presented as the mean ± standard deviation or as the median (range), whereas categorical variables are presented as percentages. Spearman's correlation was used to analyse the degree of association between apelin-12 and troponin I, whereas ROC curve analyses were used to determine a cut-off value of apelin-12 for an association with MACE. Using Kaplan-Meier estimates, we evaluated the association between apelin and future MACE after a follow-up period of 12 months. All statistical analyses were performed using SPSS statistics version 21.

Results

Patient characteristics

Baseline characteristics of the study population are displayed in Table 1. The mean age was 60.52 ± 11.50 years old (60% male). Coronary risk factors and laboratory values are presented as a mean, median or percentage. In terms of coronary angiographic findings, the culprit artery was the left anterior descending artery (LAD, 48%), right coronary artery (RCA, 40%) and circumflex (12%), whereas, in terms of vessel disease, 40% of patients had one-vessel disease, 31% had two-vessel disease and 29% had three-vessel disease.

Relationship between apelin and troponin

The degree of association between apelin-12 and troponin I in the first day of the acute phase of STEMI was

Table 1 Baseline characteristics of patients

Parameters	
Age (year), mean (±SD)	60.52 ± 11.50
Gender (male), n (%)	60 (60)
Medical history	
Hypertension, n (%)	59 (59)
Diabetes mellitus, n (%)	19 (19)
Dyslipidemia, n (%)	32 (32)
Smoking, n (%)	32 (32)
Family history of cardiovascular disease, n (%)	20 (20)
Killip class >1, n (%)	13 (13)
Ejection fraction, mean (±SD)	50.34 ± 10.20
Laboratory values	
Haemoglobin (g/dL), mean (±SD)	13.54 ± 1.39
Creatinine (umol/L), median (range)	92.90 (67.21–124.34)
Apelin 12 on the first day (ng/mL), median (range)	2.98 (0.45–15.25)
Apelin 12 on the seventh day (ng/mL), median (range)	2.33 (0.26–10.90)
Troponin I on the first day (ng/mL), mean (±SD)	54.80 ± 60.99
Troponin I on the seventh day (ng/mL), mean (±SD)	12.43 ± 24.48
Coronary angiographic findings	
Culprit lesion, n (%)	
RCA	40 (40)
LAD	48 (48)
LCx	12 (12)
Vessel disease, n (%)	
1	40 (40)
2	31 (31)
3	29 (29)

Values are n (%), mean (±SD) or median (range)
Abbreviations: *RCA* right coronary artery, *LAD* left anterior descending coronary artery, *LCx* left circumflex coronary artery

analysed with Spearman's correlation = –0.40 ($p < 0.001$). Based on the regression analysis of the relationship between apelin-12 and troponin I, one variable could be predicted from the other (Fig. 2).

Apelin and major adverse cardiac events

There was variability in the apelin values on the seventh day (Kruskal-Wallis test) in relation to major adverse cardiac events (MACE) that was significantly different ($p < 0.012$). Kaplan-Meier curves were used to show the number of MACE and the proportion of patients that survived at each event time point based on the cut-off value of apelin-12 on the seventh day (2.2 ng/mL) (Fig. 3). The log-rank test for the difference in survival resulted in a p value of 0.002.

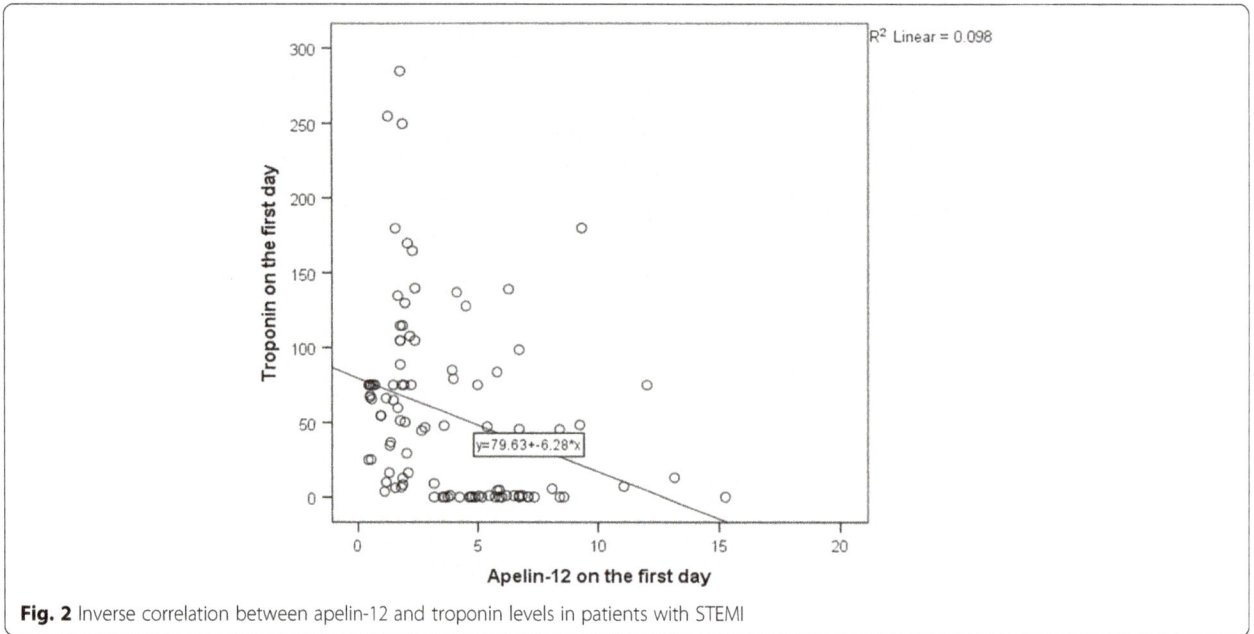

Fig. 2 Inverse correlation between apelin-12 and troponin levels in patients with STEMI

A receiver operating characteristic (ROC) curve plots the true positive rate against the false positive rate at different cut-off points. Table 2 presents the area under the curve values for biomarkers, and Fig. 4 presents the ROC curve for apelin-12 and MACE.

Discussion

In this study, we investigated the influence of apelin-12 on troponin levels and the rate of MACE in STEMI patients. The present study showed association between apelin-12 and troponin in the acute phase of myocardial

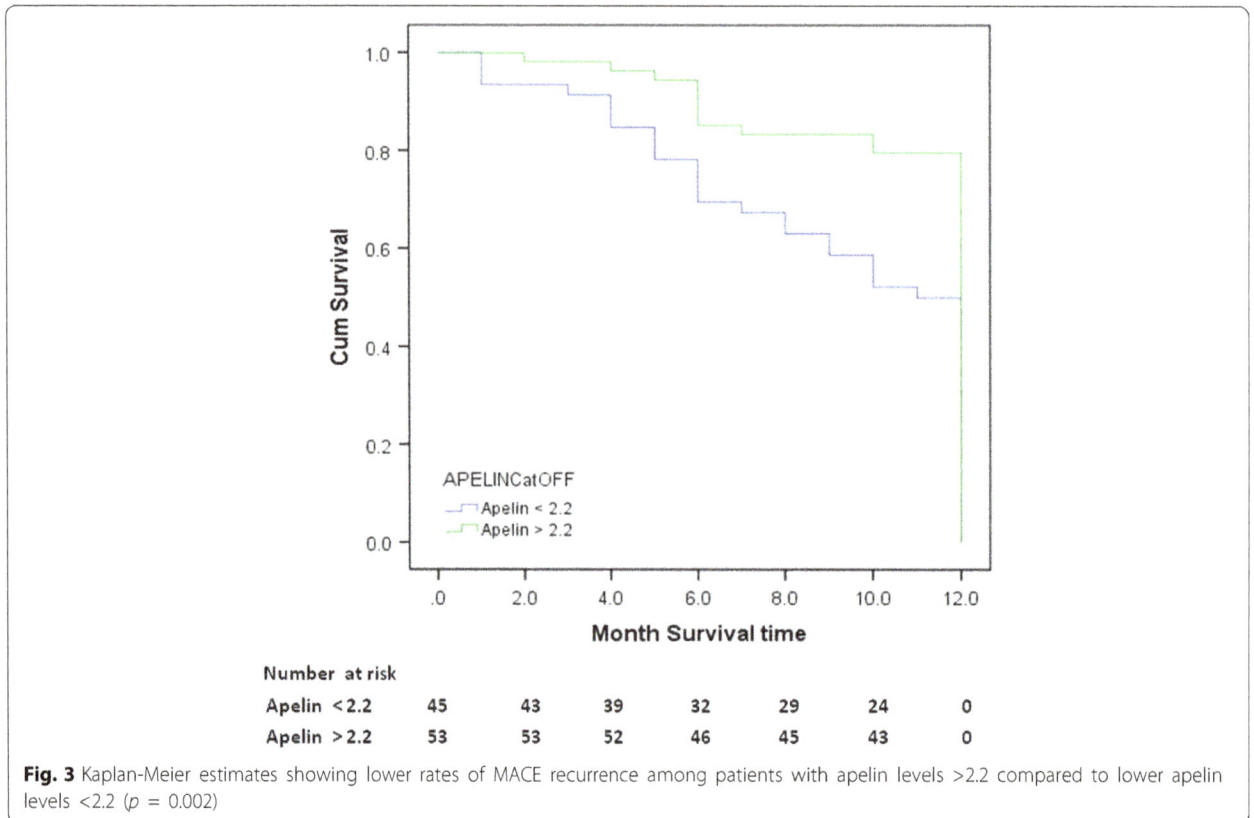

Fig. 3 Kaplan-Meier estimates showing lower rates of MACE recurrence among patients with apelin levels >2.2 compared to lower apelin levels <2.2 ($p = 0.002$)

Table 2 Area under the curve values for biomarkers

Biomarker	AUC (95% CI)	P-value
Apelin 12 on the first day	0.52 (0.37–0.67)	0.71
Apelin 12 on the seventh day	0.71 (.58–0.84)	0.004
Troponin I on the first day	0.48 (0.33–0.63)	0.8
Troponin I on the seventh day	0.41 (0.27–0.55)	0.25
Creatine kinase	0.48 (0.33–0.63)	0.84
Creatine kinase-MB	0.58 (0.43–0.73)	0.27
NT-proBNP	0.49 (0.33–0.64)	0.88
C-reactive protein	0.54 (0.39–0.69)	0.56

Abbreviations: *NT-proBNP* N-terminal pro b-type natriuretic peptide

infarction, whereas rates of MACE after STEMI were expected based on values of apelin-12 in the non-acute phase. The findings of other studies have demonstrated efficiency of myocardial protection induced by apelin limiting myocardial infarction and its action as a regulatory peptide increasing cadiac contractility [30, 31].

In the acute phase of myocardial infarction, the atheromatous plaque in the lumen suffers from complete or incomplete acute block-up, which results in ischaemia in the myocardium. During hypoxia (24 h, 2% O2), apelin gene expression and secretion are increased through the activation of hypoxia inducible factor (HIF) [10, 32, 33]. Hypoxia requires a functional mitochondrial electron transport chain for the inhibition of prolyl hydroxylases and HIF stabilization [34]. Under anoxic conditions, the stabilization of HIF is preserved due to the lack of a functioning mitochondrial respiratory chain, and thus,

the apelin gene is neither expressed nor is its expression increased [35].

Apelin activates its sites on troponin I, regulating Ca^{2+} sensitivity and ATPase activity in the myocardium through protein kinase C [23, 24]. During ischaemia/infarction, phosphorylated TnI levels, Ca^{2+} sensitivity and ATPase activity are decreased in the myocardium, and subsequently, the elevated Ca^{2+} levels activate protease I (caplain I), leading to the proteolytic degradation of troponins and ventricular dysfunction [25–28]. The degree of association between apelin-12 and troponin I in the first day of the acute phase of STEMI was analysed with Spearman's correlation = −0.40 ($p < 0.001$). The relationship between apelin-12 and troponin I was analysed by a regression analysis, predicting one variable from the other (Fig. 2).

The loss of apelin (APLN) clearly compromises the activation of the protective Akt/PI3K and extracellular signal-regulated kinase 1/2 (Erk1/2) signalling pathways both in vivo and ex vivo, resulting in increased myocardial damage and worsened heart function [36]. Low values of apelin in the non-acute phase of STEMI were associated with high rates of MACE after STEMI, with variability in the apelin values on the seventh day (Kruskal-Wallis test) based on major adverse cardiac events (MACE) that was significantly different ($p < 0.012$). A cut-off value for apelin-12 levels on the seventh day was set for the survival analysis, and a Kaplan-Meier curve was generated; the log-rank test for differences in survival resulted in a p value of 0.002. ROC curve analysis showed that the area under the curve was significantly different, with a p value of 0.004 (Fig. 4 and Table 2).

The vision for the future is potential utility of apelin-12 measurement in STEMI patients as an additional risk stratification tool and possibility for the usage as a therapy.

We were aware of some limitations to our study. This observational study had a relatively limited number of patients. Apelin levels and correlation with troponin in non-STEMI acute chest pain differential admissions to the emergency department would be interesting as control group.

Conclusion

Apelin-12 influences troponin I levels in the acute phase of STEMI, whereas during the non-acute phase, low apelin levels were associated with a high rate of MACE.

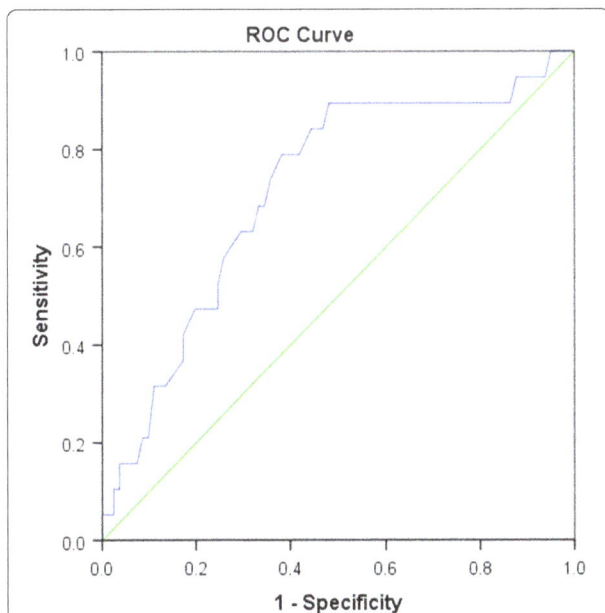

Fig. 4 ROC curve analysis of the apelin values on the seventh day for the prediction of MACE. AUC = 0.71 (95% CI, 0.58–0.84), p = 0.004

Table 3 Take home messages

Apelin-12 influences troponin I levels in the acute phase of STEMI
A high rate of MACE after STEMI was characterized with low values of apelin during non-acute phase
n the future, potential utility of apelin-12 measurement in STEMI patients as an additional risk stratification tool and possibility for the usage as a therapy

Take home message
Table 3 presents take home messages.

Abbreviations
Akt/PI3K: phosphatidylinositol 3-kinase/protein kinase B; APJ: Angiotensin receptor like-1; APLN: Apelin; ATPase: Adenosine triphosphatase; DAG: Diacylglycerol; ECG: Electrocardiography; EDTA: Ethylenediaminetetraacetic acid; ELISA: Enzyme-linked immunosorbent assay; Erk: Extracellular signal-regulated kinases; HIF: Hypoxia inducible factor; IP3: Inositol trisphosphate; LAD: Left anterior descending artery; LCx: Left circumflex; LMA: Left main artery; MACE: Major adverse cardiac events; NCX: Na^+/Ca^{2+} exchanger; NHE: Na^+/H^+ exchanger; NT-proBNP: N-terminal pro b-type natriuretic peptide; PIP2: Phosphatidyl inositol bisphosphate; PKC: Protein kinase C; PLB: Phospholamban; PLC: Phospholipase C; RCA: Right coronary artery; ROC: Receiver operating characteristic; RYRs: Ryanodine receptors; SD: Standard deviation; SERCA: Sarco/endoplasmic reticulum Ca^{2+} ATPase; STEMI: ST-Segment elevation myocardial infarction

Acknowledgements
We are grateful to the patients who participated in this study and for the follow-up data collection. We would like to thank the staff of the Dubrava University Hospital-Zagreb and the University Clinical Center of Kosova-Pristina for their assistance.

Funding
Not applicable.

Authorship declaration
All authors listed meet the authorship criteria according to the latest guidelines of the International Committee of Medical Journal Editors and are in agreement regarding the manuscript.

Authors' contributions
XK analyzed and interpreted data and was a major contributor in writing the manuscript and implementation of the study. BB analyzed the patient data and contributed in implementation of the study. MG analyzed the patient data and overview the study. DK analyzed the data and contributed in editing the manuscript. FJ analyzed the data and contributed in statistical interpretation. JV analyzed the patient data and overview the study. All authors read and approved the final manuscript.

Competing interests
The authors declare that they have no competing interests.

Author details
[1]Clinical Hospital Dubrava, Zagreb, Republic of Croatia. [2]University Clinical Center of Kosova, Mother Theresa n.n, 10000 Prishtina, Republic of Kosovo.

References
1. Chandrasekaran B, Dar O, McDonagh T. The role of apelin in cardiovascular function and heart failure. European J Heart Fail. 2008;10(8):725–32.
2. Babuin L, Jaffe A. Troponin: the biomarker of choice for the detection of cardiac injury. CMAJ. 2005;173(10):1191–202.
3. Clerico A, Emdin M. Diagnostic accuracy and prognostic relevance of the measurement of cardiac natriuretic peptides: a review. Clin Chemi. 2004;50(1):33–50.
4. Tatemoto K, Hosoya M, Habata Y, Fujii R, Kakegawa T, et al. Isolation and characterization of a novel endogenous peptide ligand for the human APJ receptor. Biochem Biophys Res Communs. 1998;251(2):471–6.
5. BF OD, Heiber M, Chan A, Heng HH, Tsui LC, et al. A human gene that shows identity with the gene encoding the angiotension receptor is located on chromosome 11. Gene. 1993;136(1–2):355–60.
6. Japp A, Newby D. The apelin-APJ system in heart failure: pathophysiologic relevance and therapeutic potential. Biochem Pharmacol. 2008;75(10):1882–92.
7. Szokodi I, Tavi P, Földes G, Voultilainen-Myllylä S, Ilves M, et al. Apelin, the novel endogenous ligand of the orphan receptor APJ, regulates cardiac contractility. Circ Res. 2002;91(5):434–40.
8. Neves SR, Ram PT, Lyengar R. G protein pathways. Science. 2002;296(5573):1636–9.
9. Karmazyn M, Gan XT, Humphreys RA, Yoshida H, Kusumoto K. The myocardial Na(+)-H(+) exchange: structure, regulation, and its role in heart disease. Cir Res. 1999;85(9):777–86.
10. Ronkainen VP, Ronkainen JJ, Hänninen SL, Leskinen H, Ruas JL, et al. Hypoxia inducible factor regulates the cardiac expression and secretion of apelin. FASEB J. 2007;21(8):1821–30.
11. Hus-Citharel A, Bodineau L, Frugière A, Joubert F, Bouby N, Llorens-Cortes C. Apelin counteracts vasopressin-induced water reabsorption via cross talk between apelin and vasopressin receptor signaling pathways in the rat collecting duct. Endocrinology. 2014;155(11):4483–93.
12. Taheri S, Murphy K, Cohen M, Sujkovic E, Kennedy A, et al. The effects of centrally administered apelin-13 on food intake, water intake and pituitary hormone release in rats. Bioch Biophys Res Commnun. 2002;291(5):1208–12.
13. Zhang Z, Yu B, Tao GZ. Apelin protects against cardiomyocytes apoptosis induced by glucose deprivation. Chin Med J. 2009;122(19):2360–5.
14. Pang H, Han B, Li ZY, Fu Q. Identification of molecular markers in patients with hypertensive heart disease accompanied with coronary artery disease. Genet Mol Res. 2015;14(1):93–100.
15. Gonzalez M, Porterfield C, Eilen D, Marzouq RA, Patel HR, et al. Quartiles of peak troponin are associated with long-term risk of death in type 1 and STEMI, but not in type 2 or NSTEMI patients. Clin Cardiol. 2009;32(10):575–83.
16. Polanczyk C, Lee T, Cook E, Walls R, Wybenga D, et al. Cardiac troponin I as a predictor of major cardiac events in emergency department patients with acute chest pain. J Am Coll Cardiol. 1998;32(1):8–14.
17. Hall TS, Hallén J, Krucoff MW, Roe MT, Brennan DM, et al. Cardiac troponin I for prediction of clinical outcomes and cardiac function through 3-month follow-up after primary percutaneous coronary intervention for ST-segment elevation myocardial infarction. Am Heart J. 2015;169(2):257–65.
18. Keller T, Zeller T, Peetz D, Tzikas S, Roth A, et al. Sensitive troponin I assay in early diagnosis of acute myocardial infarction. N Engl J Med. 2009;361(9):868–77.
19. Javed U, Aftab W, Ambrose JA, Wessel RJ, Mouanoutoua M, et al. Frequency of elevated troponin I and diagnosis of acute myocardial infarction. Am J Cardiol. 2009;104(1):9–13.
20. Auguardo C, Scalise F, Manfredi M, Casali V, Novelli E, et al. The prognostic role of troponin I elevation after elective percutaneous coronary intervention. J Cardiovasc Med (Hagerstown). 2015;16(3):149–55.
21. Yamamura K, Steenbergen C, Murphy E. Protein kinase C and preconditioning: role of sarcoplasmic reticulum. Am J Physiol Heart Circ Pysiol. 2005;289(6):2484–90.
22. Wang C, Du JF, Wu F, Wang HC. Apelin decreases the SR ca 2+ content but enhances the amplitude of [ca 2+]i transient and contractions during twitches in isolated rat cardiac myocytes. Am J Physiol Heart Circ Physiol. 2008;294(6):2540–6.
23. Farkasfalvi K, Stagg M, Coppen S, Siedlecka U, Lee J, et al. Direct effects of apelin on cardiomyocyte contractility and electrophysiology. Biochem Biophys Res Commun. 2007;357(4):889–95.
24. Pi YQ, Zhang D, Kemnitz KR, Wang H, Walker JW. Protein kinase C and a sites on troponin I regulate myofilament ca 2+, sensitivity and ATPase activity in the mouse myocardium. J Physiol. 2003;552(Pt3):845–57.
25. Bodor GS, Oakeley AE, Allen PD, Crimmins DL, Ladenson JH, et al. Troponin I phosphorylation in the normal and failing adult human heart. Circulation. 1997;96(5):1495–500.
26. Wijnker PJ, Murphy AM, Stienen GJ, van der Velden J. Troponin I phosphorylation in human myocardium in health and disease. Neth Heart J. 2014;22(10):463–9.
27. Gao WD, Liu Y, Mellgren R, Marban E. Intrinsic myofilament alterations underlying the decreased contractility of stunned myocardium. A consequence of ca 2+–dependent proteolysis? Circ Res. 1996;78(3):455–65.
28. Van der Laarse A. Hypothesis: troponin degradation is one of the factors responsible for deterioration of the left ventricular function in heart failure. Cardiovasc Res. 2002;56(1):8–14.

29. Windecker S, Kolh P, Alfonso F, Collet JP, Cremer J, et al. ESC/EACTS guidelines on myocardial revascularizations: the task force on myocardial revascularization of the European Society of Cardiology (ESC) and the European association for cardiothoracic surgery (EACTS) developed with the special contribution of the European Association of Percutaneous Cardiovascular Intervetions (EAPCI). Eur Heart J. 2014;35(46):2541–619.

30. Rastaldo R, Cappello S, Folino A, Berta GN, et al. Apelin-13 limits infarct size and improves cardiac postischemic mechanical recovery only if given after ischemia. Am J Physiol Heart Circ Physiol. 2011;300(6):2308–15.

31. Japp AG, Cruden NL, Barnes G, van Gemeren N, Mathews J, et al. Acute cardiovascular effects of apelin in humans: potential role in patients with chronic heart failure. Circulation. 2010;121(16):1818–27.

32. Jianqiang P, Ping Z, Xinmin F, Zhenhua Y, Ming Z, et al. Expression of hypoxia-inducible factor 1 alpha ameliorate myocardial ischemia in rat. Biochem Biophys Res Commun. 2015;465(4):691–5.

33. Cheng C, Li P, Wang YG, Bi MH, Wu PS. Study on the expression of VEGF and HIF-1α in infarct area of rats with AMI. Eur Rev Med Pharmacol Sci. 2016;20(1):115–9.

34. Schroedl C, McClintock DS, Budinger GRS, Chandel NS. Hypoxic but not anoxic stabilization of HIF-1α requires mitochondrial reactive oxygen species. Am J Physiol Lung Cell Mol Physiol. 2002;283(5):L922–31.

35. Vaux EC, Metzen E, Yeates KM, Ratcliffe PJ. Regulation of hypoxia-inducible factor is preserved in the absence of a functioning mitochondrial respiratory chain. Blood. 2001;98(2):296–302.

36. Wang W, McKinnie SM, Patel VB, et al. Los of Apelin exacerbates myocardial infarction adverse reomdeling and ischaemia reperfusion injury: therapeutic potential of synthetic Apelin analogues. J Am Heart Assoc. 2013;2:e000249.

21

Secondary prevention strategies after an acute ST-segment elevation myocardial infarction in the *AMI code* era: beyond myocardial mechanical reperfusion

Núria Ribas[1,2,3*], Cosme García-García[1,4], Oona Meroño[1,2], Lluís Recasens[1,2], Silvia Pérez-Fernández[5,6], Víctor Bazán[1], Neus Salvatella[1,2], Julio Martí-Almor[1,2], Jordi Bruguera[1,2] and Roberto Elosua[5,6]

Abstract

Background: The *AMI code* is a regional network enhancing a rapid and widespread access to reperfusion therapy (giving priority to primary angioplasty) in patients with acute ST-segment elevation myocardial infarction (STEMI). We aimed to assess the long-term control of conventional cardiovascular risk factors after a STEMI among patients included in the *AMI code* registry.

Design and methods: Four hundred and fifty-four patients were prospectively included between June-2009 and April-2013. Clinical characteristics were collected at baseline. The long-term control of cardiovascular risk factors and cardiovascular morbidity/mortality was assessed among the 6-months survivors.

Results: A total of 423 patients overcame the first 6 months after the STEMI episode, of whom 370 (87%) underwent reperfusion therapy (363, 98% of them, with primary angioplasty). At 1-year follow-up, only 263 (62%) had adequate blood pressure control, 123 (29%) had LDL-cholesterol within targeted levels, 126/210 (60%) smokers had withdrawn from their habit and 40/112 (36%) diabetic patients had adequate glycosylated hemoglobin levels. During a median follow-up of 20 (11–30) months, cumulative mortality of 6 month-survivors was 6.1%, with 9.9% of hospital cardiovascular readmissions. The lack of assessment of LDL and HDL-cholesterol were significantly associated with higher mortality and cardiovascular readmission rates.

Conclusions: Whereas implementation of the *AMI code* resulted in a widespread access to rapid reperfusion therapy, its long-term therapeutic benefit may be partially counterbalanced by a manifestly suboptimal control of cardiovascular risk factors. Further efforts should be devoted to secondary prevention strategies after STEMI.

Keywords: ST-segment elevation myocardial infarction, Coronary angioplasty, Secondary prevention, Prognosis, Reperfusion therapy, Cardiovascular risk factors

Background

Case-fatality and long-term mortality after an acute myocardial infarction (AMI) has manifestly decreased over the last decades. Both the use of more effective pharmacological and revascularization strategies account for this decrease [1–4]. However, coronary artery disease (CAD) continues to be the most determinant cause of mortality in high-income societies [5]. ST-segment elevation myocardial infarction (STEMI) is one of the main clinical manifestations of CAD, and rapid (<12 h) coronary reperfusion continuous to be the main therapeutic goal to enhance a favorable cardiovascular outcome after the index coronary event. In this scenario, primary percutaneous coronary intervention (PCI) is nowadys preferred over fibrinolysis, especially when the coronary intervention is performed within the first 120 min [6–8].

* Correspondence: 60055@hospitaldelmar.cat
[1]Cardiology Department, Hospital del Mar, Passeig Marítim, 25-29, 08003 Barcelona, Spain
[2]Heart Diseases Biomedical Research Group, IMIM (Hospital del Mar Medical Research Institute), Barcelona, Spain
Full list of author information is available at the end of the article

Regardless of such rapid therapeutic interventions, the readmission and mortality rates after the index AMI episode are not negligible, with an 8–20% of the patients being readmitted and 10% of them dying within the first year [9–13]. Previous reports have postulated that the suboptimal cardiovascular morbidity and mortality rates after an acute coronary event may be related to an inadequate control of the cardiovascular risk factors (secondary prevention strategies) [14–17]. However, assessment of the long-term degree of implementation and adherence to such secondary prevention strategies in STEMI patients undergoing urgent reperfusion in the era of widespread use of PCI is scarce in the literature [18–21].

In this study, we aimed to assess the long-term control of conventional cardiovascular risk factors in patients presenting with acute STEMI undergoing urgent reperfusion therapy, with urgent PCI designated as the preferred therapeutic strategy. We further analyzed the prognostic impact of an inadequate control of such risk factors.

Methods

Patient population: the AMI code program

A total of 467 consecutive STEMI patients referred to our hospital from June 2009 to April 2013 within the *AMI code* program were prospectively considered for inclusion. The *AMI code* program, created in 2009, consists of a regional network developed in Catalonia (Spain) aiming to provide a rapid and widespread access to PCI among patients presenting with an acute STEMI [8]. More precisely, it consists of an integrated assistance network for urgent action that coordinates primary health centers, 'non-PCI-available' hospitals, 'PCI-available' hospitals and mobile emergency assistance units. Upon the diagnosis of STEMI, the *AMI code* is activated and primary PCI (to be performed in a preliminary designated 'PCI-available' institution) is set up, provided that the time interval between the onset of symptoms and the percutaneous intervention is presumed to be within the therapeutic window. Additionally, the *AMI code* can be activated for those patients without apparent myocardial reperfusion after pharmacological fibrinolysis (rescue angioplasty). Twenty-four to forty-eight hours after the index STEMI episode, in the absence of acute complications, patients are planned to be discharged to their reference hospital. Patients not established in Catalonia (tourists and displaced) were excluded from the analysis upon a presumably suboptimal follow-up.

The study was designed and implemented in accordance with Guidelines for Good Clinical Practice and with the ethical principles laid down in the Declaration of Helsinki.

In-hospital data collection

Demographic (age, gender) and clinical characteristics (infarct location, systolic blood pressure, Killip class at admission and left ventricular ejection fraction), as well as history and control of cardiovascular risk factors (smoking, dyslipidemia, hypertension and diabetes mellitus) and other comorbidities (personal and family history of ischemic cardiomyopathy, chronic kidney disease, anemia) were collected at the time of patient's hospital admission during the index STEMI episode. The lipid profile, glomerular filtration rate and the glycosylated hemoglobin levels were analyzed at baseline. In-hospital morbidity and mortality, the pharmacological therapy administered during admission and the primary PCI procedure findings were also collected.

Clinical follow-up

The clinical follow-up after final hospital discharge was carried out by the primary care physician or through the cardiologist outpatient clinic/primary health center at the reference physician's discretion. After hospital discharge, assessment and control of the cardiovascular risk factors and the patient's clinical outcome were monitored and incorporated into the study database through the Catalonia's regional electronic health recording system, in which the patient's clinical status, the rate of hospital readmissions after the index STEMI event, the pharmacological intake, the laboratory test and radiology results were available for the study purposes. Overall mortality was ensured by means of consultation of the National Death Registry. Heart failure, acute coronary syndrome and stroke were considered cardiovascular readmission. Following previously reported definitions, stroke was considered a cardiovascular condition in the assessment of the clinical outcome after STEMI [22–24]. Direct telephone contact with the patient was allowed in order to fulfill any missing data from the electronic health recording system.

The long-term control of conventional cardiovascular risk factors was exclusively analyzed for those patients who survived at least the first 6 months after the index STEMI episode. By these means, any bias in the results obtained related to a suboptimal risk factor control during the very initial phases after the STEMI would be avoided. A minimum 6-months follow-up period was considered compelling for the surviving study patients in order to enhance a truly long-term assessment of the efficiency of secondary prevention strategies in this population.

Assessment of the adequate implementation secondary prevention strategies (i.e. pharmacological intake, smoking habit withdrawal, blood pressure, glycosylated hemoglobin, triglyceride and cholesterol levels) was performed 12 months after the index STEMI episode. The closest laboratory and blood pressure values were retrieved by means of manual review of the patient's electronic clinical history. A 6 to 18-month timeframe from the STEMI was allowed for the obtainment of such clinical and laboratory variables, following previously reported methodology [10, 14, 15, 18–20]. As for patients who died between the 6 months and the first year after the STEMI, the latest risk factors assessment before their decease was incorporated into the study database.

Adequate control of cardiovascular risk factors was established, following current guidelines, as follows: blood pressure <140/90 mmHg; smoking abstinence for at least 6 months; total cholesterol of <200 mg/dL, LDL-cholesterol of <70 mg/dL or ≥50% lower with respect to baseline values, HDL-cholesterol >40 mg/dL and triglycerides below 150 mg/dL [18–21, 25–28]. Glycosylated hemoglobin levels of <7.5% were pursued among diabetic study patients [18–21, 26].

Our institutional guidelines and recommendations include that all patients should undergo a cardiovascular risk factors assessment during the first year after the index STEMI event and assuming that this information was available in the regional electronic health recording system, a particular risk factor was considered: i) *controlled* when the targeted goal was achieved; ii) *not controlled* when the targeted goal was not achieved; and iii) *not assessed* when no information related to the risk factor was available in the electronic health record system.

A longer follow-up study period (beyond the 12-months study period) was allowed for the assessment of mortality and cardiovascular readmission rates.

Statistical analysis

Results are expressed as absolute and relative frequencies for categorical variables, as means and standard deviations (SD) or, when appropriate, as medians and interquartile ranges (IQR), for continuous variables. Student's T-test or Man-Whitney U test was used for the comparison of quantitative variables and the chi-squared was used for the comparison of qualitative variables. A multinomial multivariate analysis was carried out in order to identify those clinical variables associated with an adequate control of the cardiovascular risk factors in our population. Finally, in order to assess the influence of risk factors control in the long-term prognosis of our population, a Cox proportional hazard regression model was used. Those variables associated with the outcomes of interest in the univariate analysis (p-value < 0.05) were included in the multivariate models, moreover we also included age, as a

continuous variable, and sex. All analyses were performed using the R statistical package.

Results

Patient population

Out of the 467 STEMI patients consecutively admitted in our Institution upon activation of the *AMI code*, 13 were excluded because they were foreigners/displaced. Of the remaining 454 patients, 433 (95%) survived the first 30 days and 423 (93%) survived the first 6 months, the latter comprising our study population (Fig. 1). The percentage of missing data was null for the main variables of interest (control of cardiovascular risk factors and clinical outcomes in the follow-up) and < 5% for the covariates included in the multivariate analyses.

The clinical and demographic baseline characteristics of the 6-month surviving 423 patients are shown in Table 1. Of note, urgent reperfusion therapy was performed in 370 (87%) patients, in nearly all 363/370 (98%) by means of primary PCI. In the remaining seven patients (2%), fibrinolysis was preferred upon a presumably delayed access to urgent PCI. An excessively delayed time from the onset of symptoms until first medical attendance was the principal reason for reperfusion therapy not being carried out (53 out of the 423 patients not undergoing urgent reperfusion, 13%). The median time between first medical contact and reperfusion was 94 (69–128) minutes. The pharmacological treatment administered during the procedure and the hospital admission, as well as the in-hospital complications are summarized in Additional file 1: Table S1.

Cardiovascular risk factors at 1-year follow-up

Remarkably, ongoing pharmacological secondary prevention strategies was the rule among the study population, with 95% of the patients receiving statins, 90% on acetylsalicylic acid, 86% on beta-blockers and 78% on ACE inhibitors or ARBs at the end of the follow-up period.

Assessment of cardiovascular risk factors at 1-year follow-up is summarized in Fig. 2 and Table 2. Blood pressure and LDL-Cholesterol levels were not assessed in 84 (20%) and 93 (22%) patients, respectively (Fig. 2). Smoking habit withdrawal was not assessed in 41 out of the 201 smokers (20%) included

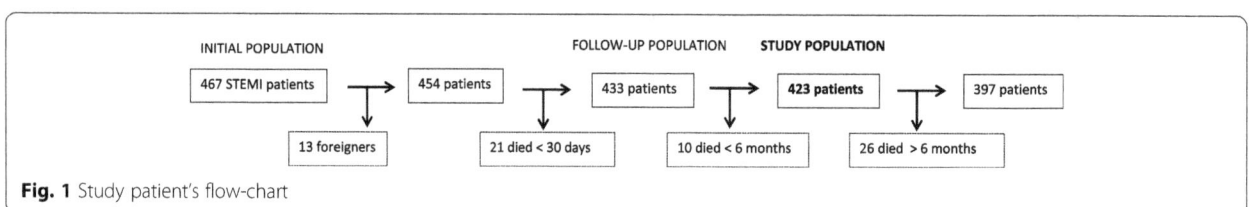

Fig. 1 Study patient's flow-chart

Table 1 Baseline characteristics of the 6-month survivors ST-elevation myocardial infarction patients included in this registry

Patient characteristics	Total (n = 423)	Men (n = 319)	Women (n = 104)	p-value
Age (years)	63 ± 13.1	60.9 ± 12.7	69.2 ± 12.4	<0.001
Current smokers	201 (47.9%)	173 (54.4%)	28 (27.5%)	<0.001
Former smokers (>1 year)	100 (23.8%)	92 (28.9%)	8 (7.8%)	<0.001
Hypertension	235 (55.5%)	165 (51.7%)	70 (67.3%)	<0.001
Dyslipidemia				0.062
Drug treatment	134 (32.5%)	94 (30.3%)	40 (39.2%)	
No drug treatment	73 (17.7%)	62 (20%)	11 (10.8%)	
Diabetes mellitus	112 (26%)	76 (24%)	36 (35%)	0.107
Family history[a]	39 (11%)	29 (10.5%)	10 (12.3%)	0.800
Previous ischemic heart disease	44 (10.4%)	35 (11%)	9 (8.7%)	0.626
Chronic kidney disease	14 (3.4%)	7 (2.3%)	7 (6.9%)	0.052
Anemia	33 (8.2%)	19 (6.3%)	14 (14.1%)	0.023
AMI data				
Systolic blood pressure at admission (mmHg)	130 [114–150]	130 [112–148]	140 [120–164]	0.003
Infarct location				0.713
Anterior	151 (35.7%)	112 (35.1%)	39 (37.5%)	
Inferior	231 (54.6%)	178 (55.8%)	53 (51%)	
Killip class				0.137
I	341 (83.2%)	264 (84.9%)	77 (77.8%)	
II	35 (8.1%)	22 (7.1%)	11 (11.1%)	
III	16 (3.9%)	9 (2.9%)	7 (7.1%)	
IV	21 (4.9%)	16 (5.1%)	4 (4.1%)	
LVEF	52.1 ± 12	52,5 ± 12	51 ± 12	0.283
Blood test at admission	Total (n = 423)	Men (n = 319)	Women (n = 104)	p-value
Hb (gr/dL)	14 ± 1.8	14.4 ± 1.7	12.9 ± 1.7	<0.001
GFR (mL/min/m2)	60 [60–60]	60 [60–60]	60 [60–60]	0.006
Basal glucose (mg/dL)	111 [98–136]	110 [98–133]	114 [97–148]	0.423
HbA1c (%) (in DM)	7.25 [6.60–8.53]	7.30 [6.60–8.53]	7.10 [6.60–8.08]	0.643
Total Cholesterol (mg/dL)	183 [150–214]	182 [151–212]	188 [150–219]	0.425
LDL-Cholesterol (mg/dL)	112 [84–139]	112 [85–138]	112 [82–142]	0.842
HDL-Cholesterol (mg/dL)	44 [37–53]	42 [36–50]	49 [41–60]	<0.001
Triglycerides (mg/dL)	120 [88–168]	124 [91–173]	112 [80–159]	0.061

Results are expressed as n (%), mean ± standard desviation or median [interquartile range]. P-value expresses the differences between men and women

AMI acute myocardial infarction, *LVEF* left-ventricular ejection fraction, *Hb* hemoglobin, *GFR* glomerular filtration rate, *HbA1c* Glycosylated hemoglobin, *LDL* low density lipoprotein, *HDL* high density lipoprotein

[a]Family history: early ischemic heart disease in first-degree relatives

in the study. Finally, in 38 out of the 112 diabetic patients (34%), the glycosylated hemoglobin was not available (Fig. 2). In those patients with a proper assessment of cardiovascular risk factors, a significant descent of total cholesterol (from 184 [179–188] to 155 [151–159] mg/dL, $p < 0.001$), LDL-cholesterol (112 [108–116] to 86 [82–89] mg/dL, $p < 0.001$) and triglycerides levels (from 120 [88–168] to 105 [81–150] mg/dL, $p < 0.001$) was observed. However, only 29% of

patients had their LDL-cholesterol values below the targeted levels 1 year after the STEMI episode (Fig. 2). No significant changes in HDL-cholesterol levels were observed ($p = 0.699$). Nearly two-thirds of patients (263 patients, 62%) had an adequate blood pressure control and a significant descent in systolic blood pressure was observed from hospital admission to 1 year after the STEMI (133 [130–136] to 126 [124–128] mmHg, $p < 0.001$). As for diabetic patients, the glycosylated

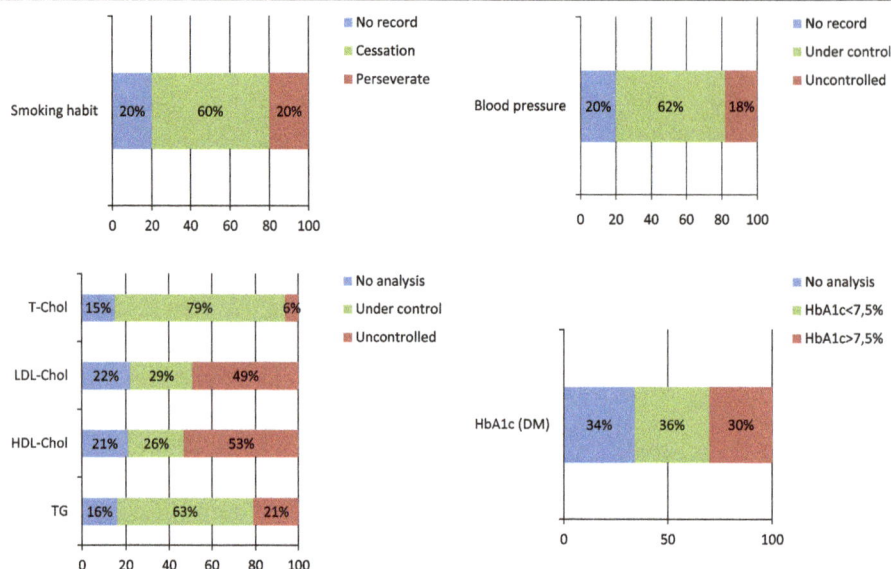

Fig. 2 Control of cardiovascular risk factors during follow-up. In *blue* it is depicted the percentage of patients in whom a particular cardiovascular risk factor was not conveniently assessed. In *green* it is depicted the percentage of patients in whom a particular cardiovascular risk factor is under control. In *red* it is depicted the percentage of patients in whom a particular cardiovascular risk factor is out of the targeted range

hemoglobin levels had significantly decreased as compared to baseline (from 7.9 [7.5–8.3] to 7.75 [7.3–8.2] %, $p = 0.02$), although with only one third of them ($n = 36$) having their glycosylated hemoglobin levels below 7.5% (Fig. 2). Finally, 120 out of the 201 smokers (60%) had given up smoking at the end of the follow-up. Altogether, only 18 out of 311 (5.8%) non-diabetic and 2 out of 112 (1.8%) diabetic patients met all the secondary prevention strategy targets at the end of the 1-year follow-up period.

No clinical variables were associated to an inadequate control of cardiovascular risk factors, with the exception of age, which was associated with a lower probability of inadequate control of HDL-cholesterol (OR = 0.96; 95% CI: 0.94–0.99; $p = 0.005$) and triglycerides (OR = 0.96; 95% CI: 0.93–0.99; $p = 0.003$). Age was also associated with lower probability of smoking habit continuation (OR = 0.93; 95% CI: 0.89–0.98; $p = 0.004$).

Impact of clinical variables and risk factor control on long-term cardiovascular outcome

Differences in baseline clinical characteristics in patients with events versus without events (cardiovascular readmission or death from any cause) during follow-up are shown in Table 3.

The median follow-up study period was 20 (11–30) months. A total of 26 patients (6.1%) died during follow-up and 42 (9.9%) were readmitted due to cardiovascular causes. Hospital readmission was due to heart failure in 21 patients, due to acute coronary syndrome in 14, and due to stroke in 7. Population who were readmitted or died during follow-up were older, had a higher prevalence of systemic hypertension and anemia, scored higher in the Killip classification and had a lower left ventricular ejection fraction at hospital-discharge (Table 3). In the multivariate analysis, hypertension, Killip class III-IV, anemia and depressed left ventricular

Table 2 Cardiovascular risk factors distribution at the end of the 1-year follow-up period

	Global	Men	Women	p-value
Systolic blood pressure (mmHg)	126 [115–137]	125 [115–136]	130 [116–137]	0.355
Total Cholesterol (mg/dL)	148 [129–175]	146 [127–167]	163 [140–191]	<0.001
LDL-Cholesterol (mg/dL)	80 [65–99]	77 [65–93]	90 [67–112]	0.005
HDL-Cholesterol (mg/dL)	44 [38–52]	44 [36–50]	49 [42–57]	<0.001
Triglycerides (mg/dL)	105 [81–150]	102 [81–146]	116 [82–158]	0.245
HbA1c (%) (in DM)	7.75 ± 1.84	7.78 ± 1.91	7.68 ± 1.71	0.824

Results are expressed as n (%), mean ± standard desviation or median [interquartile range]. P-value test differences between men and women
LDL low density lipoprotein, *HDL* high density lipoprotein, *HbA1c* glycosylated hemoglobin, DM (diabetes mellitus)

Table 3 Baseline clinical characteristics of patients with versus without events during follow-up

Patient characteristics	Event (n = 61)	No event (n = 362)	p-value
Age (years)	67 ± 15	63 ± 13	0.047
Current smokers	25 (%)	168 (46%)	0.295
Hypertension	44 (72.1%)	186 (51.4%)	0.016
Dyslipidemia	32 (52.5%)	170 (47%)	0.356
Diabetes mellitus	16 (26.2%)	72 (19.9%)	0.273
Family history*	6 (9.8%)	31 (8.6%)	0.946
Chronic kidney disease	3 (4.9%)	11 (3%)	0.448
Anemia	10 (16.4%)	23 (6.4%)	0.018
AMI data[a]	Event (n = 61)	No event (n = 362)	p-value
Infarct location			0.08
Anterior	29 (47.5%)	116 (32%)	
Inferior	28 (45.9%)	196 (54%)	
Killip class			<0.001
I	37 (60.6%)	300 (82.9%)	
II	9 (14.8%)	30 (8.3%)	
III	9 (14.8%)	13 (3.6%)	
IV	6 (9.8%)	19 (5.2%)	
LVEF[a]	46.3 ± 12.6	53.1 ± 11.3	<0.001

Event included cardiovascular readmission (due to heart failure, acute coronary syndrome or stroke) or death from any cause. Results are expressed as n (%) or mean ± standard deviation

[a]AMI acute myocardial infarction, LVEF left-ventricular ejection fraction; Family history: early ischemic heart disease in first-degree relatives

Table 4 Clinical variables associated with mortality and cardiovascular readmission in multivariate analysis

Mortality	HR [CI 95%]	p-value
Age	1.02 [0.98–1.06]	0.24
Women	0.89 [0.34–2.30]	0.81
Hypertension	3.73 [1.18–11.82]	0.03
Anemia	3.82 [1.47–9.92]	0.03
Killip class III-IV	5.40 [2.05–14.24]	<0.001
LVEF > 45%	0.22 [0.09–0.55]	<0.001
Cardiovascular readmission	HR [CI 95%]	p-value
Age	1.01 [0.98–1.04]	0.42
Women	1.34 [0.70–2.59]	0.38
Hypertension	2.72 [1.26–5.87]	0.01
Anemia	1.39 [0.59–3.29]	0.45
Killip class III-IV	3.56 [1.49–8.49]	<0.001
LVEF > 45%	0.37 [0.20–0.69]	<0.001

LVEF left-ventricular ejection fraction, HR hazard ratio, CI confidence intervals

Additionally, we have noted that an inadequate assessment of the LDL- and HDL-cholesterol levels is significantly associated with a less favorable long-term cardiovascular outcome after STEMI. Although no other prognostic impact of an adequate/inadequate risk factors control was demonstrated in our series, efficacy of secondary prevention strategies after a STEMI episode has been widely proven elsewhere [1–4, 9, 14–20]. It is suggested by this that an inadequate control of conventional cardiovascular risk factors after a STEMI episode may, at least partially, counterbalance the demonstrated prognostic benefits of current myocardial reperfusion strategies, such as urgent PCI [6–8, 10, 13]. Therefore, further efforts

ejection fraction were associated with both, mortality and cardiovascular readmissions (Table 4).

Regarding the association between inadequate assessment or control of the conventional cardiovascular risk factors and long-term cardiovascular mortality and readmission rates, the lack of assessment of LDL- cholesterol and HDL-cholesterol were significantly associated with a worse cardiovascular outcome. No other differences were noted for other *not-assessed or not controlled* variables (Table 5).

When only considering patients undergoing primary PCI (n = 363) or any reperfusion therapy (n = 370), the long-term adherence to secondary prevention strategies and its clinical impact were neither significantly different.

Discussion

In this study it is demonstrated that the long-term efficiency of conventional secondary prevention strategies after a STEMI episode in the *AMI code* era (a therapeutic strategy which enhances a rapid and widespread access to urgent PCI) is manifestly suboptimal. Impressively, less than 6% of diabetic or non-diabetic patients met all the secondary prevention strategy targets at the end of the follow-up period.

Table 5 Age, sex, hypertension, anemia and Killip adjusted *Hazard ratio* for mortality or cardiovascular readmission for those patients with no assessed or with no controlled cardiovascular risk factors (respect to patients with controlled risk factors)

		HR [CI 95%]	p-value
Total cholesterol	Not assessed	1.47 [0.74–2.93]	0.28
	Not controlled	0.18 [0.02–1.36]	0.10
LDL-cholesterol	Not assessed	2.57 [1.26–5.24]	0.01
	Not controlled	0.89 [0.44–1.81]	0.76
HDL-cholesterol	Not assessed	2.88 [1.54–5.39]	<0.001
	Not controlled	1.26 [0.61–2.61]	0.53
Triglycerides	Not assessed	1.80 [0.90–3.59]	0.09
	Not controlled	1.12 [0.56–2.21]	0.75
HbA1c	Not assessed	0.80 [0.19–3.31]	0.76
	Not controlled	0.48 [0.90–2.66]	0.40
Blood pressure	Not assessed	1.04 [0.51–2.12]	0.92
	Not controlled	0.58 [0.25–1.32]	0.19
Smoking	Not assessed	0.73 [0.38–1.40]	0.35
	Not controlled	2.05 [0.83–5.05]	0.12

HbA1c glycosylated hemoglobin

should be driven in order to enhance a more adequate accomplishment of all secondary prevention strategies after a STEMI, since these efforts should have a positive impact on the cardiovascular outcome in such patients in the long-term.

Not surprisingly, patients presenting with cardiovascular readmission or death from any cause during follow-up were older and had a higher prevalence of systemic hypertension, anemia, scored higher in Killip class classification and had lower ejection fraction. All of such conventional risk factors except for age still remain as robust predictors of a poorer cardiovascular outcome after a STEMI episode.

Long-term assessment and control of cardiovascular risk factors after STEMI

Notably, around one-sixth of our patient population did not undergo a blood test control after the index STEMI episode, with one third of the diabetic population not having glycosylated hemoglobin determinations. These figures are important and highlight the limitations of the implementation of current secondary prevention strategies among these patients. Patient education and physician awareness of this situation are some of the elements that could be implemented to decrease these poor results [21].

According to the current European clinical practice guidelines of secondary prevention, the current objective for LDL-cholesterol is to achieve a concentration inferior to 70 mg/dL or a reduction greater than 50% from the basal LDL-cholesterol levels [18, 19]. In our study, despite a high prescription rate of statins during follow-up, only one third of our patients reached the targeted levels. The EUROASPIRE IV (carried out in several European centers) and ADVANCE studies were undertaken in patients with stable coronary artery disease, and neither showed encouraging results [25, 26].

Previously reported European multicenter registers carried out over nearly two decades in a population of patients with CAD demonstrated that only half of the patients have their blood pressure under control despite of the high prescription rate of ACE inhibitors and beta blockers [25, 28]. These results are comparable with our observations, with only 62% of the patients having an adequate blood pressure control, besides the 20% percentage of the population with blood pressure control not being adequately assessed. Although a significant decrease in the systolic blood pressure values was established during follow-up as compared to the initial value upon hospital admission for the index STEMI episode ($p < 0.001$), this data has to be analyzed cautiously. The initial blood pressure value registered during an acute coronary event is not necessarily representative of the baseline patient's blood pressure control. Furthermore, the prognostic value of high systolic blood pressure values at admission in the setting of an acute STEMI remains controversial [29–32].

The observed suboptimal metabolic control of diabetic patients is in the line of previous observations reported in series of diabetic patients undergoing by-pass surgery or PCI, with around one-half of diabetic patients having inadequate and/or insufficient long-term glycosylated hemoglobin levels control [27].

Smoking cessation after STEMI is associated with improved survival rates [14, 33]. Our study confirms an unacceptably high rate of smoking habit continuation, thus suggesting that further counseling strategies pursuing smoking habit withdrawal should be rendered in this setting.

Myocardial invasive reperfusion and prognosis

The implementation of the *AMI code* program has increased the access to urgent myocardial reperfusion to an 87% of STEMI patients, nearly all of them through PCI [8]. This increase in the use of urgent reperfusion strategies is similar to that observed in another national multicenter register, with a reperfusion rate of 85.7% of patients, the difference being that, in the latter, one third of reperfusions were performed by means of fibrinolysis [3].

In our study, the 30-day mortality rate (5%) was similar to that observed in other national and international surveys in the PCI era [10, 34–39]. However, 6.1% of the STEMI 6-months survivors had deceased at the end of the 20-months (median) follow-up period, with an additional 9.9% of cardiovascular readmissions, percentages that (although low) have to be still considered suboptimal and in line with previous national series in which widespread use of urgent PCI was not yet the rule [3].

Our findings should make us reconsider the actual therapeutic yield of urgent myocardial reperfusion strategies in the setting of a STEMI: while the implementation of assistance networks (such as the *AMI code* program) has ameliorated the acute management of STEMI, the potentially beneficial impact of such strategies may be jeopardized by a suboptimal long-term implementation of the secondary prevention strategies. In the view of our results, we believe further efforts devoted to promote the cessation of smoking, periodical blood testing and blood pressure control, and to more intensively maintain LDL-cholesterol, glycosylated hemoglobin and blood pressure below the targeted levels should be undertaken. The importance of an adequate risk factors control has been highlighted also for patients with stable coronary disease, and may be specially manifest among patients with low ejection fraction and (like in our series) with a prior history of myocardial infarction [40].

Study limitations

The lack of association between cardiovascular risk factors control and cardiovascular outcome in our series is probably due to the low total number of cardiovascular events, the relatively short follow-up time and the limited sample size, reducing the statistical power of our analyses. Otherwise, dose of statins and other medication, adherence to prescribed treatment, healthy lifestyles such as diet, physical exercise, and weight control, potentially influencing the clinical outcome after a STEMI episode, were not assessed in our series due to limitations inherent to the use of the regional electronic health recording system. Finally, our single-center study may not be representative of the Spanish/European population of STEMI patients. However, its prospective nature and the consecutive inclusion appear to bestow a representative sample of real life.

Conclusions

Although implementation of the *AMI code* program has resulted in a widespread access to urgent myocardial reperfusion by means of PCI, the secondary prevention strategies after a STEMI episode are still far from being optimal, thus potentially counterbalancing the prognostic benefits of this therapy. Additional efforts to optimize the assessment and control of conventional cardiovascular risk factors should be implemented.

Acknowledgements
This work has been produced in the framework of the Doctorate in Medicine of the *Universitat Autònoma de Barcelona*.

Fundings
This work was supported by grant from Instituto de Salud Carlos III FEDER (Programa HERACLES RD12/0042/0013).

Authors' contributions
All authors made substantial contributions to conception and design, or acquisition of data, or analysis and interpretation of data. NR, CGG, VB and RE were involved in drafting the manuscript and OM, LLR, SP, NS, JMA and JB revised it critically for important intellectual content. All authors gave final approval of the version to be published and agreed to be accountable for all aspects of the work in ensuring that questions related to the accuracy or integrity of any part of the work are appropriately investigated and resolved.

Competing interests
The authors declare that they have no competing interests.

Author details
[1]Cardiology Department, Hospital del Mar, Passeig Marítim, 25-29, 08003 Barcelona, Spain. [2]Heart Diseases Biomedical Research Group, IMIM (Hospital del Mar Medical Research Institute), Barcelona, Spain. [3]Medicine Department, Program in Internal Medicine, Universitat Autònoma de Barcelona, Barcelona, Spain. [4]Hospital Universitari Germans Trias i Pujol, Badalona, Spain. [5]IMIM (Hospital del Mar Medical Research Institute). Cardiovascular Epidemiology and Genetics Group (EGEC), REGICOR Study Group, Barcelona, Spain. [6]CIBER de Enfermedades Cardiovasculares (CIBERCV), Barcelona, Spain.

References

1. Heras M, Marrugat J, Aros F, Bosch X, Enero J, Suárez MA, et al. Reduction in acute myocardial infarction mortality over a five-year period. Rev Esp Cardiol. 2006;59:200–8.
2. Ferreira-González I, Permanyer-Miralda G, Marrugat J, Heras M, Cuñat J, Civeira E, et al. MASCARA (Manejo del Síndrome Coronario Agudo. Registro Actualizado) study. General findings. Rev Esp Cardiol. 2008;61:803–16.
3. Barrabés JA, Bardají A, Jiménez-Candil J, del Nogal F, Bodí V, Basterra N, et al. Prognosis and management of acute coronary syndrome in Spain in 2012: the DIOCLES study. Rev Esp Cardiol. 2015;68:98–106.
4. García-García C, Sanz G, Valle V, Molina L, Sala J, Subirana I, et al. Trends in In-hospital mortality and six-month outcomes in patients with a first acute myocardial infarction. change over the last decade. Rev Esp Cardiol. 2010;63:1136–44.
5. Instituto Nacional de Estadística. Defunciones según la causa de muerte. http://www.ine.es. 2014. Accessed 30 Mar 2016
6. Steg PG, James SK, Atar D, Badano LP, Blömstrom-Lundqvist C, Borger MA, et al. ESC Guidelines for the management of acute myocardial infarction in patients presenting with ST-segment elevation. Eur Heart J. 2012;33:2569–619.
7. O'Gara PT, Kushner FG, Ascheim DD, Casey DE, Chung MK, Lemos JA, et al. 2013 ACCF/AHA guideline for the management of ST-elevation myocardial infarction. JACC. 2013;61:e78–149.
8. Bosch X, Curós A, Argimond JM, Faixedas M, Figueras J, Jiménez FX, et al. Modelo de intervención coronaria percutánea primaria en Cataluña. Rev Esp Cardiol Supl. 2011;11:51–60.
9. Andrés E, Cordero A, Magán P, Alegría E, León M, Luengo E, et al. Long-term mortality and hospital readmission after acute myocardial infarction, an eight-year follow-up study. Rev Esp Cardiol. 2012;65:414–20.
10. Gómez-Hospital JA, Domenico P, Sánchez JC, Ariza A, Homs S, Lorente V, et al. Impact on delay times and characteristics of patients undergoing primary percutaneous coronary intervention in the southern metropolitan area of Barcelona after implementation of the infarction code program. Rev Esp Cardiol. 2012;65:911–8.
11. Stone SG, Serrao GW, Mehran R, Tomey MI, Witzenbichler B, Guagliumi G, et al. Incidence, predictors, and implications of reinfarction after primary percutaneous coronary intervention in ST-segment-elevation myocardial infarction: the harmonizing outcomes with revascularization and stents in acute myocardial infarction trial. Circ Cardiovasc Interv. 2014;7:543–51.
12. Ng VG, Lansky AJ, Meller S, Witzenbichler B, Guagliumi G, Peruga JZ, et al. The prognostic importance of left ventricular function in patients with ST-segment elevation myocardial infarction: the HORIZONS-AMI trial. Eur Heart J Acute Cardiovasc Care. 2014;3:67–77.
13. Chan MY, Sun JL, Newby LK, Shaw LK, Lin M, Peterson ED, et al. Long-term mortality of patients undergoing cardiac catheterization for ST-elevation and non-ST-elevation myocardial infarction. Circulation. 2009;119:3110–7.
14. Wilson K, Gibson N, Willan A, Cook D. Effect of smoking cessation on mortality after myocardial infarction. meta-analysis of cohort studies. Arch Intern Med. 2000;160:939–44.
15. Cannon CP, Braunwald E, McCabe CH, Rader DJ, Rouleau JL, Belder R. Intensive versus moderate lipid lowering with statins after acute coronary syndromes. N Engl J Med. 2004;350:1495–504.
16. Ray KK, Seshasai SR, Wijesuriya S, Sivakumaran R, Nethercott S, Preiss D, et al. Effect of intensive control of glucose on cardiovascular outcomes and death in patients with diabetes mellitus: a meta-analysis of randomized controlled trials. Lancet. 2009;373:1765–72.
17. Lewington S, Clarke R, Qizilbash N, Peto R, Collins R, Collaboration PS. Age-specific relevance of usual blood pressure to vascular mortality: a meta-analysis of individual data for one million adults in 61 prospective studies. Lancet. 2002;360:1903–13.
18. Perk J, De Backer G, Gohlke H, Graham I, Reiner Z, Verschuren WMM, et al. European Guidelines on cardiovascular disease prevention in clinical practice (version 2012). Eur Heart J. 2012;33:1635–701.
19. Reiner Z, Catapano A, De Backer G, Graham I, Taskinen M, Wiklund O, et al. ESC/EAS Guidelines for the management of dyslipidaemias. Eur Heart J. 2011;32:1769–818.
20. Stone NJ, Robinson JG, Lichtenstein AH, Merz NB, Blum CB, Eckel RH, et al. 2013 ACC/AHA Guideline on the treatment of blood cholesterol to reduce atherosclerotic cardiovascular risk in adults. Circulation. 2014;129:S1–45.
21. Dennis S, Williams A, Taggart J, Newall A, Denney-Wilson E, Zwar N, et al. Which providers can bridge the health literacy gap in lifestyle risk factor

modification education: a systematic review and narrative synthesis. BMC Fam Pract. 2012;13:44.

22. Yaghi S, Pilot M, Song C, Blum CA, Yakhkind A, Silver B, et al. Ischemic stroke risk after acute coronary syndrome. J Am Heart Assoc. 2016;5, e002590.

23. Mehta SR, Eikelboom JW, Rao-Melacini P, Weitz JI, Anand SS, Pare G, et al. A risk assessment tool incorporating new biomarkers for cardiovascular events in acute coronary syndromes: the organization to assess strategies in ischemic syndromes (OASIS) risk score. Can J Cardiol. 2016;32:1332–9.

24. Jolly SS, Cairns JA, Yusuf S, Meeks B, Pogue J, Rokoss MJ, et al. Randomized trial of primary PCI with or without routine manual thrombectomy. N Engl J Med. 2015;372:1389–98.

25. Kotseva K, Wood D, De Bacquer D, De Backer G, Rydén L, Jennings C, et al. EUROASPIRE IV: A European Society of Cardiology survey on the lifestyle, risk factor and therapeutic management of coronary patients from 24 European countries. Eur J Prev Cardiol. 2016;23:636–48.

26. Borràs X, Garcia- Moll X, Gómez-Doblas JJ, Zapata A, Artigas R, et al. Stable angina in Spain and its impact on quality of life. The AVANCE registry. Rev Esp Cardiol. 2012;65:734–41.

27. Mazón-Ramos P, Cordero A, González-Juanatey JR, Bertomeu V, Delgado E, Vitale G, et al. Control of cardiovascular risk factors in revascularized patients with diabetes: a subanalysis of the ICP-bypass study. Rev Esp Cardiol. 2015;68:115–20.

28. Kotseva K, Wood D, De Backer G, De Bacquer D, Pyörälä K, Keil U, for the EUROASPIRE Study Group*. Cardiovascular prevention guidelines in daily practice: a comparison of EUROASPIRE I, II, and III surveys in eight European countries. Lancet. 2009;373:929–40.

29. Huang B, Yang Y, Zhu J, Liang Y, Tan H. Clinical characteristics and short-term outcomes in patients with elevated admission systolic blood pressure after acute ST-elevation myocardial infarction: a population-based study. BMJ Open. 2014;4, e005097.

30. Pitsavos C, Panagiotakos D, Zombolos S, Mantas Y, Antonoulas A, Stravopodis P, et al. Systolic blood pressure on admission predicts in-hospital mortality among patients presenting with acute coronary syndromes: the Greek study of acute coronary syndromes. J Clin Hypertens (Greenwich). 2008;10:362–6.

31. Stenestrand U, Wijkman M, Fredrikson M, Nystrom FH. Association between admission supine systolic blood pressure and 1-year mortality in patients admitted to the intensive care unit for acute chest pain. JAMA. 2010;303:1167–72.

32. Jonas M, Grossman E, Boyko V, Behar S, Hod H, Reicher-Reiss H. Relation of early and one-year outcome after acute myocardial infarction to systemic arterial blood pressure on admission. Am J Cardiol. 1999;84:162–5.

33. Gerber Y, Rosen LJ, Goldbourt U, Benyamini Y, Drory Y. Smoking status and long-term survival after first acute myocardial infarction. a population-based cohort study. J Am Coll Cardiol. 2009;54:2382–7.

34. Carrillo P, López-Palop R, Pinar E, Saura D, Párraga M, Picó F, et al. Treatment of acute myocardial infarction by primary angioplasty on-site compared with treatment following interhospital transfer: short- and long-time clinical outcomes. Rev Esp Cardiol. 2007;60:801–10.

35. Mingo S, Goicolea J, Nombela L, Sufrate E, Blasco A, Millán I, et al. Primary percutaneous angioplasty. An analysis of reperfusion delays, their determining factors and their prognostic implications. Rev Esp Cardiol. 2009;62:15–22.

36. Íñiguez A, Vázquez N, Trillo R, Baz JA, Vázquez JM, Amaro A, et al. Modelo de intervención coronaria percutánea primaria en la Comunidad de Galicia. Rev Esp Cardiol Supl. 2011;11:44–50.

37. Lezáun R, Alcasena MS, Basurte MT, Berjón J, Maraví C, Aleu M, et al. Modelo de intervención coronaria percutánea primaria en la Comunidad de Navarra. Rev Esp Cardiol Supl. 2011;11:21–7.

38. Dörler J, Alber HF, Altenberger J, Bonner G, Benzer W, Grimm G, et al. Primary pecutaneous intervention of ST-elevation myocardial infarction in Austria: Results from the Austrian acute PCI registry 2005–2007. Wien Klin Wochenschr. 2010;122:220–8.

39. Fassa A-A, Urban P, Radovanovic P, Duvoisin N, Gaspoz J-M, Stauffer J-C, et al. Trends in reperfusion therapy of ST segment elevation myocardial infarction in Switzerland: six year results from a nationwide registry. Heart. 2005;91:882–8.

40. Barbero U, D'Ascenzo F, Nijhoff F, Moretti C, Biondi-Zoccai G, Mennuni M, et al. Assessing risk in patients with stable coronary disease: when should we intensify care and follow-up? Results from a meta-analysis of observational studies of the COURAGE and FAME Era. Scientifica (Cairo). 2016;2016:3769152.

22

Homocysteine is a bystander for ST-segment elevation myocardial infarction

Ching-Yu Julius Chen[1,2], Tzu-Ching Yang[3], Christopher Chang[4], Shao-Chun Lu[3] and Po-Yuan Chang[1,2*] iD

Abstract

Background: Homocysteine has been long considered a risk factor for atherosclerosis. However, cardiovascular events cannot be reduced through homocysteine lowering by B vitamin supplements. Although several association studies have reported an elevation of serum homocysteine levels in cardiovascular diseases, the relationship of homocysteine with ST-segment elevation myocardial infarction (STEMI) is not well established.

Methods: We prospectively enrolled STEMI patients who were consecutively admitted to an intensive care unit following coronary intervention in a single medical center in Taiwan. Control subjects were individuals who presented to the outpatient or emergency department with acute chest pain but subsequently revealed patent coronary arteries by coronary arteriography. The association between serum homocysteine levels and STEMI was investigated. A culture system using human coronary artery endothelial cells was also established to examine the toxic effects of homocysteine at the cellular level.

Results: Patients with chest pain were divided into two groups. The STEMI group included 56 patients who underwent a primary percutaneous coronary intervention. The control group included 17 subjects with patent coronary arteries. There was no difference in serum homocysteine levels (8.4 ± 2.2 vs. 7.6 ± 1.9 μmol/L, $p = 0.142$). When stratifying STEMI patients by the Killip classification into higher (Killip III-IV) and lower (Killip I-II) grades, CRP (3.3 ± 4.1 vs. 1.4 ± 2.3 mg/L, $p = 0.032$), peak creatine kinase (3796 ± 2163 vs. 2305 ± 1822 IU/L, $p = 0.023$), and SYNTAX scores (20.4 ± 11.1 vs. 14.8 ± 7.6, $p = 0.033$) were significantly higher in the higher grades, while serum homocysteine levels were similar. Homocysteine was not correlated with WBCs, CRP, or the SYNTAX score in STEMI patients. In a culture system, homocysteine at even a supraphysiological level of 100 μmol/L did not reduce the cell viability of human coronary artery endothelial cells.

Conclusions: Homocysteine was not elevated in STEMI patients regardless of Killip severity, suggesting that homocysteine is a bystander instead of a causative factor of STEMI. Our study therefore supports the current notion that homocysteine-lowering strategies are not essential in preventing cardiovascular disease.

Keywords: Coronary artery disease, C-reactive protein (CRP), Homocysteine, ST-segment elevation myocardial infarction (STEMI), White blood cell (WBC)

_____

* Correspondence: pychang@ntu.edu.tw
[1]Cardiovascular Center and Division of Cardiology, Department of Internal Medicine, National Taiwan University Hospital, 7 Chung-Shan South Road, 100 Taipei, Taiwan
[2]Division of Cardiology, Department of Internal Medicine, National Taiwan University College of Medicine, No.1, Ren-Ai Road Section 1, 100 Taipei, Taiwan
Full list of author information is available at the end of the article

Background

Homocysteine is a highly reactive, sulfur-containing amino acid formed as a byproduct of the metabolism of the essential amino acid methionine [1], and methylenetetrahydrofolatereductase (MTHFR) is a key enzyme in this process. The serum level of homocysteine is significantly elevated in areas with dietary folate and B vitamin deficiencies as well as in subjects with the MTHFR 677 TT genotype [2], which can be lowered by B vitamins, including folic acid, B6, and B12. Homocysteine used to be considered a risk factor for atherosclerosis, which was primarily observed in children with extremely elevated serum homocysteine levels as well as premature atherothrombotic disease, and basic studies demonstrated that homocysteine can induce vascular damage by promoting platelet activation, oxidative stress, endothelial dysfunction, hypercoagulability, vascular smooth muscle cell proliferation, and endoplasmic reticulum stress [1, 3, 4]. A meta-analysis that collected large numbers of prospective studies and corrected for a regression dilution bias did show a significant association between the serum level and the incidence of cardiovascular disease (CVD) [5–10]. Serum levels were also correlated with long-term outcomes in patients with documented coronary artery disease (CAD) or acute coronary syndrome [11, 12]. However, recent studies disclosed that even though serum homocysteine levels were reduced by B vitamins in patients with stable CAD, acute coronary syndrome, or stroke, the rate of major adverse cardiac events was not reduced [13–17]. Moreover, there was no difference in early and late cardiovascular mortality among the tertiles of serum homocysteine levels in patients with ST-segment elevation myocardial infarction (STEMI) or non-ST-segment elevation acute coronary syndrome [18]. A possible explanation is the generally accepted concept of primary percutaneous coronary intervention (PCI) in STEMI, the common use of a new generation of drug-eluting stents in this era, [19, 20] and the development of a newer P2Y12 inhibitor, [21, 22] which has contributed to great improvements in survival and stent patency, thereby attenuating any potential benefits of homocysteine-lowering interventions. We tried to clarify the role of homocysteine in STEMI, an extreme entity of acute coronary syndrome, by making comparisons with subjects presenting with chest pain but proven to have patent or non-significant coronary arteries.

Methods

Study population

This study was approved by the institutional review board and conformed with the principles outlined in the *Declaration of Helsinki*. We prospectively enrolled STEMI patients who were consecutively admitted to an intensive care unit following coronary intervention in this study. The control group included individuals who presented to the outpatient or emergency department with acute chest pain but subsequently revealed patent coronary arteries by coronary arteriography. This study was carried out in a single medical center in Taiwan from March to September in 2014. STEMI was defined according to the 2013 American Heart Association (AHA)/American College of Cardiology (ACC) and European Society of Cardiology (ESC) guidelines, including persistent electrocardiographic (ECG) ST elevation and subsequent release of biomarkers of myocardial necrosis [23, 24]. All participants provided written informed consent.

Study protocol

We recorded the time elapsed from exhibition of symptoms to receipt of medical services and the door-to-balloon time; demographic data and atherosclerotic risk factors including hypertension, diabetes, dyslipidemia, cigarette smoking, a family history of premature myocardial infarction, peripheral arterial disease, stroke, and the body-mass index; serum homocysteine, complete lipid profiles, hemoglobin A1c, white cell counts, C-reactive protein (CRP), peak creatine kinase (CK), and the time elapsed to the peak value; the severity of STEMI by the Killip classification and coronary anatomy by the SYNTAX score; life-threatening conditions including ventricular tachyarrhythmias, cardiac arrest, the use of an intra-aortic balloon pump (IABP) or extracorporeal membranous oxygenation (ECMO); echocardiographic parameters including the left ventricular ejection fraction (LVEF) and E/E'; electrocardiographic parameters including the PR and QTc interval, QRS duration, existence of fragmented QRS or early repolarization; and medications for acute coronary syndrome including antiplatelets, glycoprotein IIb/IIIa inhibitor, beta-blockade, angiotensin-converting enzyme inhibitor (ACEi) or angiotensin-II receptor blocker, statins, or antiarrhythmic drugs. We compared differences between the STEMI and control groups and analyzed whether there was a correlation between the severity of STEMI and the abovementioned parameters. All live STEMI patients were followed up for at least 1 month to evaluate their short-term prognosis.

Cell cultures

Human coronary artery endothelial cells (ECs; HCAECs, Clonetics, US), at passages 4 to 7, were maintained in EGM-MV medium supplemented with 20% fetal bovine serum (FBS) and antibiotics. For the experiments, all cultures of subconfluent HCAECs were incubated with phosphate-buffered saline (PBS, as a control), homocysteine, cysteine, or electronegative L5 low-density lipoprotein (LDL) isolated from STEMI patients according to a previously described protocol [25, 26].

Cell viability 3-(4,5-dimethylthiazol-2-yl)-2,5-diphenyl-tetrazolium bromide (MTT) assay.

The chemical MTT was purchased from Sigma (St. Louis, MO) [26, 27]. HCAECs (5×10^4 cells/well) were dispensed into 24-well plates and incubated for 24 h after the addition of homocysteine or different treatments, and the index of EC viability was determined by the colorimetric MTT (tetrazolium) assay. The absorbance was measured at a wavelength of 540 nm for viable cells using a microplate reader (Thermo Electron, Waltham, MA).

Statistical analyses

A Chi-squared or Fisher exact test was used to compare categorical variables. Continuous variables were determined by either Student's t-test or a one-way analysis of variance (ANOVA). All continuous data are expressed as means ± standard deviation. A two-tailed p value of < 0.05 was considered statistically significant. Regression analysis with a linear model was used to analyze the correlation between continuous parameters. Statistical analysis was performed using IBM SPSS Statistics for Windows, Version 22.0 (Armonk, NY).

Results

We enrolled a total of 73 patients with chest pain. The STEMI group included 56 patients who underwent a primary PCI for total coronary occlusion. The control group included 17 subjects who presented with chest pain but had patent coronary arteries. In the control group, two patients visited the emergency department due to aggravating typical angina, 14 patients had stress-induced ischemia in thallium myocardial perfusion imaging, and one patient had progressive chest pain despite optimal medical treatment for reflux esophagitis; 11 patients were diagnosed as syndrome X, two patients had myocardial bridge, one patient had apical hypertrophy, one patient had coronary spasm, one patient had reflux esophagitis, and one patient had atrial fibrillation with rapid ventricular response. The demographic profile of study subjects is shown in Table 1. There was no difference in age, gender, or atherosclerosis risk factors such as hypertension, diabetes, dyslipidemia, and smoking between the two groups, as well as no differences in serum LDL and hemoglobin A1c. Two patients in the STEMI group died from cardiogenic shock; one had diabetes with multivessel coronary lesions. Among the 54 STEMI survivals, 12 were diabetes; 5 out of these 12 diabetic STEMI patients had multivessel lesions. None of our study subjects was on regular B-vitamin supplements for more than 1 year before enrollment.

White blood cell (WBC) counts ($11.9 \pm 4 \times 10^9$ vs. $6.5 \pm 2 \times 10^9$/L, $p < 0.001$), CRP (2.0 ± 3.0 vs. 0.2 ± 0.1 mg/L, $p < 0.001$), serum creatinine levels (1.2 ± 0.8 vs. 0.9 ± 0.2 mg/dL, $p = 0.004$), and QTc (441.1 ± 48 vs. 416.6 ± 21 ms, $p = 0.044$) were higher in STEMI patients. The LVEF was lower in the STEMI group ($54.1\% \pm 12\%$ vs. $69.6\% \pm 6\%$, $p < 0.001$) (Table 2). There was no significant difference in serum homocysteine levels (8.4 ± 2.2 vs. 7.6 ± 1.9 µmol/L, $p = 0.142$) after two outliers were excluded (Table 2). The two outliers (homocysteine of 36.8 and 32.3 µmol/L) were classified as Killip I and II, respectively, without renal impairment. The average follow-up time was 19.3 ± 1.9 months in the STEMI group, while one of the STEMI patients died of refractory ventricular fibrillation 4 days after the event day and another of pump failure 5 days later (Table 3). There was no difference in E/E' values in echocardiographic measurements or the percentage of early repolarization shown in electrocardiograms between the two groups, while there was a trend of greater QRS fragmentation in the STEMI group (80% vs. 53%, $p = 0.055$).

When stratifying STEMI patients by the Killip classification, CRP (3.3 ± 4.1 vs. 1.4 ± 2.3 mg/L, $p = 0.032$), peak CK (3796 ± 2163 vs. 2305 ± 1822 IU/L, $p = 0.023$), and SYNTAX scores (20.4 ± 11.1 vs. 14.8 ± 7.6, $p = 0.033$)

Table 1 Demographic data of the ST-segment elevation myocardial infarction (STEMI) and control groups

	STEMI	Control	p value
Number, n	56	17	NA
Age, yr	58.1 ± 13	57.5 ± 11	0.854
Male, n(%)	43(77)	11(65)	0.353
Hypertension, n(%)	25(45)	9(53)	0.589
Diabetes, n(%)	13(23)	3(18)	0.748
Dyslipidemia, n(%)	23(41)	8(47)	0.781
Smoking, n(%)	33(59)	6(35)	0.103
Stroke, n(%)	7(13)	1(6)	0.672
Peripheral arterial disease, n(%)	0(0)	0(0)	NA
End-stage renal disease, n(%)	1(2)	0(0)	1.000
History of congestive heart failure, n(%)	1(2)	1(6)	0.414
Family history of myocardial infarction, n(%)	7(13)	2(12)	1.000
Body-mass index, kg/m²	25.1 ± 4	25.5 ± 6	0.835
Mortality, n(%)	2(4)	0(0)	1.000
Regular B-vitamin supplements> 1 year, n(%)	0(0)	0(0)	NA

NA not available

Table 2 Comparison of laboratory, electrocardiographic, and echocardiographic parameters between the ST-segment elevation myocardial infarction (STEMI) and control groups

	STEMI	Control	p value
White cell count, ×10⁹/L	11.9 ± 4	6.5 ± 2	< 0.001*
Homocysteine, μmol/L	8.4 ± 2.2	7.6 ± 1.9	0.142[a]
C-reactive protein, mg/L	2.0 ± 3.0	0.2 ± 0.1	< 0.001*
Low-density lipoprotein, mg/dL	111.5 ± 38	95 ± 27	0.062
Creatinine, mg/dL	1.2 ± 0.8	0.9 ± 0.2	0.004*
Hemoglobin A1c, %	6.5 ± 1.6	6.1 ± 1.6	0.441
PR, ms	171.1 ± 43	173.6 ± 48	0.853
QRS, ms	94.9 ± 24	90.1 ± 12	0.273
QTc, ms	441.1 ± 48	416.6 ± 21	0.044*
QRS fragmentation, n(%)	45(80)	9(53)	0.055
Early repolarization, n(%)	18(32)	3(18)	0.362
Left ventricular ejection fraction, %	54.1 ± 12	69.6 ± 6	< 0.001*
E/E'	12.4 ± 5	12.4 ± 7	0.989

*$p < 0.05$
[a]After the two outliers of 36.8 and 32.3 μmol/L were excluded

were higher in the group with increased severity (Table 3). Serum homocysteine levels did not increase with the severity of myocardial infarction (Table 3). There was also no difference in age, time from exhibition of symptoms to hospitalization, or time elapsed to peak CK (Table 3).

When serum homocysteine levels were compared to various factors, we found that there was no correlation with WBC, CRP, or the SYNTAX score (Fig. 1a-c). In addition, the level of serum homocysteine was nearly consistent despite increases in these factors ($R^2 = 0.0008$, 0.0003, and 0.003, respectively).

The clinical bystander role of homocysteine was further confirmed at the cellular level. A culture system was established using HCAECs and an MTT assay to assess cell viability in the presence of homocysteine (Fig. 2). Exposure of HCAECs to 100 μmol/L homocysteine for up to 48 h did not decrease cell viability compared with the PBS control (Fig. 2). In contrast, treatment with L5 LDL, an electronegative molecule known as a risk marker in STEMI, resulted in a time-dependent decrease in cell viability in HCAECs. Even at concentrations of > 100 μmol/L, homocysteine still did not change cell

Table 3 Relationship between the severity of ST-segment elevation myocardial infarction (STEMI) and laboratory parameters

	Killip I	Killip II	Killip III	Killip IV	p value
Number, n	35	5	2	14	
Age, years	60.0 ± 13.5	63.6 ± 13.5	57.5 ± 12.0	51.3 ± 10.6	0.141
Symptom to hospital, h	4.6 ± 5.1	1.2 ± 1.3	0.5 ± 0.7	5.6 ± 5.4	0.249
Aborted sudden death, n(%)	1(3)	0	0	6(43)	0.001*
VT/Vf, n(%)	1(3)	0	0	5(36)	0.007*
ECMO, n(%)	0	0	0	3(21)	0.023*
IABP, n(%)	0	0	0	9(64)	< 0.001*
Follow-up time, months	19.3 ± 2.1	18.0 ± 1.1	19.0 ± 1.8	16.9 ± 7.3	0.299
Mortality, n(%)	0	0	0	2(15)	0.082
White cell count, × 10⁹/L	11.44 ± 3.5	13.7 ± 1.9	13.7 ± 6.2	12.0 ± 4.9	0.577
	11.7 ± 3.4		12.2 ± 4.9		0.704
Homocysteine, μmol/L	9.2 ± 5.3	12.9 ± 10.9	11.0 ± 3.7	8.0 ± 2.4	0.361
	9.7 ± 6.1		8.4 ± 2.6		0.256
C-reactive protein, mg/L	1.4 ± 2.3	1.4 ± 2.5	3.6 ± 3.9	3.3 ± 4.3	0.208
	1.4 ± 2.3		3.3 ± 4.1		0.032*
Low-density lipoprotein Cholesterol, mg/dL	116 ± 38	102 ± 30	127 ± 49	101 ± 41	0.574
	114 ± 37		104 ± 41		0.434
Peak creatine kinase (CK), IU/L	2100 ± 1391	3737 ± 3604	2595 ± 2773	3967 ± 2134	0.016*
	2305 ± 1822		3796 ± 2163		0.023*
Time to peak CK, h	10.4 ± 4.6	9.8 ± 4.0	6.5 ± 5.0	8.6 ± 4.0	0.460
SYNTAX score	14.2 ± 7.6	19.0 ± 6.8	20.0 ± 7.1	20.46 ± 11.7	0.123
	14.8 ± 7.6		20.4 ± 11.1		0.033*

ECMO extracorporeal membranous oxygenation, *IABP* Intra-aortic balloon pump
*$p < 0.05$

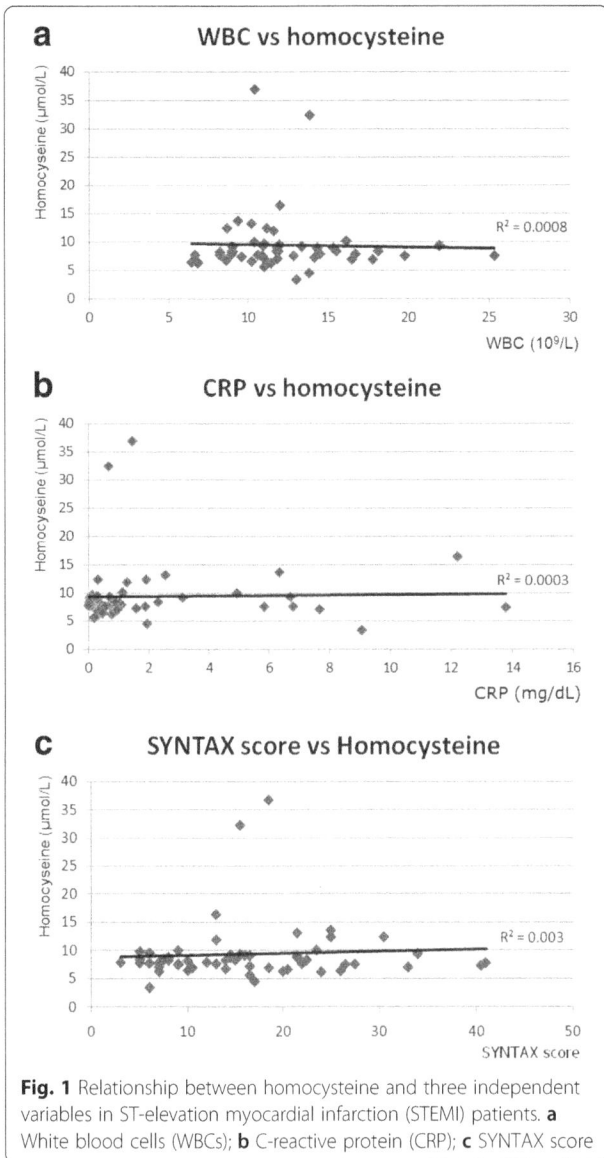

Fig. 1 Relationship between homocysteine and three independent variables in ST-elevation myocardial infarction (STEMI) patients. **a** White blood cells (WBCs); **b** C-reactive protein (CRP); **c** SYNTAX score

by coronary arteriography. This grouping contrasts with that reported in other studies in which "healthy" controls were based solely on non-invasive studies.

Although recent studies did not support the role of homocysteine as a risk factor in CVDs as previously thought, some reports have revealed an increase in homocysteine levels in CAD. A meta-analysis in 2002 reported that the mean serum homocysteine level in healthy populations at an average age of 56 years old was 11.8 μmol/L, and the odds ratio for ischemic heart disease associated with a 25% lower baseline homocysteine level was 0.83 (95% confidence interval (CI), 0.77~0.89) in prospective studies [8]. Akyurek et al. disclosed a higher serum homocysteine level in a STEMI group than in a healthy control group (19.0 ± 3.6 vs. 15.8 ± 4.2 μmol/L, $p = 0.008$) [10]. Liu C et al. found that the prevalence of hyperhomocysteinemia (> 15 μmol/L) was higher among patients with ischemic heart disease than among controls (79.1% vs. 5%) [29], and the serum homocysteine level was positively correlated with severity (acute myocardial infarction 23.44 ± 5.78 μmol/L, unstable angina 22.62 ± 6.37 μmol/L, stable angina 18.63 ± 6.73 μmol/L, and control 10.81 ± 4.62 μmol/L, $p < 0.001$) [30]. In contrast, our study showed that there was no difference in serum homocysteine levels between the control and STEMI groups, and our cohort had a mean level of homocysteine markedly lower than the levels reported in previous studies. Several public health studies have also shown a great diversity among serum homocysteine levels in different countries, ranging from 6.57 μmol/L in Kuwait [31] to 14 μmol/L in Italy [32], and folic acid fortification of grain products has already decreased the prevalence of high homocysteine levels (> 13 μmol/L) from 29.8% to 18.7% [33]. The variation in homocysteine levels may be attributed to ethnicity, socioeconomics, and nutritional status. Moreover, several studies demonstrating a neutral effect of homocysteine-lowering therapy in acute coronary syndrome have reported mean serum homocysteine levels of approximately 10 μmol/L [16, 34], relatively lower than those of previous studies, implying that the role of homocysteine in atherothrombotic heart disease may vary among populations with different average homocysteine levels. A trend of decreasing homocysteine levels in the general population also complicates the interaction of homocysteine and other established risk factors such as diabetes and smoking.

A previous study addressing the relationship of serum homocysteine levels with outcomes in patients with acute coronary syndrome showed that an elevated level on admission strongly predicted late cardiac events [12]. However, the rate of revascularization was 26.4% in that study, with an event rate of 9.3% over 28 days, which greatly differed from the current situation of acute

viability (data not shown). This bench evidence along with clinical observations in STEMI suggests that homocysteine is a bystander and not a causative factor of atherogenesis.

Discussion

Our study clearly demonstrated that homocysteine was not elevated in STEMI patients, and therefore, this long-considered risk factor for CAD was more likely a bystander rather than a causative agent in STEMI. We believe our data are trustworthy because every study subject was evaluated in detail by coronary angiography. Our control group consisted of patients with the final diagnosis of Syndrome X, myocardial bridge [28], apical hypertrophy, coronary spasm, reflux esophagitis and atrial fibrillation, whose coronary patency was confirmed

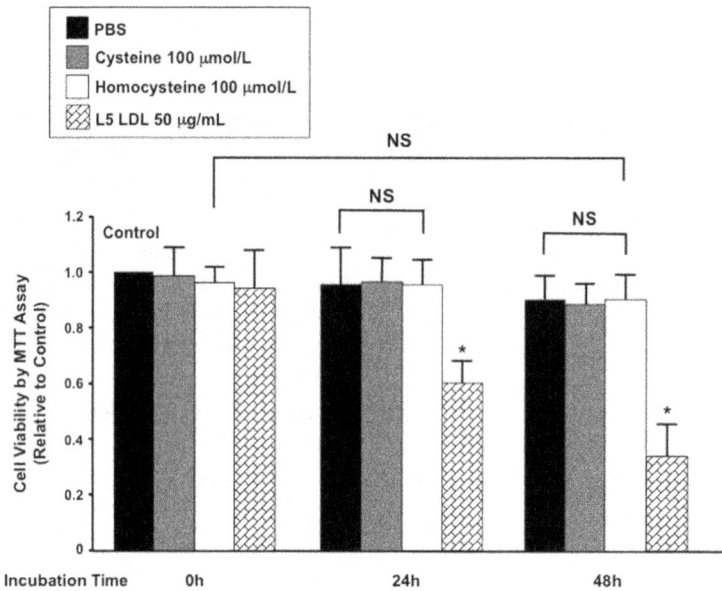

Fig. 2 Effects of homocysteine on cell viability in cultured human coronary artery endothelial cells (HCAECs). Cells were treated with the PBS control, 100 μmol/L cysteine, 100 μmol/L homocysteine, or 50 μg/mL L5 low-density lipoprotein (LDL) for 0, 24, and 48 h as indicated, and cell viability was assessed by an MTT assay. Values are the mean±SEM ($n = 3$). * $p < 0.05$ vs. the PBS control (the first black column). NS, not significant

coronary occlusion rapidly being treated through a percutaneous intervention. Because PCI has been demonstrated to be an indispensable strategy in acute coronary syndrome, the results of the abovementioned study with low revascularization rate cannot be applied to the era of aggressive and effective revascularization. Together with the findings gathered in our study, this result implies that advances in primary PCI in STEMI and the application of new-generation drug-eluting stents as well as newer P2Y12 inhibitors may attenuate the effect of serum homocysteine on cardiovascular outcomes.

One interesting finding of our study was the elevated leukocyte count in STEMI patients. It is well known that WBC counts are elevated in subjects with acute coronary syndrome [35], and leukocytosis is a predictor of major adverse cardiac events in patients with acute coronary syndrome [36, 37]. CRP is also a risk factor for cardiovascular events with a risk ratio of 1.67 (95% CI: 1.21~6.41) according to a meta-analysis of 42 prospective studies, [38] and it is an independent predictor of 30-day mortality in STEMI patients [39]. In our cohort, we observed significant increases in WBC and CRP levels in STEMI patients compared with the control group, and STEMI patients at higher Killip classes (III and IV) also had higher serum levels of these markers. However, the serum homocysteine level was consistently low regardless of the Killip class and had no correlation with WBC or CRP levels in STEMI patients. The discrepancy between our results and homocysteine's role as a cardiovascular risk factor reported in previous studies requires a thorough reevaluation of homocysteine in the

development of coronary heart disease and its prognostic value in patients with myocardial infarction.

STEMI patients had higher hemoglobin A1c levels than the control group in this prospective study, although the difference was not statistically significant. Diabetes has been known as a critical predictor of STEMI outcome. Indeed, our study showed that the diabetes% in the STEMI mortality subgroup (50%, 1 diabetes out of 2 mortality) was much higher than that in the STEMI survivals (21%, 12 diabetes out of 54 survivals). Recent studies showed that hyperglycemic stress during acute myocardial infarction (AMI) had a negative prognostic effect, [40] and diabetic patients with incretin-based therapy had a significant lower rate of all-cause mortality, cardiac death and readmission at 12 months [41]. Moreover, hyperglycemic patients with STEMI had fewer endothelial progenitor cells (EPCs) than normoglycemic patients, and an intensive glycemic control (80–140 mg/dL) group had a higher EPC number and the ability to differentiate and proportion salvaged myocardium, measured by technetium-99 m sestamibi scintigraphy [42]. These studies demonstrated that metabolic factors may directly affect the outcome of AMI and the viability of EPCs, and the latter may be a proxy for the probability of myocardial salvage.

Our in vitro experiments confirmed the bystander role of homocysteine in coronary artery cell damage (Fig. 2). As a long-considered risk factor for atherosclerosis, homocysteine can exhibit synergistic EC toxicity with modified LDL by a shared pathway related to fibroblast growth factor (FGF)-2 [26]. However, the homocysteine concentrations used in most experiments have been much higher than the physiological level, which is < 10 μmol/L, even under conditions with impaired folate metabolism [2]. In our study, under a supraphysiological concentration of 100 μmol/L, homocysteine still had no detrimental effects on HCAEC viability compared with its benign structural analog, cysteine. These results indicate that homocysteine is not the culprit molecule but instead a bystander in causing endothelial injury during cardiovascular events that arise from acute plaque rupture but not de novo thrombosis. Our findings have complicated the existing notions of the relationship between homocysteine and thrombosis [43] and may explain why homocysteine-lowering therapy has failed to reduce the risk of cardiovascular events. These observations offer a potential explanation for the negative results obtained from most clinical outcome trials on homocysteine reduction and raise a new topic of future homocysteine research.

Conclusions

Unlike the leukocyte count and CRP, homocysteine was not elevated in STEMI patients regardless of Killip severity, suggesting that homocysteine is a bystander instead of a causative factor of STEMI. Our study therefore supports the current notion that homocysteine-lowering strategies are not essential in CVD prevention. Larger prospective studies are warranted to reevaluate the role of homocysteine in CAD.

Abbreviations
CAD: Coronary artery disease; CRP: C-reactive protein; CVD: Cardiovascular disease; ECMO: Extracorporeal membranous oxygenation; IABP: Intra-aortic balloon pump; LDL: Low-density lipoprotein; LVEF: Left ventricular ejection fraction; PCI: Percutaneous coronary intervention; STEMI: ST-segment elevation myocardial infarction; WBC: White blood cell

Acknowledgements
Not applicable

Funding
This study was supported by grant NSC101-2320-B-002-026 from the National Science Council, Taipei, Taiwan (to Dr. Chang).

Authors' contributions
CYC analyzed and interpreted the patient data and wrote the manuscript. TCY performed the cell experiments. CC assisted in cell experiments. SCL analyzed the results of cell and biochemical assays. PYC coordinated the basic and clinical study and wrote the manuscript. All authors read and approved the final manuscript.

Competing interests
The authors declare that they have no competing interests.

Author details
[1]Cardiovascular Center and Division of Cardiology, Department of Internal Medicine, National Taiwan University Hospital, 7 Chung-Shan South Road, 100 Taipei, Taiwan. [2]Division of Cardiology, Department of Internal Medicine, National Taiwan University College of Medicine, No.1, Ren-Ai Road Section 1, 100 Taipei, Taiwan. [3]Department of Biochemistry and Molecular Biology, National Taiwan University College of Medicine, No.1, Ren-Ai Road Section 1, 100 Taipei, Taiwan. [4]Taipei American School, 800 Chung Shan North Road Section 6, Taipei 11152, Taiwan.

References
1. Mangoni AA, Jackson SH. Homocysteine and cardiovascular disease: current evidence and future prospects. Am J Med. 2002;112:556–65.
2. Crider KS, Zhu JH, Hao L, Yang QH, Yang TP, Gindler J, Maneval DR, Quinlivan EP, Li Z, Bailey LB, Berry RJ. MTHFR 677C->T genotype is associated with folate and homocysteine concentrations in a large, population-based, double-blind trial of folic acid supplementation. Am J Clin Nutr. 2011;93:1365–72.
3. De Bree A, Verschuren WM, Kromhout D, Kluijtmans LA, Blom HJ. Homocysteine determinants and the evidence to what extent homocysteine determines the risk of coronary heart disease. Pharmacol Rev. 2002;54:599–618.
4. Werstuck GH, Lentz SR, Dayal S, Hossain GS, Sood SK, Shi YY, Zhou J, Maeda N, Krisans SK, Malinow MR, Austin RC. Homocysteine-induced endoplasmic reticulum stress causes dysregulation of the cholesterol and triglyceride biosynthetic pathways. J Clin Invest. 2001;107:1263–73.
5. Wald DS, Law M, Morris JK. Homocysteine and cardiovascular disease: evidence on causality from a meta-analysis. BMJ. 2002;325:1202.
6. Moller J, Nielsen GM, Tvedegaard KC, Andersen NT, Jorgensen PE. A meta-analysis of cerebrovascular disease and hyperhomocysteinaemia. Scand J Clin Lab Invest. 2000;60:491–9.
7. Bautista LE, Arenas IA, Penuela A, Martinez LX. Total plasma homocysteine level and risk of cardiovascular disease: a meta-analysis of prospective cohort studies. J Clin Epidemiol. 2002;55:882–7.
8. Choe S. Potassium channel structures. Nat Rev Neurosci. 2002;3:115–21.
9. Verhoef P, Stampfer MJ, Buring JE, Gaziano JM, Allen RH, Stabler SP, Reynolds RD, Kok FJ, Hennekens CH, Willett WC. Homocysteine metabolism and risk of myocardial infarction: relation with vitamins B6, B12, and folate. Am J Epidemiol. 1996;143:845–59.
10. Akyurek O, Akbal E, Gunes F. Increase in the risk of ST elevation myocardial infarction is associated with homocysteine level. Arch Med Res. 2014;45:501–6.
11. Anderson JL, Muhlestein JB, Horne BD, Carlquist JF, Bair TL, Madsen TE, Pearson RR. Plasma homocysteine predicts mortality independently of traditional risk factors and C-reactive protein in patients with angiographically defined coronary artery disease. Circulation. 2000;102:1227–32.
12. Stubbs PJ, Al-Obaidi MK, Conroy RM, Collinson PO, Graham IM, Noble IM. Effect of plasma homocysteine concentration on early and late events in patients with acute coronary syndromes. Circulation. 2000;102:605–10.
13. Toole JF, Malinow MR, Chambless LE, Spence JD, Pettigrew LC, Howard VJ, Sides EG, Wang CH, Stampfer M. Lowering homocysteine in patients with ischemic stroke to prevent recurrent stroke, myocardial infarction, and death: the vitamin intervention for stroke prevention (VISP) randomized controlled trial. JAMA. 2004;291:565–75.
14. Albert CM, Cook NR, Gaziano JM, Zaharris E, MacFadyen J, Danielson E, Buring JE, Manson JE. Effect of folic acid and B vitamins on risk of cardiovascular events and total mortality among women at high risk for cardiovascular disease: a randomized trial. JAMA. 2008;299:2027–36.
15. Armitage JM, Bowman L, Clarke RJ, Wallendszus K, Bulbulia R, Rahimi K, Haynes R, Parish S, Sleight P, Peto R, Collins R. Effects of homocysteine-lowering with folic acid plus vitamin B12 vs placebo on mortality and major morbidity in myocardial infarction survivors: a randomized trial. JAMA. 2010;303:2486–94.
16. Ebbing M, Bleie O, Ueland PM, Nordrehaug JE, Nilsen DW, Vollset SE, Refsum H, Pedersen EK, Nygard O. Mortality and cardiovascular events in patients treated with homocysteine-lowering B vitamins after coronary angiography: a randomized controlled trial. JAMA. 2008;300:795–804.
17. Lonn E, Held C, Arnold JM, Probstfield J, McQueen M, Micks M, Pogue J, Sheridan P, Bosch J, Genest J, Yusuf S. Rationale, design and baseline characteristics of a large, simple, randomized trial of combined folic acid

and vitamins B6 and B12 in high-risk patients: the heart outcomes prevention evaluation (HOPE)-2 trial. Can J Cardiol. 2006;22:47–53.

18. Foussas SG, Zairis MN, Makrygiannis SS, Manousakis SJ, Patsourakos NG, Adamopoulou EN, Beldekos DJ, Melidonis AI, Handanis SM, Manolis AJ, et al. The impact of circulating total homocysteine levels on long-term cardiovascular mortality in patients with acute coronary syndromes. Int J Cardiol. 2008;124:312–8.

19. Palmerini T, Biondi-Zoccai G, Della Riva D, Mariani A, Sabate M, Smits PC, Kaiser C, D'Ascenzo F, Frati G, Mancone M, et al. Clinical outcomes with bioabsorbable polymer- versus durable polymer-based drug-eluting and bare-metal stents: evidence from a comprehensive network meta-analysis. J Am Coll Cardiol. 2014;63:299–307.

20. D'Ascenzo F, Iannaccone M, Saint-Hilary G, Bertaina M, Schulz-Schupke S, Wahn Lee C, Chieffo A, Helft G, Gili S, Barbero U, et al. Impact of design of coronary stents and length of dual antiplatelet therapies on ischaemic and bleeding events: a network meta-analysis of 64 randomized controlled trials and 102 735 patients. Eur Heart J. 2017;38:3160–72.

21. Andell P, James SK, Cannon CP, Cyr DD, Himmelmann A, Husted S, Keltai M, Koul S, Santoso A, Steg PG, et al. Ticagrelor versus Clopidogrel in patients with acute coronary syndromes and chronic obstructive pulmonary disease: an analysis from the platelet inhibition and patient outcomes (PLATO) trial. J Am Heart Assoc. 2015;4:e002490.

22. Wiviott SD, Braunwald E, McCabe CH, Montalescot G, Ruzyllo W, Gottlieb S, Neumann FJ, Ardissino D, De Servi S, Murphy SA, et al. Prasugrel versus clopidogrel in patients with acute coronary syndromes. N Engl J Med. 2007; 357:2001–15.

23. O'Gara PT, Kushner FG, Ascheim DD, Casey DE Jr, Chung MK, de Lemos JA, Ettinger SM, Fang JC, Fesmire FM, Franklin BA, et al. ACCF/AHA guideline for the management of ST-elevation myocardial infarction: a report of the American College of Cardiology Foundation/American Heart Association task force on practice guidelines. Circulation. 2013;2013(127):e362–425.

24. Ibanez B, James S, Agewall S, Antunes MJ, Bucciarelli-Ducci C, Bueno H, Caforio ALP, Crea F, Goudevenos JA, Halvorsen S, et al. ESC guidelines for the management of acute myocardial infarction in patients presenting with ST-segment elevation: the task force for the management of acute myocardial infarction in patients presenting with ST-segment elevation of the European Society of Cardiology (ESC). Eur Heart J. 2017;2018(39):119–77.

25. Chang PY, Chen YJ, Chang FH, Lu J, Huang WH, Yang TC, Lee YT, Chang SF, Lu SC, Chen CH. Aspirin protects human coronary artery endothelial cells against atherogenic electronegative LDL via an epigenetic mechanism: a novel cytoprotective role of aspirin in acute myocardial infarction. Cardiovasc Res. 2013;99:137–45.

26. Chang PY, Lu SC, Lee CM, Chen YJ, Dugan TA, Huang WH, Chang SF, Liao WS, Chen CH, Lee YT. Homocysteine inhibits arterial endothelial cell growth through transcriptional downregulation of fibroblast growth factor-2 involving G protein and DNA methylation. Circ Res. 2008;102:933–41.

27. Chang PY, Luo S, Jiang T, Lee YT, Lu SC, Henry PD, Chen CH. Oxidized low-density lipoprotein downregulates endothelial basic fibroblast growth factor through a pertussis toxin-sensitive G-protein pathway: mediator role of platelet-activating factor-like phospholipids. Circulation. 2001;104:588–93.

28. Cerrato E, Barbero U, D'Ascenzo F, Taha S, Biondi-Zoccai G, Omede P, Bianco M, Echavarria-Pinto M, Escaned J, Gaita F, Varbella F. What is the optimal treatment for symptomatic patients with isolated coronary myocardial bridge? A systematic review and pooled analysis. J Cardiovasc Med (Hagerstown). 2017;18:758–70.

29. Liu C, Yang Y, Peng D, Chen L, Luo J. Hyperhomocysteinemia as a metabolic disorder parameter is independently associated with the severity of coronary heart disease. Saudi Med J. 2015;36:839–46.

30. Ma Y, Peng D, Liu C, Huang C, Luo J. Serum high concentrations of homocysteine and low levels of folic acid and vitamin B12 are significantly correlated with the categories of coronary artery diseases. BMC Cardiovasc Disord. 2017;17:37.

31. Akanji AO, Thalib L, Al-Isa AN. Folate, vitamin B(1)(2) and total homocysteine levels in Arab adolescent subjects: reference ranges and potential determinants. Nutr Metab Cardiovasc Dis. 2012;22:900–6.

32. Zappacosta B, Persichilli S, Iacoviello L, Di Castelnuovo A, Graziano M, Gervasoni J, Leoncini E, Cimino G, Mastroiacovo P. Folate, vitamin B12 and homocysteine status in an Italian blood donor population. Nutr Metab Cardiovasc Dis. 2013;23:473–80.

33. Jacques PF, Selhub J, Bostom AG, Wilson PW, Rosenberg IH. The effect of folic acid fortification on plasma folate and total homocysteine concentrations. N Engl J Med. 1999;340:1449–54.

34. Doshi SN, McDowell IF, Moat SJ, Payne N, Durrant HJ, Lewis MJ, Goodfellow J. Folic acid improves endothelial function in coronary artery disease via mechanisms largely independent of homocysteine lowering. Circulation. 2002;105:22–6.

35. Takeda Y, Suzuki S, Fukutomi T, Kondo H, Sugiura M, Suzumura H, Murasaki G, Okutani H, Itoh M. Elevated white blood cell count as a risk factor of coronary artery disease: inconsistency between forms of the disease. Jpn Heart J. 2003;44:201–11.

36. Hatmi ZN, Saeid AK, Broumand MA, Khoshkar SN, Danesh ZF. Multiple inflammatory prognostic factors in acute coronary syndromes: a prospective inception cohort study. Acta Med Iran. 2010;48:51–7.

37. Cabrerizo García SJL, Zalba EB, Pérez CJI, Ruiz RF. Leukocyte count as a risk factor for coronary adverse events among patients admitted for an acute coronary syndrome. Rev Med Chil. 2010;138:274–80.

38. Barbero U, D'Ascenzo F, Nijhoff F, Moretti C, Biondi-Zoccai G, Mennuni M, Capodanno D, Lococo M, Lipinski MJ, Gaita F. Assessing risk in patients with stable coronary disease: when should we intensify care and follow-up? Results from a meta-analysis of observational studies of the COURAGE and FAME era. Scientifica (Cairo). 2016;2016:3769152.

39. Ribeiro DR, Ramos AM, Vieira PL, Menti E, Bordin OL Jr, Souza PA, Quadros AS, Portal VL. High-sensitivity C-reactive protein as a predictor of cardiovascular events after ST-elevation myocardial infarction. Arq Bras Cardiol. 2014;103:69–75.

40. Marfella R, Sardu C, Balestrieri ML, Siniscalchi M, Minicucci F, Signoriello G, Calabro P, Mauro C, Pieretti G, Coppola A, et al. Effects of incretin treatment on cardiovascular outcomes in diabetic STEMI-patients with culprit obstructive and multivessel non obstructive-coronary-stenosis. Diabetol Metab Syndr. 2018;10:1.

41. Marfella R, Sardu C, Calabro P, Siniscalchi M, Minicucci F, Signoriello G, Balestrieri ML, Mauro C, Rizzo MR, Paolisso G, Barbieri M. Non-ST-elevation myocardial infarction outcomes in patients with type 2 diabetes with non-obstructive coronary artery stenosis: effects of incretin treatment. Diabetes Obes Metab. 2017. https://doi.org/10.1111/dom.13122. [Epub ahead of print].

42. Marfella R, Rizzo MR, Siniscalchi M, Paolisso P, Barbieri M, Sardu C, Savinelli A, Angelico N, Del Gaudio S, Esposito N, et al. Peri-procedural tight glycemic control during early percutaneous coronary intervention up-regulates endothelial progenitor cell level and differentiation during acute ST-elevation myocardial infarction: effects on myocardial salvage. Int J Cardiol. 2013;168:3954–62.

43. Undas A, Brozek J, Szczeklik A. Homocysteine and thrombosis: from basic science to clinical evidence. Thromb Haemost. 2005;94:907–15.

23

In-hospital prognosis and long-term mortality of STEMI in a reperfusion network "Head to head" analisys: invasive reperfusion vs optimal medical therapy

C . García-García[1,2,3]*[iD], N. Ribas[1,4,5], L. L. Recasens[1,5], O. Meroño[1,5], I. Subirana[3,6], A. Fernández[1], A. Pérez[1], F. Miranda[1], H. Tizón-Marcos[1,5], J. Martí-Almor[1,5], J. Bruguera[1,5] and R. Elosua[4,6]

Abstract

Background: ST Segment Elevation Acute myocardial infarction (STEMI) preferred treatment is culprit artery reperfusion with primary percutaneous coronary intervention (PPCI). We ought to analyze the benefit of early reperfusion vs. optimal medical therapy in STEMI before and after the set-up of a regional STEMI network that prioritizes PPCI.

Methods: Between January 2002 and December 2013, 1268 STEMI patients were consecutively admitted in a University Hospital. Patients were classified in two groups: pre-STEMI Network (January 2002–June 2009; $n = 670$) and post-STEMI network (July 2009–December 2013; $n = 598$). Vital status was available at 2-year follow-up.

Results: The STEMI network increased reperfusion (89.2% vs 64.4%, $p < 0.001$) mainly using PCI (99.0% vs 43.9%, $p < 0.001$). In univariate analysis, in-hospital mortality was significantly lower in the post-STEMI network period (2.51% vs. 7.16%, $p < 0.001$). After multivariate adjustment, including age, sex, comorbidities, severity and reperfusion therapy, a trend to a lower in-hospital mortality was observed (post-Network OR: 0.50, 95% CI:0.16–1.59, $p = 0.24$); this trend disappeared when optimal medical therapy was included in the model (post-Network OR: 1.14, 95% CI:0.32–4.08, $p = 0.840$). No differences in 2-year mortality were observed (post-Network HR: 0.83; CI 95%: 0.55–1.25, $p = 0.37$).

Conclusion: A STEMI network with PPCI 24/7 improved reperfusion therapy, resulting in an increase on PPCI. Despite in-hospital mortality decreased with a STEMI network, 2-year mortality remained similar in both periods, pre- and post-Network. Optimal medical therapy could be as important as reperfusion therapy in a STEMI reperfusion network.

Keywords: Reperfusion network, AMI prognosis, Long-term mortality, Optimal medical therapy, Reperfusion therapy

Background

Primary percutaneous coronary intervention (PPCI) is the choice reperfusion therapy for ST-elevation acute myocardial infarction (STEMI) when performed at the right time [1, 2]. Reperfusion networks, which have been defined and established to optimize reperfusion therapy in STEMI patients [3–5], have achieved a reduction in reperfusion times and an increase in the proportion of patients receiving PPCI [6, 7]. However, the information about short- and long-term prognosis of patients included in a "real life" STEMI network and about the predictors of prognosis in these patients is scarce. The mortality of acute coronary syndromes has been reduced in the last years, and this decrease has been related not only to invasive or revascularization procedures but also to pharmacological treatments [8–11]. In stable coronary artery disease patients, optimal medical therapy (OMT)

* Correspondence: cosmecg7@gmail.com
[1]Cardiology Department, Hospital del Mar, Parc de Salut Mar-IMIM, Barcelona, Spain
[2]Cardiology Department, Hospital Universitari Germans Trias i Pujol, Carretera Canyet s/n, 08916 Badalona, Spain
Full list of author information is available at the end of the article

and angioplasty have similar beneficial effects [12–14], but the relative benefits of OMT in STEMI patients compared to those related to reperfusion therapy have not been well established. The aim of our study was: 1) to analyze the STEMI Reperfusion Network on in-hospital prognosis and 2-year mortality and 2) to compare the relative benefits of improving reperfusion therapy vs. optimal medical therapy in a consecutive population of STEMI patients in the last 11 years.

Methods

Study design

This is a prospective hospital register of STEMI patients with a long-term vital status follow up. All STEMI patients aged >18 admitted in the Coronary Care Unit of a University hospital from January 2002 to December 2013 were prospectively and consecutively included. The study was designed and implemented in accordance with Guidelines for Good Clinical Practice and with the ethical principles laid down in the Declaration of Helsinki. All participants gave their written consent to participate in the study. The study was approved by our institution Ethics Committee, the CEIC-Parc de Salut Mar with reference number 2012/4806/I.

Variables of interest and STEMI management

Demographic variables and comorbidities such as history of hypertension, diabetes, hypercholesterolemia, smoking, and previous angina were prospectively collected. Clinical characteristics of the event were recorded, including ischemia times, AMI location and complications such as the development of pulmonary edema or cardiogenic shock or the presence of malignant arrhythmias. In addition, information about the management of the acute event, including medical treatments during the hospital stay, reperfusion therapy (including both thrombolysis or PPCI), type of reperfusion therapy (thrombolysis or PPCI) and invasive procedures (coronary angiography, mechanical ventilation), was also collected.

Patients' care followed the current clinical practice guidelines for STEMI patients at the time of the study [15–17], but reperfusion therapy was applied according to the STEMI Code instruction [4] as a regional Reperfusion Network. In our study there was no standard care for patients. All treatments were performed under the physicians' medical criteria depending on clinical patients' situation.

STEMI Reperfusion Network was initiated in Catalonia in June 2009 with the purpose of reaching an optimal reperfusion therapy with PPCI [4]. Before the establishment of the STEMI Network (June 1st, 2009– pre-Network period), PPCI was performed in our hospital in STEMI patients only during working hours;

thrombolytic therapy during on-duty time. After June 2009 (post-Network period), PPCI was the elective reperfusion therapy in STEMI patients. During working hours (8 am-20 pm), PPCI was performed in our hospital and patients first admitted in our hospital during on-duty time were transferred to another PPCI capable centre near our institution. Depending on the period of admission, patients were classified in two groups: pre-Network (January 2002 to May 2009) and post-Network (June 2009 to December 2013).

Events of interest

Events of interest were defined as in-hospital and 2-year mortality. In order to identify long-term fatal cases, we accessed the National Death Registry. This is an exhaustive and mandatory official database which collects individual data of all the deceased in Spain from 1987 up to now. This database, promoted by the Spanish Health Ministry, provides public institutions (healthcare administrations, research centers) with information regarding vital status and date of death, although it does not indicate the specific cause of death. We linked our data with the National Death Registry. We assumed that study participants who did not appear in this registry were alive at the end of the follow-up.

Statistical analysis

In the comparison of study groups (pre and post-Code), analysis of variance or Kruskall-Wallis test were used for continuous variables and the Chi-square test for categorical variables. Unconditional logistical regression and Cox regression were used to determine the association between comorbidities, reperfusion therapy and in-hospital or long-term mortality, with adjustment to the identified confusing variables. We tested the interaction between the use of reperfusion therapy, medical therapy and period of admission in order to evaluate in-hospital prognosis as well as after 2 years. P values lower than 0.05 were considered statistically significant.

In order to evaluate a mortality time trend along the period, day of admission was also incorporated in the Cox regression model as a spline term to accommodate a possible non-linear effect.

Results

The study included 1268 consecutive STEMI patients. These patients were classified in two groups: pre-Code (n = 670) and post-Code (n = 598). The patients' demographic and clinical characteristics are shown in Table 1. The proportion of smokers and peripheral artery disease was higher in the post-Network period whereas the proportion of diabetes mellitus was higher in the pre-Network period.

Table 1 Demographic and clinical characteristics of patients included in the study according to the two periods analyzed

	Pre-network N = 670	Post-network N = 598	P value
Age* (SD)	62.6 (13.6)	63.6 (13.1)	0.189
Men	76.1%	75.7%	0.929
Smoker	41.0%	48.0%	0.029
Hypertension	51.9%	57.3%	0.062
Dyslipidaemia	47.4%	50.7%	0.267
Diabetes mellitus	26.9%	23.9%	0.001
Peripheral vascular disease	4.9%	8.6%	0.013
Family history of CAD	11.2%	10.8%	0.789
Previous AMI	10.7%	11.2%	0.865
Killip III-IV at admission	10.3%	8.3%	0.075

SD standard deviation, AMI acute myocardial infarction, CAD coronary artery disease

STEMI management

Reperfusion therapy increased in the post-Network period (89.2% vs. 64.4%). Among those treated with reperfusion there was an important increase in the use of PPCI (99% in the post-Network vs. 43.9% in the pre-Network period) with a subsequent decrease in the use of thrombolytics (1% vs. 56.1%). The changes in the reperfusion therapy strategy were associated with a slight increase in the ischemia time: median time from pain onset to reperfusion performance was 165 min (105–325 min) vs. 186 min (130–284 min) in pre- and post-Network periods respectively, $p < 0.001$. There were no changes in time from pain onset to monitoring: pre-Code 130 (60–258 min) vs. post-Network 90 (45–201 min), $p = 0.254$.

Medical therapy and procedures during hospital stay are shown in Table 2. There was an important increase in the use of evidence-based drugs such as statins, betablockers or angiotensin converting enzyme inhibitors. Above all, an increase in the use of dual antiplatelet therapy (clopidogrel and the new adenosine phosphate inhibitors), which could be associated to the extended use of PPCI in the post-Network period, was also observed. Although comprehensive data about length of dual antiplatelet therapy were not available for all patients, European Society of Cardiology STEMI guidelines recommendation about length of antiplatelet therapy (1) were systematic followed in all patients. Dual antiplatelet therapy (aspirin plus clopidogrel, ticagrelor or prasugrel) were prescribed during 1 year in all patients (either bare metal or drug eluting stents). After the first year, aspirin was the only antiplatelet therapy in treatment.

In-hospital prognosis

In-hospital prognosis and complications are shown in Table 3. There was a reduction in complete atrioventricular block and a non significant trend to a lower Killip

Table 2 Medical therapy and procedures used in the two periods

Drugs	Pre-network N = 670	Post-network N = 598	P value
Aspirin	96.6%	99.3%	0.001
Clopidogrel	54.3%	79.9%	<0.001
Ticagrelor	——	27.9%	——
Prasugrel	——	3.3%	——
GP IIb/IIIa Inhibitors	16.1%	13.1%	0.252
Heparin	82.1%	93.9%	<0.001
Betablockers	69.3%	81.2%	<0.001
Statins	89.7%	98.0%	<0.001
ACE inhibitors	70.1%	77.8%	0.003
Nitroglicerin	40.6%	37.2%	0.241
Eplerenone	——	17.9%	——
Mecanichal ventilation	8.5%	8.0%	0.870
Echocardiogram	40.3%	56.0%	<0.001
Coronary angiography	55.2%	99.5%	<0.001
IABP	4.8%	4.1%	0.680
Swan-Ganz cathether	7.8%	5.1%	0.080
Reperfusion	64.4%	89.2%	<0.001
PPCI	43.9%	99.0%	<0.001
Thrombolysis	56.1%	1.0%	<0.001

ACE angiotensin converting enzyme, IABP intra-aortic balloon pump, PPCI primary percutaneous coronary intervention

grade III-IV in the post-Nework period. An important decrease in in-hospital mortality (65%) was observed in the post-Network period (2.51% vs. 7.16%, $p < 0.001$).

However, a significant decrease trend in in-hospital mortality was observed in the period analyzed (Fig. 1). Therefore, in order to analyze the effect of the reperfusion network on in-hospital mortality and the potential variables that could be involved in this effect, we included this mortality decreasing trend in the multivariate models. We observed a trend towards a decrease in in-

Table 3 In-hospital complications and prognosis in the two periods analyzed

	Pre-network N = 670	Post-network N = 598	P value
Reinfarction	2.5%	1.5%	0.450
Ventricular fibrillation	4.5%	5.8%	0.327
Complete AV block	8.7%	5.5%	0.040
Flutter/Atrial fibrillation	6.3%	4.5%	0.211
Septal rupture	1.2%	0.7%	0.501
Papillar muscle rupture	0.7%	0.5%	0.729
Free wall rupture	0.7%	0.7%	1.000
Killip -Maximum, III-IV	13.7%	11.6%	0.349
In-hospital mortality	7.16%	2.51%	<0.001

AV atrio-ventricular

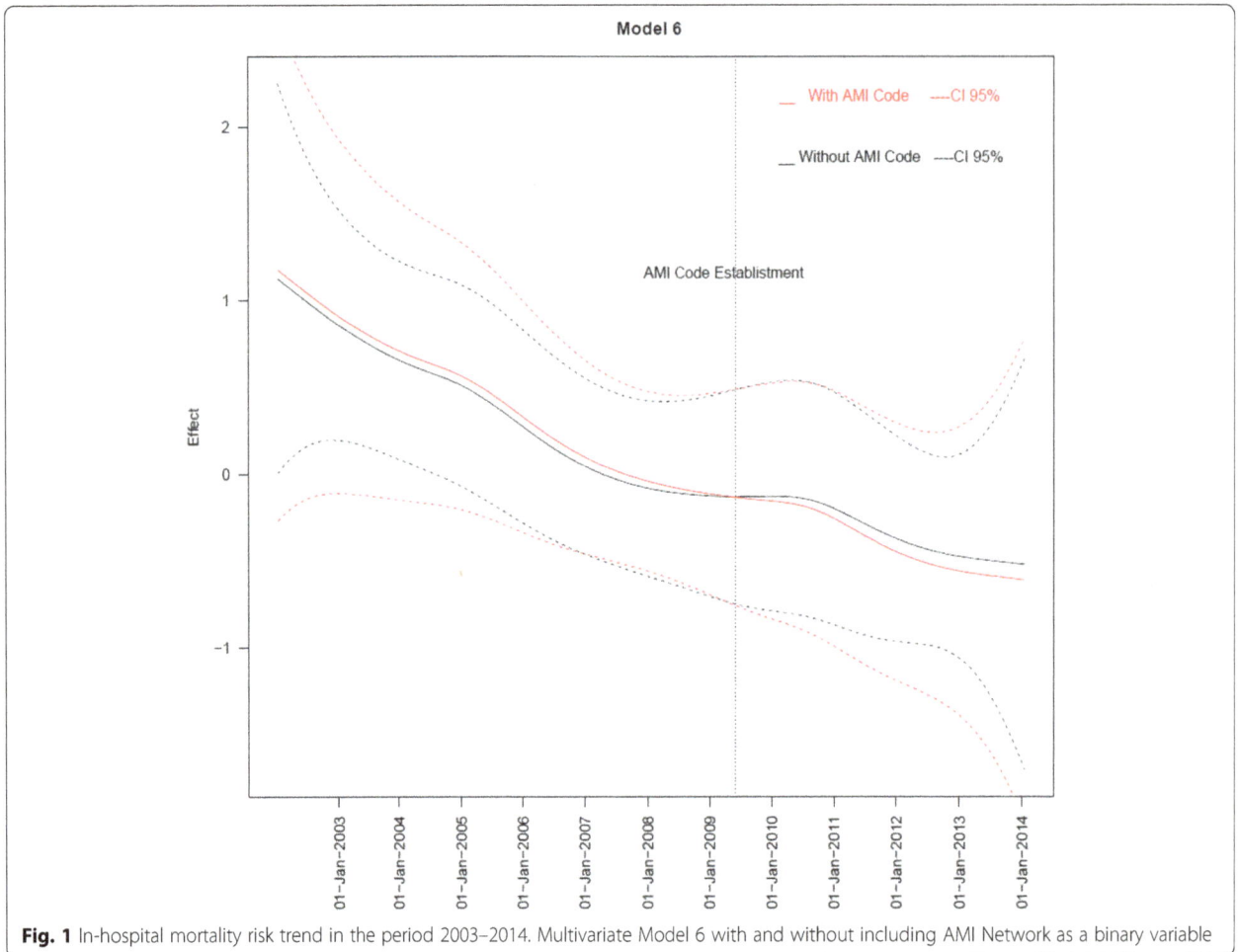

Fig. 1 In-hospital mortality risk trend in the period 2003–2014. Multivariate Model 6 with and without including AMI Network as a binary variable

hospital mortality in the post-Network period compared to the pre-Network period even when the model was adjusted by age, sex (Model 1), comorbidities (Model 2), severity (Model 3) and reperfusion (Model 4) with ORs ranged between 0.45 and 0.59 (Table 4). Noteworthy, when the model was further adjusted by optimal medical therapy (aspirin, statins, beta-blockers and angiotensin converting enzyme inhibitors), the benefit of the post-Network period disappeared totally (Table 4).

Long-term mortality

There was no difference in 2-year mortality among acute phase survivors between the two analyzed periods (10% pre-Network vs. 8.5% post-Network, $p = 0.467$). Kaplan Maier curves with cumulative 2-year mortality rates are shown in Fig. 2.

Discussion

We analyzed the impact of the establishment of a reperfusion network, the STEMI Code, on the management and prognosis of STEMI patients in a prospective and consecutive hospital registry. In the post-Network

period, reperfusion therapy was performed in almost 90% of STEMI patients, a significant increase compared to the pre-Network period, mainly due to an increase in the practice of PPCI. Furthermore, an important improvement in evidence-based medical treatment use (antiplatelet therapy, statins, beta-blockers or angiotensin converting enzyme inhibitors) was observed in the post-Network period. In-hospital mortality decreased after the establishment of the STEMI Network. This decrease seems to be mainly related to the optimization of medical treatment rather than to the increase of reperfusion. Two-year mortality was similar in both periods.

Reperfusion therapy and ischemia times

In our series, the STEMI Network had an important impact on the reperfusion therapy rate and strategy. Reperfusion therapy was performed in nearly 90% of all STEMI patients, more than other national registries [18] and similar to the best European countries in STEMI acute phase reperfusion [19] like Czech Republic, a small country with a huge and experienced AMI network. Moreover, we also observed a change in the reperfusion

Table 4 Association between the STEMI-Code period and in-hospital mortality in different multivariate models

	Pre-network N = 670	Post-network N = 598 OR (CI 95%)	P value
Model 1	1	0.45 (0.15; 1.37)	0.160
Model 2	1	0.48 (0.16; 1.49)	0.207
Model 3	1	0.59 (0.18; 1.95)	0.385
Model 4a	1	0.57 (0.16; 1.97)	0.375
Model 4b	1	0.50 (0.16; 1.59)	0.239
Model 5	1	1.19 (0.30; 4.76)	0.805
Model 6	1	1.14 (0.32; 4.08)	0.840

Model 1: Adjusted by age and sex
Model 2: Model 1 plus hypertension, diabetes and smoke
Model 3: Model 2 plus Killip grade III-IV at admission
Model 4a: Model 3 plus reperfusion (including both thrombolysis or PPCI)
Model 4b: Model 2 plus reperfusion (including both thrombolysis or PPCI)
Model 5: Model 4a plus medical therapy (Aspirin, beta-blocker, ACE-inhibitors and statins)
Model 6: Model 2 plus medical therapy (Aspirin, beta-blocker, ACE-inhibitors and statins)

strategy that was almost exclusively based on PPCI in the post-Network period, similar to what occurred in the Czech Republic registry [19].

Reperfusion therapy strategy is one of the most important factors to improve AMI prognosis, but time to reperfusion therapy is a main pillar too [20]. In our study we report an important increase in reperfusion rate and in the use of PPCI instead of thrombolysis, with a slight increase in time from pain onset to reperfusion performance (21 min). Our global ischemia time is similar to that reported in other European countries [21] or better than that reported in other recent studies [19]. Although some registries have confirmed the benefit of minimizing total ischemia time to improve in-hospital and long term prognosis [20], other studies have recently shown that short variations in ischemia time were not enough to modify in-hospital STEMI prognosis [22].

In-hospital mortality

The establishment of the STEMI Network was associated with an in-hospital mortality decrease among the lowest compared to most developed European countries [23]. When we tried to identify the variables which caused that decrease, reperfusion therapy was not the main factor. The use of evidence-based medical therapy could be another potential explanation as has been reported in other recent STEMI registers [18]. The use of aspirin, beta-blockers, ACE inhibitors and statins in our

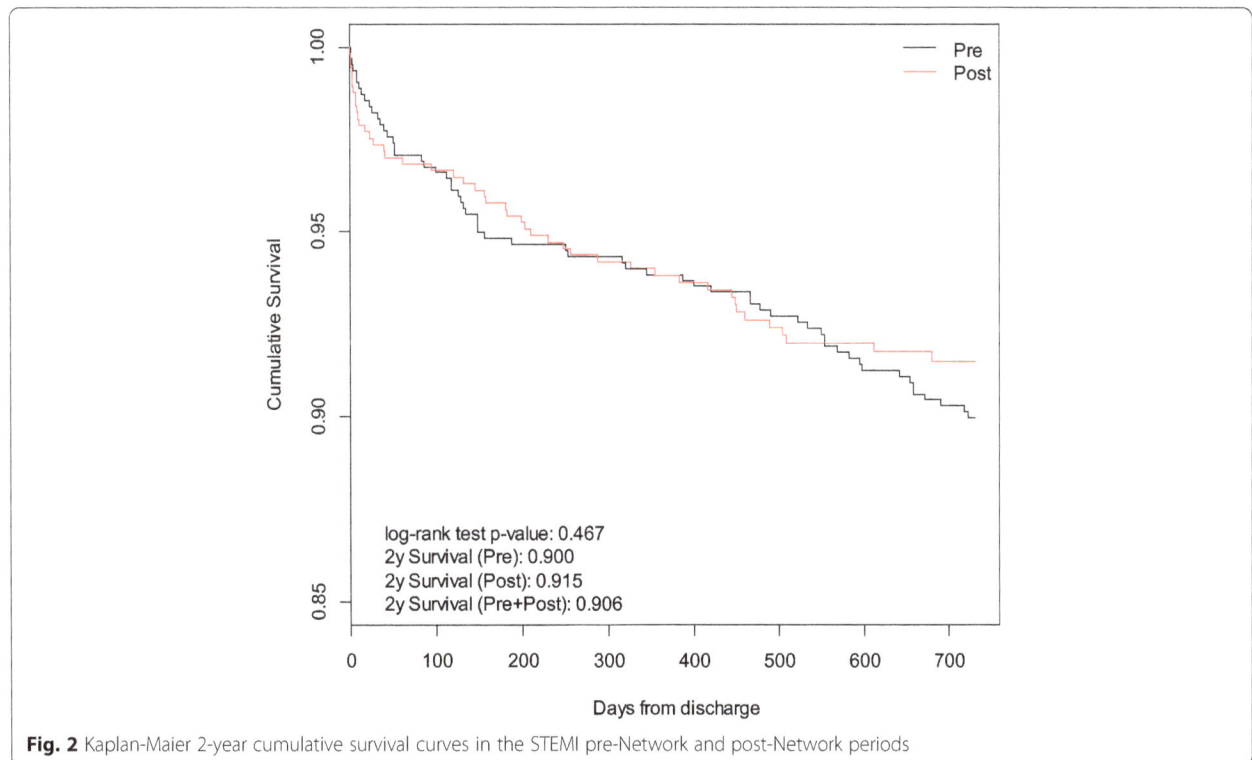

Fig. 2 Kaplan-Maier 2-year cumulative survival curves in the STEMI pre-Network and post-Network periods

series increased and could be considered at least as optimal as those prescribed in the Courage Trial [12], a study that proved a similar benefit of this optimal medical therapy compared to angioplasty in stable patients with angina. Both the introduction of this medical therapy in the multivariate model (model 5 and 6; Table 4) and the decrease of the benefit in the post-Code period imply that optical medical therapy could be one of the main variables related to the lower mortality of STEMI patients in the post-Code period. This fact suggests that optimal medical therapy could be as important as both the observed reperfusion therapy rate increase and the PPCI reperfusion strategy. These findings need careful validation in bigger observational studies.

Long-term mortality

There were no differences in 2-year mortality rate among survivors to the STEMI acute phase between both periods, although our 2-year mortality is similar to the 1-year mortality rate reported in other recent studies [24]. Unfortunately, we had only information related to the vital status but not to the cause of death in fatal cases. No information about other prognosis variables, such as re-infarction or the need of revascularization was available. However, the main cause of death in the first year after an AMI is mainly related to cardiovascular events, as we can see in recent registries or important randomized studies [24, 25].

On the other hand, the benefits of PPCI vs thrombolytic therapy out of the acute phase could be more related to a lower re-infarction rate or to the need of revascularization than to prevent cardiovascular death. The reduction in long-term mortality could be due to optimal control of cardiovascular risk factors and the use of evidence-based medical therapy [26], especially in high risk patients [27].

Study limitations

This is a single centre register that includes a limited number of patients, which limits the statistical power of the study and the capability to show statistically significant results. However, our results suggest a significant clinical association between the STEMI-Network and lower in-hospital mortality. Although the data come from a single centre and could limit the external validity of the results, the internal validity is guaranteed by the accuracy, homogeneity and consecutiveness of the data collection. Other study limitations are related to the long term follow-up; we had information concerning the discharge treatment but we lack information on long-term compliance to medical therapy and on the type of stent used during PPCI (bare metal or drug eluting stent) that could also be associated with the outcomes of interest of the study.

Conclusions

The STEMI Code network increases reperfusion therapy rate and changes the reperfusion strategy that is mainly based on PPCI. In-hospital mortality of STEMI patients has decreased in the last 11 years probably due to the improvement in reperfusion therapy and evidence-based medical therapy optimization. Even in the setting of STEMI reperfusion networks, our results emphasize the relevance of optimal medical therapy. The establishment of STEMI Code network does not seem to be enough to reduce long-term mortality of STEMI patients.

Abbreviations

OMT: Optimal medical therapy; PPCI: Primary percutaneous coronary intervention; STEMI: ST-elevation acute myocardial infarction

Acknowledgements

The authors thank Dr. Antoni Bayés-Genís for the support and final review of the manuscript and Montserrat Navarro for the support in proofreading.

Fundings

This work has been produced in the framework of the Doctorate in Medicine of the Universitat Autònoma de Barcelona. The study was partially funded by Fondo Europeo de Desarrollo Regional (FEDER).

Authors' contributions

CGG: substantial contributions to conception and design, acquisition of data, analysis and its interpretation; manuscript drafting; final approval of the version to be published; accountability on all aspects of the work in ensuring that questions related to the accuracy or integrity of any part of the work are appropriately investigated and resolved. NR: substantial contributions to conception and design, acquisition of data, analysis and its interpretation; manuscript drafting; final approval of the version to be published; accountability on all aspects of the work in ensuring that questions related to the accuracy or integrity of any part of the work are appropriately investigated and resolved. LR: substantial contributions to conception and design, acquisition of data, analysis and its interpretation; manuscript drafting; final approval of the version to be published; accountability on all aspects of the work in ensuring that questions related to the accuracy or integrity of any part of the work are appropriately investigated and resolved. OM: substantial contributions to conception and design, acquisition of data, analysis and its interpretation; manuscript drafting; final approval of the version to be published; accountability on all aspects of the work in ensuring that questions related to the accuracy or integrity of any part of the work are appropriately investigated and resolved. IS: substantial contributions to conception and design, acquisition of data, analysis and its interpretation; manuscript drafting; final approval of the version to be published; accountability on all aspects of the work in ensuring that questions related to the accuracy or integrity of any part of the work are appropriately investigated and resolved. AF: substantial contributions to conception and design and acquisition of data; manuscript drafting; final approval of the version to be published; accountability on all aspects of the work in ensuring that questions related to the accuracy or integrity of any part of the work are appropriately investigated and resolved. AP: substantial contributions to conception and design and acquisition of data; manuscript drafting; final approval of the version to be published; accountability on all aspects of the work in ensuring that questions related to the accuracy or integrity of any part of the work are appropriately investigated and resolved. FM: substantial contributions to conception and design, data analysis and its interpretation; manuscript drafting; final approval of the version to be published; accountability on all aspects of the work in ensuring that questions related to the accuracy or integrity of any part of the work are appropriately investigated and resolved. HTM: substantial contributions to conception and design, data analysis and its interpretation; manuscript drafting; final approval of the version to be published; accountability on all aspects of the work in ensuring that questions related to the accuracy or integrity of any part of the work are appropriately investigated and resolved. JMA: substantial contributions to conception and design, data analysis and its interpretation; manuscript drafting; final approval of the version to be published; accountability on all aspects of the work in ensuring that questions related to the accuracy or integrity of any part of the work are appropriately investigated and resolved. JB: substantial contributions to conception and design, data analysis and its interpretation; manuscript drafting; final approval of the version to be published; accountability on all aspects of the work in ensuring that questions related to the accuracy or integrity of any part of the work are appropriately investigated and resolved. RE: substantial contributions to conception and design, data analysis and its interpretation; manuscript drafting; final approval of the version to be published; accountability on all aspects of the work in ensuring that questions related to the accuracy or integrity of any part of the work are appropriately investigated and resolved.

Authors' information
C. García-García takes responsibility for all aspects of the reliability and freedom from bias of the data presented and their discussed interpretation.

Competing interests
The authors declare that they have no competing interests.

Author details
[1]Cardiology Department, Hospital del Mar, Parc de Salut Mar-IMIM, Barcelona, Spain. [2]Cardiology Department, Hospital Universitari Germans Trias i Pujol, Carretera Canyet s/n, 08916 Badalona, Spain. [3]CIBER de Enfermedades Cardiovasculares (CIBERCV), Barcelona, Spain. [4]Ph Program in Internal Medicine, Universitat Autònoma de Barcelona, Barcelona, Spain. [5]Heart Diseases Biomedical Research Group, IMIM (Hospital del Mar Medical Research Institute), Barcelona, Spain. [6]IMIM (Hospital del Mar Medical Research Institute), Cardiovascular Epidemiology and Genetics Group (EGEC), REGICOR Study Group, Barcelona, Spain.

References
1. Steg G, James DK, Atar D, Badano L, Lundqvist C, Borger M, et al. ESC Guidelines for the management of acute myocardial infarction in patients presenting with ST-segment elevation: the Task Force on the management of ST-segment elevation acute myocardial infarction of the European Society of Cardiology. Eur Heart J. 2012;33:2569–619.
2. O'Gara PT, Kushner FG, Aschein DD, Casey D Jr, Chung M, de Lemos J, et al. ACCF/AHA guideline for the management of ST-segment elevation myocardial infarction: executive summary: a report of The American College of Cardiology Foundation/American Heart Association Task Force on Practice Guideline. J Am Coll Cardiol. 2013;61:485–510.
3. Jacobs AK, Antman EM, Faxon DP, Gregory T, Solis P. Development of systems of care for ST-elevation myocardial infarction patients: executive summary. Circulation. 2007;116:217–30.
4. Bosch X, Curós A, Argimon JM, Faixedas M, Figueras J, Jiménez JX, et al. Model of primary percutaneous intervention in Catalonia. Rev Esp Cardiol. 2011;11:51–60.
5. Huber K, Gersh BJ, Goldstein P, Granger CB, Armstrong PW. The organization, function, and outcomes of ST-elevation myocardial infarction networks worldwide: current state, unmet needs and future directions. Eur Heart J. 2014;35:1526–32.
6. Rodriguez-Leor O, Fernandez-Nofrerias E, Mauri J, Carrillo X, Salvatella N, Curós A, et al. Integration of a local into a regional primary angioplasty action plan (the Catalan Codi Infart network) reduces time to reperfusion. Int J Cardiol. 2013;168:4354–7.
7. Fosbol EL, Granger CB, Jollis JG, Monk L, Lin L, Lytle BL, et al. The impact of a statewide pre-hospital STEMI strategy to bypass hospitals without percutaneous coronary intervention capability on treatment times. Circulation. 2013;127:604–12.
8. Ford ES, Ajani UA, Croft JB, Critchley JA, Labarthe DR, Kottke TE, et al. Explaining the decrease in U.S. deaths from coronary disease, 1980–2000. N Engl J Med. 2007;356:2388–98.
9. García-García C, Sanz G, Valle V, Molina L, Sala J, Subirana I, et al. Trends in in-hospital mortality and 6-months outcomes in patients with a first acute myocardial infarction. Change over the last decade. Rev Esp Cardiol. 2010;63:1136–44.
10. Flores-Mateo G, Grau M, O'Flaherty M, Ramos R, Elosua R, Violan-Fors C, et al. Analyzing the coronary heart disease mortality decline in a Mediterranean population: Spain 1988–2005. Rev Esp Cardiol. 2011;64:988–96.
11. García-García C, Subirana I, Sala J, Bruguera J, Sanz G, Valle V, et al. Long-term prognosis of first myocardial infarction according to the electrocardiographic pattern (ST elevation myocardial infarction, non-ST elevation myocardial infarction and non-classified myocardial infarction) and revascularization procedures. Am J Cardiol. 2011;108:1061–7.
12. Boden WE, O'Rourke RA, Teo KK, Hartigan PM, Maron DJ, Kostuk WJ, et al. Optimal medical therapy with or without PCI for stable coronary disease. N Engl J Med. 2007;356:1503–16.
13. Boden WE, O'Rourke RA, Teo KK, Maron DJ, Hartigan PM, Sedlis SP, et al. Impact of optimal medical therapy with or without percutaneous coronary intervention on long-term cardiovascular end points in patients with stable coronary artery disease (from the COURAGE Trial). Am J Cardiol. 2009;104:1–4.
14. Epstein SE, Waksman R, Pichard AD, Kent KM, Panza JA. Percutaneous coronary intervention versus medical therapy in stable coronary artery disease: the unresolved conundrum. JACC Cardiovasc Interv. 2013;6:993–8.
15. Braunwald E, Antman EM, Beasley JW, Califf RM, Cheitlin MD, Hochman JS, et al. ACC/AHA guideline update for the management of patients with unstable angina and non-ST-segment elevation myocardial infarction-2002. Summary article: a report of the American College of Cardiology/American Heart Association Task Force on practice guidelines. Circulation. 2002;106:1893–900.
16. Van de Werf F, Bax J, Betriu A, Blomstrom-Lundqvist C, Crea F, Falk V, et al. Management of acute myocardial infarction in patients presenting with persistent ST-segment elevation: the Task Force on the Management of ST-segment elevation acute myocardial infarction of the European Society of Cardiology. Eur Heart J. 2008;29:2909–45.
17. Antman EM, Hand M, Armstrong PW, Bates ER, Green LA, Halasyamani LK, et al. 2007 Focused Update of the ACC/AHA 2004 Guidelines for the management of patients with ST-elevation myocardial infarction: a report of the American College of Cardiology/American Heart Association Task Force on Practice Guidelines: developed in collaboration with the Canadian Cardiovascular Society endorsed by the American Academy of Family Phisicians: 2007 Writing Group to review new evidence and update the ACC/AHA 2004 Guidelines for the management of patients with ST-elevation myocardial infarction, writing on behalf of the 2004 Writing Committee. Circulation. 2008;117:296–329. Erratum in: Circulation. 2008;117:e162.
18. Barrabés JA, Bardají A, Jiménez-Candil J, del Nogal SF, Bodí V, Basterra N, et al. Prognosis and management of acute coronary syndrome in Spain in 2012: the DIOCLES study. Rev Esp Cardiol. 2015;68:98–106.
19. Widimsky P, Zelizko M, Jansky P, Tousek F, Holm F, Aschermann M, et al. The incidence, treatment strategies and outcomes of acute coronary syndromes in the "reperfusion network" of different hospital types in the Czech Republic: results of the Czech evaluation of acute coronary syndromes in hospitalized patients (CZECH) registry. Int J Cardiol. 2007;119:212–9.
20. Polańska-Skrzypczyk M, Karcz M, Bekta P, Kępka C, Sielatycki P, Rużyłło W, et al. Total ischaemic time and 9-year outcomes in STEMI patients treated with pPCI. Int J Cardiol. 2015;184:184–9.
21. Widimsky P, Wijns W, Fajadet J, de Belder M, Knot J, Aaberge L, et al. Reperfusion therapy for ST elevation acute myocardial infarction in Europe: description of the current situation in 30 countries. Eur Heart J. 2010;31:943–57.
22. Menees D, Peterson E, Wanhg Y, Curtis JP, Messenger JC, Rumsfeld JS, et al. Door-to-Balloon time and mortality among patients undergoing primary PCI. N Engl J Med. 2013;369:901–9.
23. Kristensen S, Laut K, Fajadet J, Kaifoszova Z, Kala P, Di Mario C, et al. Reperfusion therapy for ST elevation acute myocardial infarction 2010/2011: current status in 37 ESC countries. Eur Heart J. 2014;35:1957–70.
24. Pedersen F, Butrymovich V, Kelbæk H, Wachtell K, Helqvist S, Kastrup J, et al. Short- and long-term cause of death in patients treated with primary PCI for STEMI. J Am Coll Cardiol. 2014;64:2101–8.
25. Wallentin L, Becker RC, Budaj A, Cannon CP, Emanuelsson H, Held C, et al. Ticagrelor versus clopidogrel in patients with acute coronary syndromes. N Engl J Med. 2009;361:1045–57.

24

Thrombus aspiration in patients with ST-elevation myocardial infarction: results of a national registry of interventional cardiology

Hélder Pereira[1,2*†], Daniel Caldeira[1,2,3†] (iD), Rui Campante Teles[4,5], Marco Costa[6], Pedro Canas da Silva[7], Vasco da Gama Ribeiro[8], Vítor Brandão[9], Dinis Martins[10], Fernando Matias[11], Francisco Pereira-Machado[12], José Baptista[13], Pedro Farto e Abreu[14], Ricardo Santos[15], António Drummond[16], Henrique Cyrne de Carvalho[17], João Calisto[18], João Carlos Silva[19], João Luís Pipa[20], Jorge Marques[21], Paulino Sousa[22], Renato Fernandes[23], Rui Cruz Ferreira[24], Sousa Ramos[25], Eduardo Infante Oliveira[5,7], Manuel de Sousa Almeida[26] and on behalf of the investigators of Portuguese Registry on Interventional Cardiology (Registo Nacional de Cardiologia de Intervenção)

Abstract

Background: We aimed to evaluate the impact of thrombus aspiration (TA) during primary percutaneous coronary intervention (P-PCI) in 'real-world' settings.

Methods: We performed a retrospective study, using data from the National Registry of Interventional Cardiology (RNCI 2006–2012, Portugal) with ST-elevation myocardial infarction (STEMI) patients treated with P-PCI. The primary outcome, in-hospital mortality, was analysed through adjusted odds ratio (aOR) and 95% confidence intervals (95%CI).

Results: We assessed data for 9458 STEMI patients that undergone P-PCI (35% treated with TA). The risk of in-hospital mortality with TA (aOR 0.93, 95%CI:0.54–1.60) was not significantly decreased. After matching patients through the propensity score, TA reduced significantly the risk of in-hospital mortality (OR 0.58, 95%CI:0.35–0.98; 3500 patients).

Conclusions: The whole cohort data does not support the routine use of TA in P-PCI, but the results of the propensity-score matched cohort suggests that the use of selective TA may improve the short-term risks of STEMI.

Keywords: Thrombectomy, Thrombus aspiration, Mortality, Portugal, Primary PCI, Angioplasty

Background

The impact of thrombus aspiration (TA) during primary percutaneous coronary intervention (P-PCI) has been widely discussed in the recent years. The removal of the thrombus before stent deployment has shown to improve myocardial blush grade [1], but evidence has been heterogeneous regarding pragmatic outcomes, namely mortality. Survival benefits were previously supported by the TAPAS trial [1], as well as subsequent meta-analyses [2], including of patient level meta-analysis [3]. Both European and American guidelines for the management of patients with ST-Elevation Myocardial Infarction (STEMI) recommended that routine TA should be considered, based on evidence of moderate robustness (Class IIa, level of evidence B) [4, 5]. However, the results of larger trials did not show significant improvements in the mortality. Moreover, the existing evidence does not exclude the possibility of TA benefit in high-risk patients or in selected cases.

We intended to assess the impact of TA outside of the randomized controlled trial setting, to evaluate whether

---

* Correspondence: helder@netcabo.pt
†Equal contributors
[1]Serviço de Cardiologia, Hospital Garcia de Orta EPE, Avenida Prof. Torrado da Silva, 2801-951 Almada, Portugal
[2]Centro Cardiovascular da Universidade de Lisboa (CCUL), CAML, Faculdade de Medicina, Universidade de Lisboa, Avenida Professor Egas Moniz, Lisboa 1649-028, Portugal
Full list of author information is available at the end of the article

the findings of randomized controlled trials (RCTs) are similar to those occurring in the 'real-world'.

Methods

Data was retrieved from the Registo Nacional de Cardiologia de Intervenção (RNCI, Portuguese Registry on Interventional Cardiology) between January 2006 and December 2012 [6].

This is a continuous, prospective and observational registry, which includes all consecutive patients undergoing coronary angiography in multiple centers with interventional cardiology. Until December 2012 there were overall 58,434 procedures registered.

All included patients gave informed consent for the intervention and data collection for CNCDC (Centro Nacional de Colecção de Dados em Cardiologia from the Portuguese Society of Cardiology; http://www.spc.pt/CNCDC/) and the registry procedures are in accordance with the rules of CNPD (Comissão Nacional de Protecção de Dados – National Committee of Data Protection; https://www.cnpd.pt/). The registry was approved by the Portuguese Society of Cardiology ethics committee and local ethics committees.

Inclusion criteria was P-PCI within less than 12 h of symptom in the context of persistent (> 30 min) ST-segment elevation or new left bundle branch block [7–9]. Exclusion criteria were facilitated and rescue PCI as well stable coronary disease and non-ST elevation acute coronary syndromes.

Patients were stratified in two groups per the presence or absence of TA in the index procedure. TA was performed at the discretion of the operator. Demographic, clinical, patient management-related characteristics, as well as clinical outcomes were assessed.

Our primary outcome was all-cause mortality during the index hospitalization.

The risk was determined by odds ratio (OR) and 95% confidence intervals (CIs) were calculated for the primary outcome. Differences between patients treated with both TA and P-PCI, and those with PCI-PCI alone were adjusted through multivariable regression analysis.

All demographic information, comorbidities and TIMI flow pre-PCI data were included in a multivariable logistic regression to estimate a propensity score for the likelihood of being treated with thrombus aspiration. Matching was performed in a 1:1 fashion using with a 0.05 calliper width of the propensity score [10].

The analyses were further adjusted to residual confounding through multivariable logistics regression, to derive adjusted OR and 95%CIs. Statistical analyses were performed with SPSS version 19.0 (SPSS Inc., Chicago, IL, USA).

Results

A total of 9458 procedures fulfilled the inclusion criteria and 35% of them had adjunctive thrombus aspiration. Time trends show that this procedure had been increasing overtime (Fig. 1).

In the whole cohort, patients treated with TA were overall younger and had lower proportion of cardiovascular risk factors, with exception of smoking, as well as lower proportion of major comorbidities (Table 1). Patients in the group of TA had more frequently a left anterior descending artery occlusion. In the patients with TA the radial access was more common than other accesses, as well as stenting and use of GpIIbIIIa inhibitors (Table 1).

The overall in-hospital mortality was non-significantly lower (2.2% vs 2.8%) in the TA group (Fig. 2). Differences between important baseline characteristics were adjusted to confounders and the estimate of TA impact on mortality remained non-significant (OR 0.93, 95%CI 0.54–1.60, $p = 0.79$) (Fig. 2).

The stroke rate was low and thrombus aspiration was unlikely to affect its risk in our cohort (TA + P-PCI vs. P-PCI: 0.1% vs. 0.2%, $p = 0.77$).

We conducted a sub-analysis among the 7.692 patients that full fielded the inclusion criteria and had full information about the TIMI flow of coronary arteries.

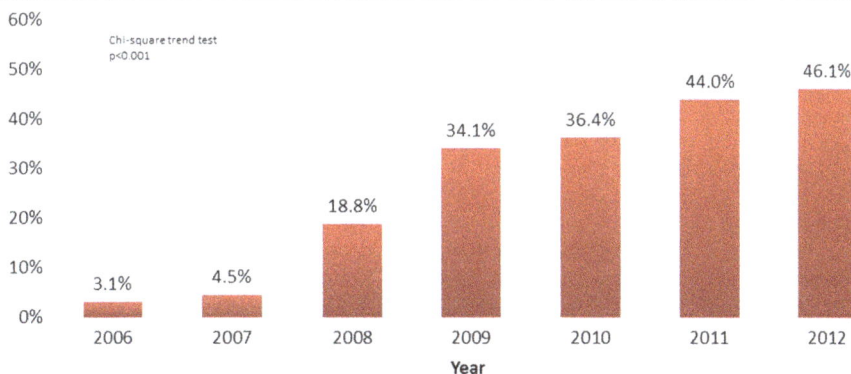

Fig. 1 The trend of use of thrombus aspiration in Portugal from 2006 to 2012

Table 1 Clinical characteristics of included patients according to the use of thrombus aspiration during P-PCI

	Before Matching			After Matching		
	Thrombus aspiration and P-PCI (n = 3311)	P-PCI only (n = 6247)	p-value	Thrombus aspiration and P-PCI (n = 1750)	P-PCI only (n = 1750)	p-value
Age	60 ± 13	63 ± 13	< 0.001	61 ± 13	60 ± 13	0.10
Male	77.4%	74.6%	0.002	77.7%	78.6%	0.59
Risk factors						
Dyslipidemia	44.7%	44.6%	0.95	45.0%	46.2%	0.50
DM	18.7%	24.0%	< 0.001	19.0%	18.9%	0.93
Smoking	43.1%	36.4%	< 0.001	41.8%	45.0%	0.38
Hypertension	53.3%	59.7%	< 0.001	54.1%	54.5%	0.87
Previous history						
MI	11.3%	14.2%	< 0.001	12.1%	12.3%	0.84
PCI	12.3%	14.0%	0.035	12.9%	13.8%	0.46
CABG	1.3%	1.7%	0.188	1.3%	1.1%	0.64
Stroke	3.9%	5.2%	0.009	4.0%	4.1%	1.00
PAD	1.9%	3.1%	0.002	1.9%	1.9%	1.00
HF	0.9%	1.9%	< 0.001	0.8%	0.6%	0.69
CKD	3.2%	3.4%	0.56	3.7%	4.6%	0.21
Admission						
KK IV class	6.3%	6.6%	0.57	7.3%	6.4%	0.43
Infarction-related artery						
LM	1.0%	1.3%	0.20	3.6%	3.5%	0.86
LAD	42.4%	35.7%	< 0.001	69.1%	69.4%	0.86
Circumflex	13.4%	17.5%	< 0.001	39.5%	46.8%	< 0.001
RCA	42.8%	45.1%	0.03	58.8%	57.3%	0.36
Radial access	40.2%	22.9%	< 0.001	40.3%	20.3%	< 0.001
Stenting / DES	79.4% / 47.5%	75.9% / 50.9%	< 0.001	91.6% / 45.4%	90.9% / 46.9%	0.50 / 0.40
GpIIb/IIIa	36.9%	18.9%	< 0.001	51.9%	31.0%	< 0.001

CABGCoronary artery bypass graft, CKD Chronic kidney disease, DES Drug-eluting stent, DM Diabetes Mellitus, HF heart failure, KK Killip-Kimball, LAD Left Anterior Descending Artery, LM Left Main Artery, MI Myocardial infarction, PAD peripheral artery disease, PCI angioplasty/percutaneous coronary intervention, P-PCI Primary angioplasty. RCA Right Coronary Artery, TA Thrombus aspiration

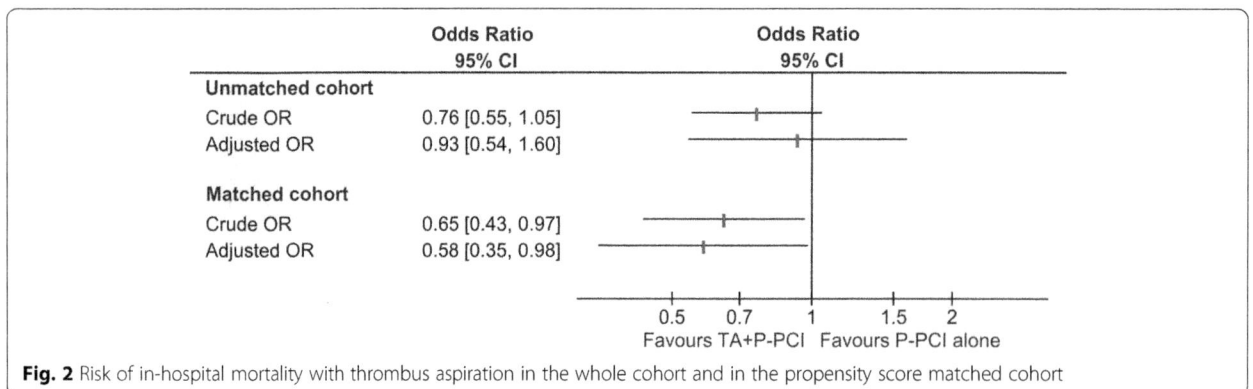

Fig. 2 Risk of in-hospital mortality with thrombus aspiration in the whole cohort and in the propensity score matched cohort

Patients with TA had more frequently post-PCI TIMI flow< 3 compared to those without TA (14.0% vs.10.6%).

After propensity score matching, 1750 patients remained in each group. The details of patients' characteristics are depicted in Table 1. The risk of in-hospital mortality was significantly increased (OR 0.65, 95%CI 0.43–0.97, p = 0.03), and remained after the multivariable logistic regression (OR 0.58, 95%CI 0.35–0.98, p = 0.04) (Fig. 2).

Discussion

This data based on a large real-world prospective registry, showed that TA decreased the risk of mortality among patients with STEMI that underwent P-PCI after matching the patients' characteristics for the likelihood of being treated with TA. In Portugal we observed an increase in the use of TA but more than 50% of P-PCI evaluated were performed without this technique. It is possible that in some case TA was used as a bail-out procedure because the use of inhibitors of GpIIbIIIa was higher in the TA group. Our results are distinct from those obtained in largest RCTs, the TASTE and TOTAL trials [11, 12]. Despite the matching and the multivariable adjustments, our data is still retrospective, underpowered and with possible residual cofounding bias.

Improving the microvascular perfusion in patients with STEMI is attractive, particularly when large macroscopic thrombi are retrieved. It provides the feeling that operators interfere directly with the pathophysiologic mechanics and improve the prognostic of patients. The RCT data show that routine thrombus aspiration does not seem to influence the mortality of patients with STEMI. However, our data suggests that 'selective' TA may be useful to improve outcomes in patients with STEMI. The recognition of the type of patients in which TA is likely to be successful may be the key to the obtained results.

Due to limited data accuracy for other outcomes, our study only covered the in-hospital mortality. Similarly to the results regarding the short-term outcomes, the major trials also showed that TA did not improve 1-year outcomes [13, 14]. The results of observational data are heterogeneous. In a cohort with more than 10,000 patients with STEMI (about 3500 of STEMI patients treated with TA and P-PCI), TA did not show improvement in the risk of mortality [15]. Inversely, other observational studies showed that a 'selective' TA in P-PCI can improve outcomes, mortality included [16, 17]. The best available evidence, based on RCTs, is robust for not using 'routinely' the TA in P-PCI but do not preclude the use of TA in selected cases, as occurs with other interventions available for acute cardiac care setting [18].

In this cohort the rates of stroke were very low, and no differences were found between the groups, despite the cumulative evidence regarding this adverse event which is known to have a small increase in the absolute risk with TA [19].

Limitations

Our results are limited because this is a consecutive all-comers procedural registry that has inherently limitations due to the lack of randomization and blinding effect. Despite the adjustment to multiple clinical and angiographic characteristics, it is worth noting that the data may not adjust to all potential confounders and thus increase the risk of bias in the analyses. The propensity score matching partially improves some of these limitations. However, this matching occurs with a decrease of the sample size which increases the risk of type II errors [20, 21]. Unfortunately, there are no data regarding the types of devices used in the TA as well as additional details of operators and procedures, which also hampers the conclusions.

Conclusion

The use of thrombus aspiration did not have a significant impact in the short-term prognosis of STEMI patients that underwent primary percutaneous coronary intervention in the whole cohort. The results of the propensity-score matched cohort suggests a potential role for selective thrombus aspiration.

Abbreviations

95%CI: 95% confidence interval; CNCDC: Centro nacional de colecção de dados em cardiologia; CNPD: Comissão nacional de proteccção de dados – national committee of data protection; GpIIbIIIa: Glycoproteins IIb/IIIa; OR: Odds ratio; P-PCI: Primary percutaneous coronary intervention; RCT: Randomized controlled trials; RNCI: Registo nacional de cardiologia de intervenção - portuguese registry on interventional cardiology; STEMI: ST-elevation myocardial infarction; TA: Thrombus aspiration; TASTE: Thrombus aspiration in myocardial infarction; TOTAL: A trial of routine aspiration thrombectomy with Percutaneous Coronary Intervention (PCI) versus PCI alone in patients with ST-Segment Elevation Myocardial Infarction (STEMI) Undergoing Primary PCI

Acknowledgments

We would like to acknowledge Dra. Adriana Belo for performing the statistical analyses presented in this manuscript.

Funding

None.

Authors' contributions

HP and DC: Contributed to the concept and design, data acquisition, data analysis, and interpretation of the data; wrote the first draft of the manuscript; critically revised the manuscript; and gave final approval of the submitted manuscript; RCT, MC, PCS, VGR, VB, DM, FM, FPM, JB, PFA, RC, AD, HCC, JC, JCS, JLP, JM, PS, RF, RCF, SR, EIO, MA: contributed to the data analysis and interpretation; critically revised the manuscript; and gave final approval of the submitted manuscript.

Competing interests

The authors declare that they have no competing interests.

Author details

[1]Serviço de Cardiologia, Hospital Garcia de Orta EPE, Avenida Prof. Torrado da Silva, 2801-951 Almada, Portugal. [2]Centro Cardiovascular da Universidade de Lisboa (CCUL), CAML, Faculdade de Medicina, Universidade de Lisboa, Avenida Professor Egas Moniz, Lisboa 1649-028, Portugal. [3]Unidade de Farmacologia Clínica, Instituto de Medicina Molecular; Laboratório de Farmacologia Clínica e Terapêutica, Faculdade de Medicina, Universidade de Lisboa, Avenida Professor Egas Moniz, Lisboa 1649-028, Portugal. [4]Hospital de Santa Cruz, Centro Hospitalar de Lisboa Ocidental, EPE, Lisboa, Portugal. [5]Registo Nacional de Cardiologia de Intervenção, APIC-CNCDC, Lisboa, Portugal. [6]Centro Hospitalar e Universitário de Coimbra – CHC, Coimbra, Portugal. [7]Hospital de Santa Maria, Centro Hospitalar de Lisboa Norte EPE, Lisboa, Portugal. [8]Centro Hospitalar de Vila Nova de Gaia/Espinho - Hospital Eduardo Santos Silva, Porto, Portugal. [9]Hospital de Faro EPE, Faro, Portugal. [10]Hospital do Divino Espírito Santo de Ponta Delgada EPE, Açores, Portugal. [11]Hospital da Cruz Vermelha Portuguesa, Lisboa, Portugal. [12]Hospital da Luz, Lisboa, Portugal. [13]Unidade de Intervenção Cardiovascular – Alvor, Portimão, Portugal. [14]Hospital Professor Doutor Fernando da Fonseca EPE, Amadora, Portugal. [15]Hospital de São Bernardo, Centro Hospitalar de Setúbal EPE, Setúbal, Portugal. [16]Hospital do Funchal, Madeira, Portugal. [17]Hospital de Santo António, Centro Hospitalar do Porto, Porto, Portugal. [18]Centro Hospitalar e Universitário de Coimbra – HUC, Coimbra, Portugal. [19]Centro Hospitalar de São João EPE, Porto, Portugal. [20]Hospital de São Teotónio, Viseu, Portugal. [21]Hospital de São Marcos, Braga, Portugal. [22]Hospital de Vila Real, Centro Hospitalar de Trás-os-Montes e Alto Douro EPE, Vila Real, Portugal. [23]Hospital do Espírito Santo, Évora, Portugal. [24]Hospital de Santa Marta, Centro Hospitalar Lisboa Central EPE, Lisboa, Portugal. [25]Hospital CUF Infante Santo, Lisboa, Portugal. [26]Hospital de Santa Cruz. CHLO; Departamento de Fisiopatologia Nova Medical School, Lisboa, Portugal.

References

1. Svilaas T, Vlaar PJ, van der Horst IC, Diercks GF, de Smet BJ, van den Heuvel AF, Anthonio RL, Jessurun GA, Tan ES, Suurmeijer AJ, et al. Thrombus aspiration during primary percutaneous coronary intervention. N Engl J Med. 2008;358(6):557–67.
2. Kumbhani DJ, Bavry AA, Desai MY, Bangalore S, Bhatt DL. Role of aspiration and mechanical thrombectomy in patients with acute myocardial infarction undergoing primary angioplasty: an updated meta-analysis of randomized trials. J Am Coll Cardiol. 2013;62(16):1409–18.
3. Burzotta F, De Vita M, Gu YL, Isshiki T, Lefevre T, Kaltoft A, Dudek D, Sardella G, Orrego PS, Antoniucci D, et al. Clinical impact of thrombectomy in acute ST-elevation myocardial infarction: an individual patient-data pooled analysis of 11 trials. Eur Heart J. 2009;30(18):2193–203.
4. Steg PG, James SK, Atar D, Badano LP, Blömstrom-Lundqvist C, Borger MA, Di Mario C, Dickstein K, Ducrocq G, Fernandez-Aviles F, et al. ESC Guidelines for the management of acute myocardial infarction in patients presenting with ST-segment elevation. Eur Heart J. 2012;33(20):2569-19.
5. O'Gara PT, Kushner FG, Ascheim DD, Casey DE, Chung MK, De Lemos JA, Ettinger SM, Fang JC, Fesmire FM, Franklin BA. 2013 ACCF/AHA guideline for the management of ST-elevation myocardial infarction: a report of the American College of Cardiology Foundation/American Heart Association task force on practice guidelines. J Am Coll Cardiol. 2013;61(4):e78–e140.
6. Cale R, de Sousa L, Pereira H, Costa M, de Sousa Almeida M. Primary angioplasty in women: data from the Portuguese registry of interventional cardiology. Rev Port Cardiol. 2014;33(6):353–61.
7. Thygesen K, Alpert JS, Jaffe AS, Simoons ML, Chaitman BR, White HD, Thygesen K, Alpert JS, White HD, Jaffe AS, et al. Third universal definition of myocardial infarction. Eur Heart J. 2012;33(20):2551–67.
8. Mendis S, Thygesen K, Kuulasmaa K, Giampaoli S, Mahonen M, Ngu Blackett K, Lisheng L. World Health Organization definition of myocardial infarction: 2008-09 revision. Int J Epidemiol. 2011;40(1):139–46.
9. Thygesen K, Alpert JS, White HD. Universal definition of myocardial infarction. J Am Coll Cardiol. 2007;50(22):2173–95.
10. Portugal G, Cunha P, Valente B, Feliciano J, Lousinha A, Alves S, Braz M, Pimenta R, Delgado AS, Oliveira M, et al. A link to better care: the effect of remote monitoring on long-term adverse cardiac events in a propensity score-matched cohort. Rev Port Cardiol. 2017;36(3):189–95.
11. Frobert O, Lagerqvist B, Olivecrona GK, Omerovic E, Gudnason T, Maeng M, Aasa M, Angeras O, Calais F, Danielewicz M, et al. Thrombus aspiration during ST-segment elevation myocardial infarction. N Engl J Med. 2013;369(17):1587–97.
12. Jolly SS, Cairns JA, Yusuf S, Meeks B, Pogue J, Rokoss MJ, Kedev S, Thabane L, Stankovic G, Moreno R, et al. Randomized trial of primary PCI with or without routine manual thrombectomy. N Engl J Med. 2015;372(15):1389–98.
13. Lagerqvist B, Frobert O, Olivecrona GK, Gudnason T, Maeng M, Alstrom P, Andersson J, Calais F, Carlsson J, Collste O, et al. Outcomes 1 year after thrombus aspiration for myocardial infarction. N Engl J Med. 2014;371(12):1111–20.
14. Jolly SS, Cairns JA, Yusuf S, Rokoss MJ, Gao P, Meeks B, Kedev S, Stankovic G, Moreno R, Gershlick A, et al. Outcomes after thrombus aspiration for ST elevation myocardial infarction: 1-year follow-up of the prospective randomised TOTAL trial. Lancet. 2016;387(10014):127–35.
15. Jones DA, Rathod KS, Gallagher S, Jain AK, Kalra SS, Lim P, Crake T, Ozkor M, Rakhit R, Knight CJ, et al. Manual Thrombus aspiration is not associated with reduced mortality in patients treated with primary percutaneous coronary intervention: an observational study of 10,929 patients with ST-segment elevation myocardial infarction from the London heart attack group. JACC Cardiovasc Interv. 2015;8(4):575–84.
16. Javaid A, Siddiqi NH, Steinberg DH, Buch AN, Slottow TL, Roy P, Sammee S, Okabe T, Suddath WO, Kent KM, et al. Adjunct thrombus aspiration reduces mortality in patients undergoing percutaneous coronary intervention for ST-elevation myocardial infarction with high-risk angiographic characteristics. Am J Cardiol. 2008;101(4):452–6.
17. Shiraishi J, Kohno Y, Nakamura T, Yanagiuchi T, Hashimoto S, Ito D, Kimura M, Matsui A, Yokoi H, Arihara M, et al. Clinical impact of thrombus aspiration during primary percutaneous coronary intervention in acute myocardial infarction with occluded culprit. Cardiovasc Interv Ther. 2015;30(1):22–8.
18. Caldeira D, Pereira H, Costa J, Vaz-Carneiro A. Cochrane corner: intra-aortic balloon pump in patients with cardiogenic shock following myocardial infarction. Rev Port Cardiol. 2016;35(4):229–31.
19. Barkagan M, Steinvil A, Berchenko Y, Finkelstein A, Keren G, Banai S, Halkin A. Impact of routine manual aspiration thrombectomy on outcomes of patients undergoing primary percutaneous coronary intervention for acute myocardial infarction: a meta-analysis. Int J Cardiol. 2016;204:189–95.
20. Akobeng AK. Understanding type I and type II errors, statistical power and sample size. Acta Paediatr. 2016;105(6):605–9.
21. Carneiro AV. Estimating sample size in clinical studies: basic methodological principles. Rev Port Cardiol. 2003;22(12):1513–21.

25

Ticagrelor versus clopidogrel in real-world patients with ST elevation myocardial infarction: 1-year results by propensity score analysis

Matteo Vercellino[1]* [iD], Federico Ariel Sànchez[2], Valentina Boasi[3], Dino Perri[4], Chiara Tacchi[5], Gioel Gabrio Secco[1], Stefano Cattunar[4], Gianfranco Pistis[6] and Giovanni Mascelli[7]

Abstract

Background: European guidelines recommend the use of ticagrelor versus clopidogrel in patients with ST elevation myocardial infarction (STEMI). This recommendation is based on inconclusive results and subanalyses from clinical trials. Few data are available on the effects of ticagrelor in a real-world population.

Methods: To compare the effects of ticagrelor and clopidogrel in a real-world STEMI population, we conducted a pre-post case-control study examining all patients with STEMI included in the Cardio-STEMI Sanremo registry between February 2011 and June 2013. Cases and controls were defined according to $P2Y_{12}$ inhibitors, correcting the bias due to lack of randomization by propensity score analysis. Ticagrelor was introduced in 2012 in both in-hospital and pre-hospital settings independently of this study.

Results: Of the 416 patients enrolled in the Cardio-STEMI registry, 401 with a definite diagnosis of STEMI were included in this study. One hundred forty-two patients received ticagrelor and 259 received clopidogrel. Regarding clinical presentation and procedural data, those in the ticagrelor group had lower CRUSADE scores (23 [14–36] vs 27 [18–38]; $p = 0.015$] but a higher proportion of radial access (33% vs 14%; $p < 0.001$), percutaneous coronary intervention (PCI; 92% vs 81 %; $p = 0.002$) and primary PCI $\leq$ 12 h (82% vs 66%; $p = 0.001$). The patients in the ticagrelor group had a higher procedural success rate (100% vs. 96%; $p = 0.044$). There was no difference in Bleeding Academic Research Consortium bleeding and in unadjusted incidence of hospital major adverse cardiovascular events (MACE; cardiac death, myocardial infarction, or stroke) but there was a significant reduction in unadjusted cardiac hospital death in the ticagrelor group (0.7% vs 5.4%; $p = 0.024$). After correcting for propensity score, hospital death ($p = 0.22$) and hospital MACE ($p = 0.96$) did not differ in both groups. The unadjusted survival at 1 year after STEMI was higher in the ticagrelor group (97.8% vs 87.8%; $p = 0.024$), and this result was confirmed by propensity score analysis (hazard ratio = 0.29 [0.08–0.99]; $p = 0.048$).

Conclusions: In this real-word propensity score analysis, ticagrelor did not affect the risk of MACE during the hospital phase, or the incidence of hospital bleeding in patients with STEMI. However, in this mono-centric experience, ticagrelor resulted in improved 1-year survival, even after correction by propensity score.

Keywords: Acute coronary syndrome, ST elevation myocardial infarction, Clopidogrel, Ticagrelor, Registry

* Correspondence: matteovrc@gmail.com; matteo.vercellino@ospedale.al.it
[1]Interventional Cardiology, Santi Antonio, Biagio e Cesare Arrigo Hospital, Alessandria, AL, Italy
Full list of author information is available at the end of the article

Background

Patients with ST elevation myocardial infarction (STEMI) represent 32% of patients with acute coronary syndrome (ACS), with in-hospital mortality ranging from 5% to 15% according to geographic and baseline differences [1]. Each year in the United States alone, hospital costs related to acute myocardial infarction (AMI) are estimated to be as high as US$11.5 billion [2].

Dual antiplatelet therapy (DAPT) is a cornerstone of therapy for patients with STEMI. Clopidogrel has been used extensively worldwide for more than a decade; more recently, new antiplatelet agents, prasugrel and ticagrelor, have been developed and tested clinically, resulting in faster, more potent and consistent antiplatelet action [3–6].

Clopidogrel, a second-generation thienopyridine, is now available as a low-cost generic drug, with a favourable cost-effectiveness ratio. A drawback of clopidogrel is that as a pro-drug, it needs liver metabolism to be activated. In patients with STEMI, drug metabolism is hampered by specific circulatory conditions, resulting in a delayed effect of the drug compared with the time frame needed for percutaneous coronary intervention (PCI) [7, 8]. Moreover, this pathway is susceptible to genetic polymorphism, which may lead to unexpected variations in drug activity.

Ticagrelor is a novel oral, reversible P2Y12 inhibitor belonging to the cyclopentyltriazolopyrimidine class. It has a plasma half-life of 12 h. It is an active drug with more rapid onset and offset of action than clopidogrel, so that inhibition and recovery of platelet function is faster [4, 9].

A large randomized controlled trial (RCT) showed the superiority of ticagrelor compared with clopidogrel in ACS in patients with STEMI and non-ST-segment elevation myocardial infarction (NSTEMI) [6]. This large RCT led to a change in guideline recommendations in favour of ticagrelor in patients with STEMI undergoing primary PCI, largely reducing clopidogrel use in this setting. The beneficial effects of ticagrelor were demonstrated to be independent from the clinical presentation of STEMI, because no interaction has been demonstrated in the PLATO (Platelet Inhibition and Patient Outcomes) [8]. However, no specific randomized trial was designed to detect the effect of ticagrelor in patients with STEMI, leading to inconclusive and underpowered data [5, 10].

Although results from large real-world registries are important to better understand the effectiveness, use and outcomes of novel therapies [11–16], data on the benefits of ticagrelor in a real-world population of patients with STEMI are lacking. The sole large observational registry about ticagrelor in STEMI population yielded results that were in contrast with the PLATO trial, with no improvement in ischaemic events and a higher rate of bleeding for ticagrelor versus clopidogrel [17].

The safety and efficacy of drug-eluting stents (DESs) based on the generation of the device and the duration of DAPT have recently been examined. A recent meta-analysis showed that patients treated with short DAPT (<12 months) have similar survival (all-cause mortality and cardiovascular mortality) than patients treated with long DAPT (≥12 months). However, the RCTs collected in the meta-analysis examined DAPT duration, not the type of DAPT (ticagrelor vs clopidogrel), and the prevalence of ACS was widely heterogeneous (32–77%). To date, we have few data about the differences related to the type of DAPT in a population of STEMI patients treated with second-generation DESs.

We thus performed the present study to compare the effect of ticagrelor and clopidogrel in a real-world population of patients with STEMI.

Methods

A pre-post case-control study was performed using data from the Cardio-STEMI Sanremo registry, a single-centre, ongoing, observational cohort study conducted in Sanremo Hospital, the hub for a population of 210,000 inhabitants, with 2 spokes. Every adult patient (>18 years old) admitted to the hub with a diagnosis of STEMI [18] was enrolled in the registry.

Exclusion criteria were: type 4a or 5 AMI according to the universal definition of myocardial infarction [19]; high probability of being unavailable for follow-up visits because of limited ability to cooperate or severe comorbidity with very short life expectancy.

For this study, all patients enrolled between February 2011 and June 2013 were examined. Ticagrelor became available in addition to clopidogrel in May 2012, in both in-hospital and pre-hospital settings. Since then, the choice between the two drugs has been left to the cardiologist who first makes the diagnosis of STEMI. Ticagrelor was introduced into clinical practice independently from this observational study and in accordance with European guidelines for the treatment of STEMI patients published in 2012 [20]. Patients were divided into the ticagrelor group and the clopidogrel group according to the P2Y12 inhibitor received. Local guidelines recommend the early administration of 2PY12 inhibitors, acetylsalicylic acid and unfractionated heparin immediately after a STEMI diagnosis. Therefore, in most patients presenting through the ambulance service, 2PY12 inhibitors were administered during the ambulance journey, usually after transmission of the electrocardiogram report to the hub. Patients were treated according to usual clinical practice at each institution, and PCI was performed using standard techniques. All patients received indication to continue DAPT for at least 1 year after discharge, according to the current European and American guidelines [20, 21]. Study endpoints were: (1) TIMI flow grade before and after PCI [22] and ST resolution 90 min after PCI; (2) the rate of hospital major adverse cardiovascular events (MACE; cardiovascular death, AMI and stroke) and bleeding; (3) the 12-month survival. MACE were defined according to the PLATO trial criteria, with stroke defined as focal loss of neurologic function caused by ischaemic or haemorrhagic events, with symptoms lasting at least 24 h or leading to death [6]. Myocardial infarction (MI) was defined according to the universal definition reported in the literature [19]. Bleeding Academic Research Consortium (BARC) criteria were used for bleeding assessment [23].

A paper-based case report form was prospectively collected for each patient by the referring physician. All the data were entered into an electronic database by 4 trained researchers, and the data entries were checked periodically by a data manager. The validation of in-hospital study outcomes was performed through the periodic revision of medical documents. Follow-up was performed with the support of a local health registry and a telephone interview with the patient, family physician or relatives [24]. Only mortality was inquired about during post-discharge follow-up, because this endpoint can be reliably and easily collected, and it is a surrogate for the most severe sequelae such as re-infarction, stroke or bleeding occurring during follow-up.

The Cardiology Department of Sanremo Hospital served as the data analysis centre. The study was conducted in accordance with the principles of the Helsinki Declaration and received local ethical committee approval before recruitment.

Statistical analysis

Baseline patient and procedural characteristics are presented as means ± standard deviation, median (inter-quartile range), or frequency (percentage) as appropriate. The normal distribution of continuous variables in the study was determined by Shapiro-Wilks and Kolmogorov-Smirnov tests. Normally distributed continuous variables were compared using the Student t test and those with skewed distributions using the Mann-Whitney U test. Categorical variables were compared using the $\chi2$ test or Fisher exact test. In-hospital nominal outcomes are presented as proportions and odds ratios (OR) with relative 95% confidence intervals (CI). We used Kaplan-Meier curves for survival analysis and the log-rank test to compare the treatment groups. With the aim of reducing bias related to the lack of randomization, a propensity score was calculated [25, 26] using a non-parsimonious, multivariate, binary logistic regression model.

Variables presenting a p value ≤0.2 for the univariate analysis and those judged to be of clinical importance, biologically plausible or supported by previously published data in the literature, were tested for inclusion in the multivariable model building process. Variables with a missing rate ≥ 5% were excluded.

Model discrimination was measured by the C statistic and calibration by the Hosmer-Lemeshow goodness-of-fit test [27]. The propensity score was used as a correction factor in a binary logistic regression to calculate the adjusted hospital outcomes and in a Cox regression analysis to examine the adjusted 1-year survival. The Cox regression results were expressed by hazard ratios (HR) with 95% CIs. All tests were two-sided. A p value ≤0.05 was considered statistically significant. Statistics were calculated using SPSS version 22.0 (SPSS Inc., Chicago, IL, USA).

Results

A total of 416 patients were enrolled in the Cardio-STEMI Sanremo registry during the study period. Fifteen patients (3.6%) were subsequently ruled out with conditions mimicking MI, and were therefore excluded from this study. The study flowchart is shown in Fig. 1. The study population included 401 patients, 259 patients in the clopidogrel group and 142 patients in the ticagrelor group. From its introduction into clinical practice in May 2012, its use had peaked at 83% by the end of 2012. Data on the adoption of ticagrelor in clinical practice are reported in Fig. 2.

Demographic and baseline data are reported in Table 1. Comparing the baseline data of the 2 groups, there were no significant differences between ticagrelor and clopidogrel, except for a lower proportion of patients aged over 75 years (21% vs 32%, respectively; p = 0.037), with no difference in median age.

In the ticagrelor group, all patients received the loading dose, administered in 98% of cases before the cardiac catheterization laboratory; in the clopidogrel group, 236 patients (91%) received the loading dose (42% >300 mg as reported in Fig. 3), administered in 94% before the cardiac catheterization laboratory.

With regard to clinical presentation and reperfusion strategy, a lower CRUSADE score (23 [14–36] vs 27 [18–38]; p = 0.015), a higher rate of PCI (92% vs 80%; p = 0.002) and primary PCI within 12 h (82% vs 66%; p = 0.001) were found in the ticagrelor group compared with the clopidogrel group. (Table 2). The laboratory tests were similar between the 2 groups (Additional file 1).

Procedural data and times are reported in Table 3. The only significant difference was a higher frequency of the radial access approach for PCI in the ticagrelor group (33% vs 14%; p < 0.001). For patients undergoing primary PCI, the frequency of thrombus aspiration (45% vs 37%; p = 0.22) and the use of glycoprotein (GP) IIb/IIIa receptor antagonists (13% vs 17%; p = 0.41) were comparable in the ticagrelor and clopidogrel groups. With regard to the type of stent used, there were no significant differences between the clopidogrel and tica-grelor groups, although the use of bare metal stents was nominally higher in the clopidogrel group (27% vs 15%).

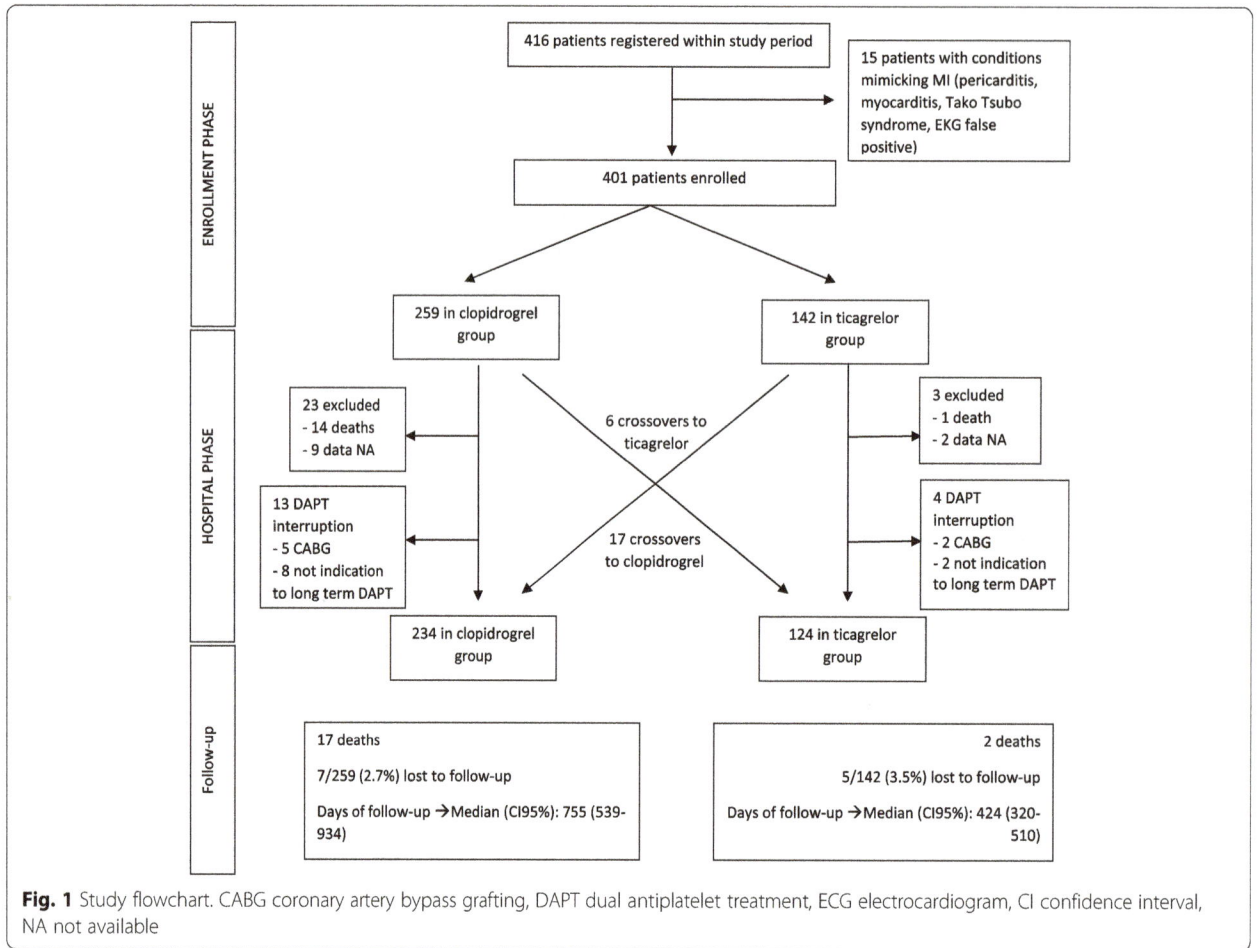

Fig. 1 Study flowchart. CABG coronary artery bypass grafting, DAPT dual antiplatelet treatment, ECG electrocardiogram, CI confidence interval, NA not available

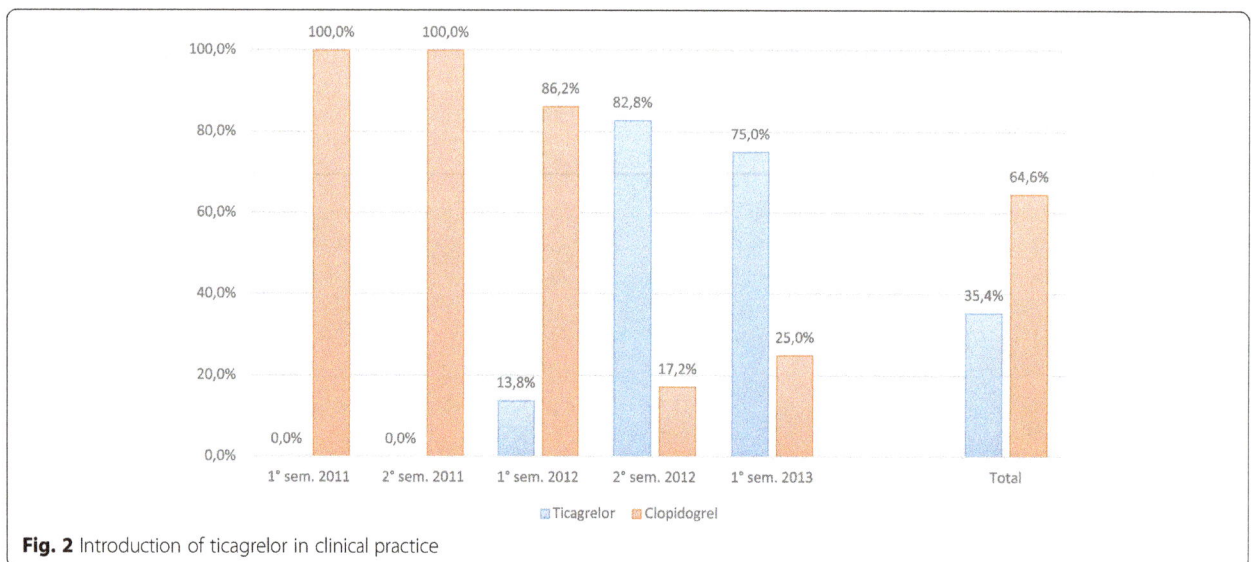

Fig. 2 Introduction of ticagrelor in clinical practice

Table 1 Baseline and demographic data. Data are expressed as percentage (frequency) or median (IQR)

	Ticagrelor (n = 142)	Clopidogrel (n = 259)	p
Age (years)	66 (56–73)	67 (56–67)	0.206
Age ≥ 75 years	21.8 (31)	32.0 (83)	*0.037*
Sex male	73.9 (105)	69.9 (81)	0.420
BMI (kg/m²)[a]	26 (24–30)	26 (24–29)	0.772
Hypertension	52.8 (75)	56.0 (145)	0.600
Dyslipidemia	36.6 (52)	39.0 (101)	0.668
Active smoke	45.8 (65)	37.8 (98)	0.137
Diabetes mellitus	22.5 (32)	18.5 (48)	0.362
Familiar of CAD	21.1 (30)	24.7 (64)	0.461
Previous stable angina	11.3 (16)	6.6 (17)	0.128
Previous unstable angina	3.5 (5)	4.6 (12)	0.797
Previous AMI	11.3 (16)	11.2 (29)	1.000
Previous PCI	7.0 (10)	9.3 (24)	0.574
Previous CABG	1.4 (2)	0.0 (0)	0.125
Previous CVA	4.9 (7)	7.3 (19)	0.403
PVD	16.2 (23)	11.2 (29)	0.164
Chronic kidney disease	7.0 (10)	4.6 (12)	0.361
COPD	8.5 (12)	8.9 (23)	1.000
Previous bleeding	0.7 (1)	3.9 (10)	0.106
Previous neoplasia	10.6 (15)	15.8 (41)	0.175

Italics: *p* value ≤0.05

BMI body mass index, *CAD* coronary artery disease, *AMI* acute myocardial infarction, *PCI* percutaneous coronary intervention, *CABG* coronary artery bypass grafting, *CVA* cerebrovascular accident, *PVD* peripheral vascular disease, *COPD* chronic obstructive pulmonary disease
[a]*n* = 139 for ticagrelor, 258 for clopidogrel

In each group, most of the DESs were second-generation devices.

The system-related delay, patient-related delay and the time intervals were not different between the 2 groups.

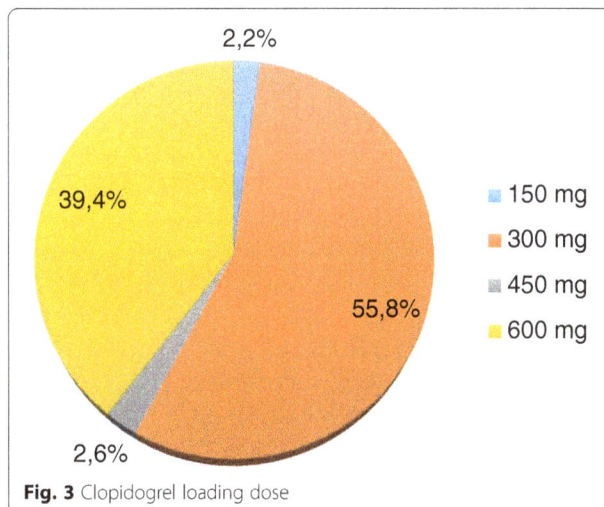

Fig. 3 Clopidogrel loading dose

2,2%
39,4%
2,6%
55,8%
■ 150 mg
■ 300 mg
■ 450 mg
■ 600 mg

Table 2 Clinical presentation and reperfusion strategy. Data are expressed as percentage (frequency), median (IQR), or mean (SD)

	Ticagrelor	Clopidogrel	p
Call to emergency service	43.0 (61/142)	41.3 (107/259)	0.75
Secondary transfer by emergency service	40.8 (58/142)	40.3 (104/258)	0.92
Hub vs spoke	67.1 (94/140)	64.5 (167/259)	0.65
Anterior AMI	46.5 (66/142)	39.8 (103/259)	0.21
New LBBB at first EKG	2.3 (5/142)	3.5 (6/256)	0.53
Cardiac frequency (bpm)	75 (65–88)	77 (63–94)	0.28
Systolic blood pressure (mmHg)	140 (120–160)	140 (120–160)	0.76
Killip class ≥ 3	5.6 (8/142)	8.1 (21/259)	0.42
Cardiac arrest	2.1 (3/142)	3.1 (8/259)	0.75
LV ejection fraction (%)	46 (40–55)	45 (40–55)	0.83
GFR Cockroft Gault (mL/min/m²)	72 (55–90)	67 (52–86)	0.08
GFR MDRD (mL/min/m²)	76 ± 25	72 ± 23	0.09
GRACE-in-hospital mortality	139 (122–157)	141 (121–167)	0.32
GRACE 6-month mortality	106 (86–128)	106 (87–125)	0.96
TIMI risk score	3 (2–5)	4 (2–5)	0.18
CRUSADE	23 (14–36)	27 (18–38)	*0.015*
Thrombolysis	1.8 (4/142)	4.6 (12/259)	0.44
Coronary angiography	100.0 (142/142)	93.1 (241/259)	*0.001*
PCI	92.3 (131/142)	80.7 (209/259)	*0.002*
Primary PCI (≤12 h after first medical contact)	82.4 (117/142)	66.4 (172/259)	*0.001*
IABP	0.7 (1/142)	3.1 (8/259)	0.17

Italics: *p* value ≤0.05

AMI acute myocardial infarction, *LBBB* left bundle branch block, *EKG*, electrocardiogram, *LV* left ventricle, *GFR* glomerular filtration rate, *MDRD* modification of diet in renal disease, *GRACE* global registry of acute coronary events, *TIMI* thrombolysis in myocardial infarction, *CRUSADE* can rapid risk stratification of unstable angina patients suppress adverse outcome with early implementation of ACC/AHA Guidelines, *PCI* percutaneous coronary intervention, *IABP* intra-aortic balloon pump

Discharge therapy was not significantly different between the ticagrelor and clopidogrel groups (Additional file 2).

Procedural success, defined either as TIMI 3 or TIMI 2–3 with stenosis <50% after primary PCI, was higher in the ticagrelor group than in the clopidogrel group (99% vs 90%, *p* = 0.001; 100.0% vs. 96%, *p* = 0.044), whereas the proportion of patients with ≥50% ST resolution (78% vs 78%; *p* = 0.879) or ≥70% ST resolution (60% vs 67%; *p* = 0.294) was similar between the groups. Data on procedural outcomes are reported in Table 4.

In the unadjusted analysis, there was no difference in hospital MACE (cardiovascular death, non-fatal MI, stroke) between the ticagrelor and clopidogrel groups (4.9% vs 6.9%; *p* = 0.520; OR, 0.69 [95% CI, 0.28–1.70]). However, the use of ticagrelor resulted in a significant reduction of cardiovascular mortality (0.7% vs 5.4%; *p* = 0.024; OR, 0.12 [95% CI, 0.02–0.95]). No difference was found in new hospital non-fatal AMI (3.5% vs 1.2%,

Table 3 Procedural data in patients with STEMI and in primary PCI. Data are expressed as percentage (frequency) or median (IQR)

	Ticagrelor	Clopidogrel	p
Radial vs femoral	33.1 (47/142)	14.5 (35/241)	<0.001
Left main	1.4 (2/142)	2.1 (5/241)	1.00
Multi-vessel CAD	36.6 (52/142)	36.5 (88/241)	1.00
Culprit vessel			0.19
RCA	38.7 (53/137)	38.9 (91/234)	
CX	10.9 (15/137)	17.9 (42/234)	
LAD	48.9 (67/137)	41.5 (97/234)	
Other	1.5 (2/137)	1.7 (4/234)	
Complete revascularization	58.0 (76/131)	56.9 (119/234)	0.91
Total contrast amount (mL)	200 (147–268)	203 (148–284)	0.89
Primary PCI			
Multi-vessel CAD	35.9 (42/117)	34.9 (88/241)	0.90
Culprit vessel			0.44
RCA	38.8 (45/116)	39.0 (67/172)	
CX	11.2 (13/116)	15.7 (27/172)	
LAD	48.2 (56/116)	43.0 (74/172)	
Others	1.8 (2/116)	2.3 (4/172)	
TIMI flow pre-PCI	1 (0–3)	1 (0–3)	0.09
Reperfusion before PCI (TIMI 3)	26.5 (31/117)	16.9 (29/172)	0.047
Reperfusion before PCI (TIMI 2 o 3)	45.3 (53/117)	37.8 (65/172)	0.22
Type B2-C ACC/AHA lesion classification	73.6 (81/110)	74.5 (117/155)	0.78
Thrombus aspiration	44.8 (52/116)	37.2 (64/172)	0.22
GPIIb/IIIa receptor antagonist	12.8 (15/117)	16.9 (29/172)	0.41
Stent type			0.15
BMS	14.7 (17/116)	27.1 (46/170)	
First-generation DES	0.9 (1/116)	0.6 (1/170)	
Second-generation DES	75.0 (86/116)	61.8 (104/170)	
BMS and DES	2.6 (3/116)	2.4 (4/170)	
No stent	7.8 (9/116)	8.8 (15/170)	
Symptom onset to EKG (hh:min)	1:25 (0:40–2:26)	1:19 (0:50–2:41)	0.84
EKG to door hub (hh:min)	1:26 (1:14–2:10)	1:21 (1:06–1:51)	0.25
Transfer time (hh:min)	0:42 (0:36–0:52)	0:38 (0:34–0:48)	0.11
DTB min (hh:min)	1:46 (1:35–2:37)	1:49 (1:34–2:30)	0.75
DTB ≤60 min	3.5 (4/114)	3.0 (5/166)	1.00
DTB ≤90 min	20.2 (23/114)	21.7 (36/166)	0.88
DTB ≤120 min	52.6 (60/114)	52.4 (87/166)	1.00
Total ischaemic time(hh:min)	3:50 (2:45–5:34)	3:30 (2:42–5:39)	0.37

Italics: p value ≤0.05
CAD coronary artery disease, RCA right coronary artery, CX circumflex coronary artery, LAD left anterior descending, ACC/AHA American College of Cardiology/American Heart Association, GPIIb/IIIa glycoprotein IIb/IIIa, PCI percutaneous coronary intervention, TIMI thrombolysis in myocardial infarction, BMS bare metal stent, DES drug-eluting stent, EKG electrocardiogram, DTB door to balloon

Table 4 Procedural and hospital outcomes. Data are expressed as percentage (frequency) or median (IQR)

	Ticagrelor (n = 142)	Clopidogrel (n = 259)	p
Procedural outcomes (unadjusted analysis)			
TIMI flow post-PCI	3 (3–3)	3 (3–3)	0.002
Procedural success (TIMI 3 and stenosis <50%)	99.0 (115/116)	89.9 (151/168)	0.001
Procedural success (TIMI 2–3 and stenosis <50%)	100.0 (116/116)	95.8 (161/168)	0.044
STR%	89 (50–100)	100 (50–100)	0.482
STR ≥ 50%	78.1 (82/105)	78.2 (122/156)	0.879
STR% ≥ 70%	60.0 (63/105)	66.7 (104/156)	0.294
Hospital outcomes (unadjusted analysis)			
In-hospital all-cause death	0.7 (1)	5.4 (14)	0.024
In-hospital CV death	0.7 (1)	5.4 (14)	0.024
In-hospital non-fatal AMI	3.5 (5)	1.2 (3)	0.14
Ischaemic CVA	0.4 (1)	0.7 (1)	1.00
Total CVA (ischaemic or haemorrhagic)	0.4 (1)	0.7 (1)	1.00
Hospital MACE	4.9 (7)	6.9 (18)	0.52
Definite stent thrombosis	1.4 (2)	0.8 (2)	0.62
Final LVEF [%]	50 (40–55)	48 (40–55)	0.55
CPK peak [UI/L]	1347 (535–2590)	1376 (677–2491)	0.77
Hospital stay [days]	4 (4–6)	5 (4–6)	0.84

Italics: p value ≤0.05
TIMI thrombolysis in myocardial infarction, STR ST resolution, CV cardiovascular, AMI acute myocardial infarction, CVA cerebrovascular accidents, LVEF left ventricular ejection fraction, CPK creatine phosphokinase

$p = 0.14$) or in cerebrovascular accidents (0.4% vs 0.7% vs 0.8%; $p = 1.000$) (Table 4). No significant difference between the ticagrelor and clopidogrel groups was found in stent thrombosis (1.4% vs 0.8%, $p = 0.62$) and infarct size, estimated by the peak creatine kinase value (1347 vs 1372 UI/L, $p = 0.77$), or for left ventricular ejection fraction (50% vs 48%, $p = 0.55$) before hospital discharge. The causes of cardiovascular death are reported in Additional file 3.

BARC bleeding was similar between the 2 groups; there was no difference in BARC categories for BARC ≥2 and BARC ≥3. The lowest median haemoglobin value (12.2 vs 12.2 g/dL; $p = 0.8$) and the difference between the highest and lowest haemoglobin value during hospital stay (2.2 vs 2.1 g/dL; $p = 0.9$) were similar between the ticagrelor and clopidogrel groups. The risk of transfusion and the amount of packed red blood cell units did not show any significant difference (Additional file 4).

In the Kaplan-Meier analysis, unadjusted 1-year survival probability was higher in the ticagrelor group than in the clopidogrel group (97.8% vs 87.8%; log-rank $p = 0.024$) (Fig. 4), as was the probability of 1-year survival free from

MORTALITY

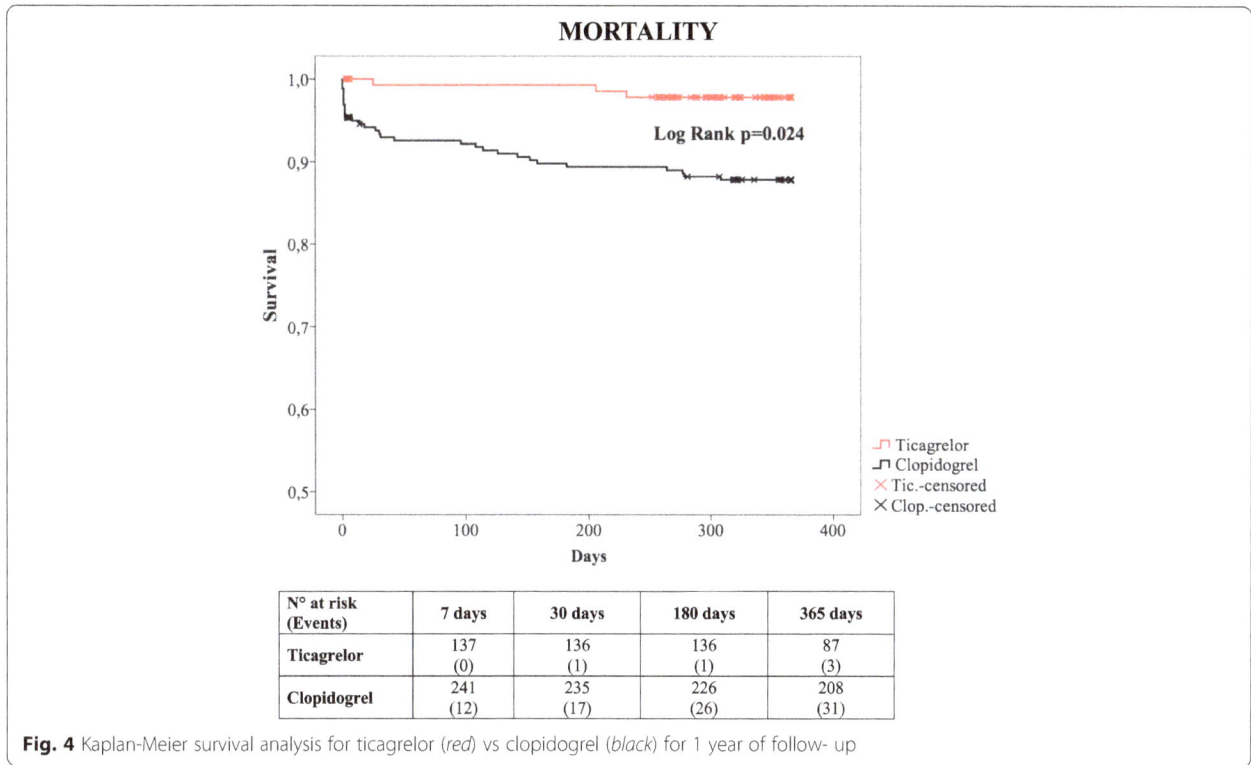

Log Rank p=0.024

Legend:
- Ticagrelor
- Clopidogrel
- × Tic.-censored
- × Clop.-censored

N° at risk (Events)	7 days	30 days	180 days	365 days
Ticagrelor	137 (0)	136 (1)	136 (1)	87 (3)
Clopidogrel	241 (12)	235 (17)	226 (26)	208 (31)

Fig. 4 Kaplan-Meier survival analysis for ticagrelor (*red*) vs clopidogrel (*black*) for 1 year of follow- up

cardiovascular death (97.8% vs 90.2%; log-rank p = 0.005) (Additional file 5).

Propensity score analysis

A total of 21 interfering variables were included in the propensity score and are reported in Additional file 6. Candidate variables included sex, age, BMI, smoking, diabetes, dyslipidemia, familiar history of coronary artery disease, cerebrovascular accident (CVA), bleeding, previous AMI or PCI, glomerular filtration rate, TIMI risk score, CRUSADE score, anterior AMI, first medical contact through the ambulance service, admission to hub vs spoke, left ventricular ejection fraction, Killip class III-IV, radial access, primary PCI ≤12 h.

The propensity score was calculated for 368 patients (missing for 33, 8.2%) and showed good discrimination (area under the curve =0.695 [0.640–0.751]; p < 0.01) and good calibration (p = 0.355). Using propensity score regression, there were no differences in mortality, ischaemic or haemorrhagic events during the hospital stay. As showed in Fig. 5, after adjusting for the propensity score, hospital cardiovascular mortality (OR, 0.27 [95% CI, 0.03–2.19]; p = 0.218) and hospital MACEs (OR, 1.02 [95% CI, 0.38–2.79];], p = 0.963) were similar in the ticagrelor and clopidogrel groups.

However, the survival analysis adjusted by propensity score demonstrated that all-cause mortality at 1 year after STEMI remained significantly lower for the ticagrelor group (HR, 0.29 [0.08–0.99]; p = 0.048).

Variable	OR (CI95%)	p
MACE	0.69 (0.28-1.70)	0.520
CV death	0.12 (0.02-0.95)	0.024
BARC≥2	0.49 (1.94-0.98)	1.000

Variable	OR (CI95%)	p
MACE	1.02 (0.38-2.79)	0.963
CV death	0.27 (0.03-2.19)	0.218
BARC≥2	1.45 (0.65-3.21)	0.365

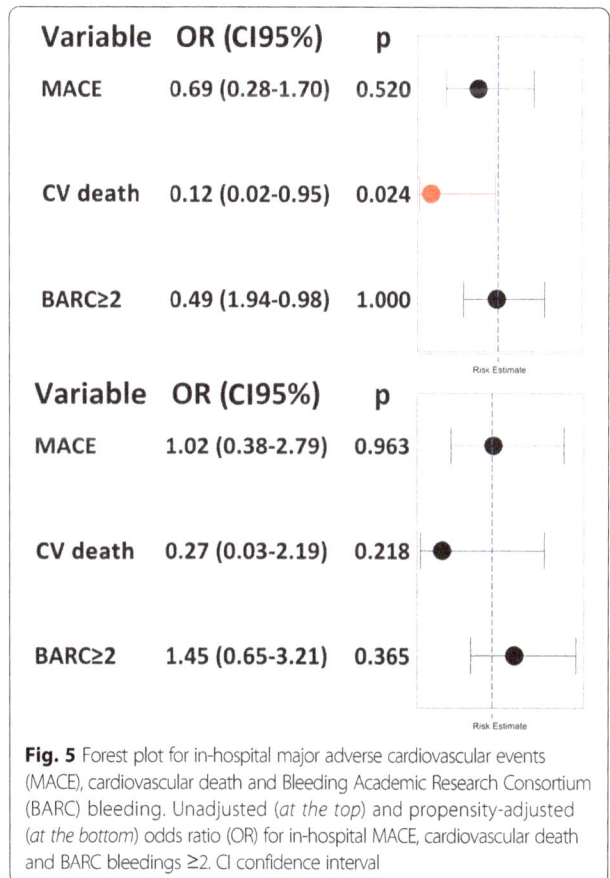

Fig. 5 Forest plot for in-hospital major adverse cardiovascular events (MACE), cardiovascular death and Bleeding Academic Research Consortium (BARC) bleeding. Unadjusted (*at the top*) and propensity-adjusted (*at the bottom*) odds ratio (OR) for in-hospital MACE, cardiovascular death and BARC bleedings ≥2. CI confidence interval

There were 6 crossovers from clopidogrel to ticagrelor (3 for STEMI occurring on clopidogrel therapy, 3 for unknown cause), and 17 crossovers from ticagrelor to clopidogrel (4 for high bleeding risk or vitamin K antagonist [VKA], 2 for dyspnoea, 2 for low patient compliance, 4 for low ischaemic risk after coronary angiography, 4 for unknown cause). Seven of 401 patients were proposed for elective coronary artery bypass graft (1.7%) during hospitalization, 5 in the clopidogrel group and 2 in the ticagrelor group. Ten patients were discharged without DAPT for high bleeding risk or contemporary VKA therapy (Fig. 1).

Discussion

In real-world populations of patients with STEMI admitted to an Italian hospital, treatment with ticagrelor reduced the mortality rate at 1 year compared with clopidogrel, with a risk of mortality 3.4 times higher for clopidogrel than for ticagrelor. This was confirmed when propensity analysis was used to reduce the risk of bias because of lack of randomization. Ticagrelor did not reduce hospital MACE after propensity score correction, and it did not affect hospital bleeding according to the BARC classification.

The new 2PY12 inhibitors, ticagrelor and prasugrel, are known to have more favourable pharmacologic proprieties for ACS than clopidogrel. Because of more predictable pharmacokinetics and a more potent and constant effect with faster onset, there is strong rationale for their use in patients with STEMI [4, 9]. However, despite promising pharmacological data and European guidelines recommendations to administer the new 2PY12 inhibitors in patients with STEMI [28], there is still uncertainty about their real clinical efficacy compared with the older and more widely adopted clopidogrel.

The STEMI population differs from the larger ACS population in several respects, because it is composed of younger patients with less comorbidities and lower procedural haemorrhage risk, but higher incidence of hemodynamic instability at presentation. Moreover, conditions affecting drug bioavailability, such as reduced gastrointestinal absorption, vomiting and morphine administration, can reduce the effect of P2Y12 more in patients with STEMI than other ACS [8, 29]. In an RCT directly comparing ticagrelor and clopidogrel, patients with STEMI had a delayed onset of both these P2Y12 inhibitors [30]. A delayed onset of action for ticagrelor was also confirmed in a small randomized trial measuring platelet reactivity after a loading dose of ticagrelor and prasugrel in patients with STEMI [9].

With no randomized trial focusing on the effect of ticagrelor or prasugrel versus clopidogrel in a STEMI population and the uncertainties about pharmacokinetics, the source of evidence on the new 2PY12 inhibitors in the STEMI population is still the subgroup analysis in the PLATO and TRITON-TIMI 38 trials [10].

The TRITON-TIMI trial subgroup analysis showed that prasugrel was superior to clopidogrel (300 mg loading dose/75 mg maintenance dose) in 3534 patients with STEMI undergoing primary or secondary PCI when considering cardiovascular death, non-fatal MI, or non-fatal stroke at 30 days (115 [6.5%] vs 166 [9.5%]; 0.68 [0.54–0.87]; p = 0.0017] and at 15 months (174 [10.0%] vs 216 [12.4%]; 0.79 [0.65–0.97]; p = 0.0221). A subanalysis in the PLATO trial on 7544 patients with STEMI has shown no superiority in MACE (cardiovascular death, non-fatal MI and stroke) for ticagrelor versus clopidogrel at 12 months follow-up, although there was a nominal trend in favour of ticagrelor (HR, 0.87 [0.75–1.01]; p = 0.07). However, in this analysis, ticagrelor significantly reduced secondary endpoints such as total mortality (HR 0.82; p = 0.05), MI (HR, 0.8; p = 0.03), and definite stent thrombosis (HR 0.66; p = 0.03).

Because the PLATO and TRITON-TIMI 38 trials are heterogeneous with regard to patient characteristics and treatments, their results could not be compared. The TRITON-TIMI 38 trial enrolled clopidogrel-naive patients undergoing primary and secondary PCI, whereas in PLATO almost 50% of patients were preloaded with open-label clopidogrel (300 or 600 mg), reducing the benefit of ticagrelor in the early phase of follow-up. Considering the PLATO subgroup analysis, ticagrelor did not reduce the primary endpoint at 12 months but conferred a survival advantage after 30 days, and this may be the result of a mechanism that differs from antiplatelet activity. Type 1 equilibrative nucleoside transporter (ENT1) protects adenosine from intercellular metabolism. Inhibiting ENT1 increases the concentration and biological activity of adenosine, particularly at sites of ischemia and tissue injury where it is formed [31]. Furthermore, in patients with STEMI, the beneficial effect of ticagrelor may be more pronounced in a subpopulation of high-risk patients characterized by high on-treatment platelet reactivity even after large loading doses of clopidogrel [32]. In these patients, even a double dose of clopidogrel did not reduce cardiovascular events compared with the standard dose, as demonstrated by the CURRENT-OASIS trial [33].

Despite the large number of patients included, PLATO and TRITON-TIMI 38 were not designed specifically to assess the effect of P2Y12 in patients with STEMI, and both trials are underpowered to reach a definitive conclusion; the low quality of this conclusion is summarized in the B level of evidence in the European guidelines [28].

In the absence of high-quality RCTs, however, there is increasing interest in prospective observational registries. The Swiss ATACS registry analysed the effect of prasugrel on a STEMI population, demonstrating that it is advantageous over clopidogrel (in-hospital mortality 1.7% vs 4.4%)

at the expense of an increased bleeding risk (significantly superior for prasugrel on adjusted but not crude analysis) [15]. Another Swiss observational study, the Swiss ACS bleeding score, demonstrated that clopidogrel and prasugrel had similar safety profiles at 30 days (BARC 3, 4, 5 adjusted HR, 0.75 [0.42–136]) and at 1 year (BARC 3, 4, 5 adjusted HR, 0.67 [0.38–1.20]), without considering efficacy [14]. The SCAAR registry from Sweden demonstrated that ticagrelor increased survival and reduced bleeding risk in selected patients with ACS at low risk of bleeding [11]. Conversely, there is no European registry on the effect of ticagrelor in the STEMI population. The Greek GRAPE registry considered the clinical effect of clopidogrel, prasugrel, and ticagrelor in the general ACS population, hindering conclusions on the STEMI population. The GRAPE study demonstrated that ticagrelor does not reduce the rate of MACE at 1 year (HR, 0.78 [0.54–1.12]), whereas the bleeding rate increased (HR, 1.81 [1.55–2.10]) [16].

Our study is one of the few available registries on the effect of ticagrelor in a STEMI population and is the first to focus on the European setting. It has confirmed the findings from the PLATO trial. Our study demonstrated no benefit for ticagrelor with regard to cardiovascular death, AMI and stroke during the hospital phase. The risk reduction observed for in-hospital unadjusted cardiovascular mortality was not confirmed after propensity score analysis. This may be because of the use of a high clopidogrel loading dose (over 42% patients ≥300 mg) in the pre-hospital phase through the ambulance service. These results are concordant with the PLATO trial, where the beneficial effect of ticagrelor on MACE was achieved only after 30 days.

In our data, ticagrelor did not increase the risk of bleeding according to the BARC classification. This may depend on the lower haemorrhagic risk of the STEMI population compared with the general ACS population. The low haemorrhagic risk could have reduced the rate of clinically relevant bleeding even if the drug demonstrated a larger antiplatelet effect. Both these findings are in accordance with the PLATO subanalysis on STEMI.

A recent meta-analysis found a 20% reduced rate of MACE in patients on the new P2Y12 compared with clopidogrel [34], at the expense of a 50% increase in the risk of stroke. This was not confirmed in our study, where the proportions of MACE and stroke were similar in the 2 groups.

The main result of the present study, a reduction in 1-year mortality for ticagrelor, is concordant with the results of the PLATO study and the substudy in the STEMI population. In our registry, limited by the small sample size, this finding may be the result of statistical chance; however, it may also result from pharmacodynamic proprieties of ticagrelor that are distinct from its antiplatelet function, such as adenosine mimetic action [31]. Moreover, it may result from a favourable ratio between the unavoidable haemorrhagic risk and protection from ischaemic events. The observational registry by Park et al. [17] on ticagrelor in a STEMI population yielded contrasting results, showing that it did not reduce the risk of ischaemic events but was associated with an increased risk of bleeding compared with clopidogrel after controlling for propensity score. That study was conducted in Korea, thus it may lack external validity in Europe due to genetic variations and difference in patient characteristics, such as BMI or age. Furthermore, Park et al. considered only patients with STEMI undergoing PCI, excluding patients with STEMI undergoing medical therapy, where the beneficial effect of ticagrelor vs clopidogrel is increased [35].

In the present study, there was a 10% improvement in the success rate of primary PCI in patients on ticagrelor, with improvement in post-PCI TIMI 3 score ($p = 0.001$). This result came from crude data, without randomization or propensity score correction. Therefore, the better angiographic results in patients treated with ticagrelor could be secondary to chance. The PLATO angiographic substudy [36] showed that neither coronary flow nor myocardial perfusion demonstrated a difference with ticagrelor versus clopidogrel. However, in this substudy, the time interval between randomization and angiography or PCI was really short, particularly in the STEMI patients. In our institution, many patients were pretreated before arrival at the catheterization laboratory and the time for the pharmacological effect was longer. This fact, associated with greater platelet inhibition with ticagrelor, could have improved angiographic outcomes. Ticagrelor is also known to inhibit cell uptake of adenosine [31], and it could also be hypothesized that ticagrelor might increase the concentration of adenosine in the myocardium more than clopidogrel, inducing hyperemia and vasodilation, which is inconsistent with the results of the PLATO angiographic subgroup, where there was no improvement in coronary flow after percutaneous revascularization [36]. We should underline that this finding came from crude analysis and it could be biased by the lack of randomization or propensity score correction. However, in our sample, as in the PLATO angiographic subgroup, ticagrelor and clopidogrel achieved a similar proportion of ST resolution after PCI, with no effects on cardiac reperfusion.

Ticagrelor was discontinued in 2% of patients due to dyspnoea, a previously reported complication [6]. Other patients were converted to clopidogrel because of compliance problems, increased haemorrhagic risk or contemporary VKA treatment. There was only one intra-hospital death in the ticagrelor group (caused by cardiogenic shock), compared with 14 intra-hospital deaths in the clopidogrel group; this difference is relevant but it was not significant after controlling for the propensity score.

Limitations

This study has the limitations of a prospective case-control study. There were some differences between baseline and procedural data. Cases and controls were enrolled in different time periods, and this may contribute to confounding and to the different sizes of the study groups. However, we used propensity scores to minimize the bias related to lack of randomization, a strategy commonly used in other studies based on similar prospective registries. Power may be limited by sample size, however to our knowledge this study is the largest real-world registry on ticagrelor in Europe, even though the study was not powered for hard endpoints. The use of radial access was lower than the current standard and this issue could have had an unfavorable impact, increasing the bleeding risk in our sample. However, the type of access was included in the propensity score model in order to reduce the interference related to the differences between ticagrelor and clopidogrel groups. One further limitation is the lack of data collection on MACE and bleeding after the hospital phase. This may have influenced the perception of the favourable effects on the rate of MACE, which may become apparent only after 30 days [6]. However, this choice is often used during follow-up data collection within observational registries, as mortality is more easily and reliably collected after discharge, and it may be considered a surrogate outcome of complications including MACE and bleeding. Although the 2012 ESC guidelines recommended the use of ticagrelor or prasugrel in place of clopidogrel, in our institution prasugrel was not introduced during the time window examined in this study. This is mainly because prasugrel should not be administered in patients older than 75 years, with low body weight (≤60 kg) or with a history of previous CVA. So its introduction in our STEMI network, particularly in the pre-hospital setting, was considered difficult. We have no data on the duration of DAPT; however, each patient received indication to continue DAPT for at least 12 months after STEMI.

Conclusions

In this real-world single-centre experience, ticagrelor resulted in improved survival at 1 year versus clopidogrel in patients with STEMI, even after propensity score correction. Ticagrelor did not reduce the composite outcome of in hospital MACE, and it did not increase the risk of in-hospital bleeding. Although these results confirm data from previous subanalysis in STEMI patients, large RCTs are warranted to confirm the positive effect of ticagrelor shown in this population.

Additional files

Additional file 1: Baseline laboratory data. (DOCX 15 kb)

Additional file 2: Discharge therapy. Data are expressed as percentage (frequency). (DOCX 11 kb)

Additional file 3: Intra-hospital causes of death. Data are expressed as percentage (frequency). (DOCX 11 kb)

Additional file 4: Data on BARC bleeding. Data are expressed as percentage (frequency) or median (IQR). (DOCX 12 kb)

Additional file 5: Unadjusted Kaplan-Maier analysis on cardiovascular mortality at 1 year. (DOCX 51 kb)

Additional file 6: Interfering variables retained in the propensity score model. (DOCX 11 kb)

Abbreviations

ACS: Acute coronary syndrome; AMI: Acute myocardial infarction; BARC: Bleeding Academic Research Consortium; BMI: Body mass index; CI: Confidence interval; CRUSADE: Can rapid Risk stratification of Unstable angina patients Suppress ADverse outcome with Early implementation of ACC/AHA Guidelines; CVA: Cerebrovascular accident; DAPT: Dual antiplatelet treatment; DES: Drug-eluting stent; HR: Hazard ratio; IQR: Interquartile range; MACE: Major adverse cardiovascular event; MI: Myocardial infarction; NSTEMI: Non-ST-segment elevation myocardial infarction; OR: Odds ratio; PCI: Percutaneous coronary intervention; RCT: Randomized controlled trial; STEMI: ST-segment elevation myocardial infarction; TIMI score: Thrombolysis in myocardial infarction score; VKA: Vtamin K antagonist

Acknowledgements
None.

Funding
Cardio-STEMI is an independent study.
English language editing and styling assistance was provided by Edra spa, and unconditionally funded by AstraZeneca.

Authors' contributions
FAS and MV contributed to conception and study design. FAS designed the software to support data collection and acted as data manager. FAS, MV, VB, CT, DP, SC collected data. FAS, MV, VB and GGS helped in data analysis and interpretation. MV performed statistical analysis and acted as corresponding author. MV, FAS, VB were the major contributors in drafting the manuscript. GM and GP revised the manuscript critically for important intellectual content and supervised the development of the work. All authors read and approved the final manuscript.

Competing interests
Cardio-STEMI is an independent study.
The authors declare that they have no competing interests.
Editorial support, in the form of technical editing and language editing and proofreading was provided by Edra spa, and unconditionally funded by AstraZeneca, manufacturer of ticagrelor.

Author details
[1]Interventional Cardiology, Santi Antonio, Biagio e Cesare Arrigo Hospital, Alessandria, AL, Italy. [2]Coronary Care Unit, Sanremo Hospital, Sanremo, IM, Italy. [3]Interventional Cardiology, Sanremo Hospital, Sanremo, IM, Italy. [4]Sanremo Hospital, Sanremo, IM, Italy. [5]Emergency Room, Sanremo Hospital, Sanremo, IM, Italy. [6]Cardiology Unit, Santi Antonio, Biagio e Cesare Arrigo Hospital, Alessandria, AL, Italy. [7]Cardiology Unit, Sanremo Hospital, Sanremo, IM, Italy.

References

1. André R, Bongard V, Elosua R, Kirchberger I, Farmakis D, Häkkinen U, et al. International differences in acute coronary syndrome patients' baseline characteristics, clinical management and outcomes in Western Europe: the EURHOBOP study. Heart Br Card Soc. 2014;100:1201–7.

2. Mozaffarian D, Benjamin EJ, Go AS, Arnett DK, Blaha MJ, Cushman M, et al. Heart disease and stroke statistics - 2016 update: a report from the American Heart Association. Circulation. 2016;133:e38–360.

3. Wallentin L, Varenhorst C, James S, Erlinge D, Braun OO, Jakubowski JA, et al. Prasugrel achieves greater and faster P2Y12 receptor-mediated platelet inhibition than clopidogrel due to more efficient generation of its active metabolite in aspirin-treated patients with coronary artery disease. Eur Heart J. 2008;29:21–30.

4. Gurbel PA, Bliden KP, Butler K, Tantry US, Gesheff T, Wei C, et al. Randomized double-blind assessment of the ONSET and OFFSET of the antiplatelet effects of ticagrelor versus clopidogrel in patients with stable coronary artery disease: the ONSET/OFFSET study. Circulation. 2009;120:2577–85.

5. Wiviott SD, Braunwald E, McCabe CH, Montalescot G, Ruzyllo W, Gottlieb S, et al. Prasugrel versus clopidogrel in patients with acute coronary syndromes. N Engl J Med. 2007;357:2001–15.

6. Wallentin L, Becker RC, Budaj A, Cannon CP, Emanuelsson H, Held C, et al. Ticagrelor versus clopidogrel in patients with acute coronary syndromes. N Engl J Med. 2009;361:1045–57.

7. Morici N, Colombo P, Mafrici A, Oreglia JA, Klugmann S, Savonitto S. Prasugrel and ticagrelor: is there a winner? J Cardiovasc Med. 2014;15:8–18.

8. Alexopoulos D, Xanthopoulou I, Goudevenos J. Effects of P2Y12 receptor inhibition in patients with ST-segment elevation myocardial infarction. Am J Cardiol. 2014;113:2064–9.

9. Parodi G, Valenti R, Bellandi B, Migliorini A, Marcucci R, Comito V, et al. Comparison of prasugrel and ticagrelor loading doses in ST-segment elevation myocardial infarction patients. J Am Coll Cardiol. 2013;61:1601–6.

10. Steg PG, James S, Harrington RA, Ardissino D, Becker RC, Cannon CP, et al. Ticagrelor versus clopidogrel in patients with ST-elevation acute coronary syndromes intended for reperfusion with primary percutaneous coronary intervention: A Platelet Inhibition and Patient Outcomes (PLATO) trial subgroup analysis. Circulation. 2010;122:2131–41.

11. Damman P, Varenhorst C, Koul S, Eriksson P, Erlinge D, Lagerqvist B, et al. Treatment patterns and outcomes in patients undergoing percutaneous coronary intervention treated with prasugrel or clopidogrel (from the Swedish Coronary Angiography and Angioplasty Registry [SCAAR]). Am J Cardiol. 2014;113:64–9.

12. Bhatt DL. Prasugrel in clinical practice. N Engl J Med. 2009;361:940–2.

13. Bae JP, Faries DE, Ernst FR, Lipkin C, Zhao Z, Moretz C, et al. Real-world observations with prasugrel compared to clopidogrel in acute coronary syndrome patients treated with percutaneous coronary intervention in the United States. Curr Med Res Opin. 2014;30:2207–16.

14. Klingenberg R, Heg D, Räber L, Carballo D, Nanchen D, Gencer B, et al. Safety profile of prasugrel and clopidogrel in patients with acute coronary syndromes in Switzerland. Heart Br Card Soc. 2015;101:854–63.

15. Zeymer U, Hochadel M, Lauer B, Kaul N, Wöhrle J, Andresen D, et al. Use, efficacy and safety of prasugrel in patients with ST segment elevation myocardial infarction scheduled for primary percutaneous coronary intervention in clinical practice. Results of the prospective ATACS-registry. Int J Cardiol. 2015;184:122–7.

16. Alexopoulos D, Xanthopoulou I, Deftereos S, Hamilos M, Sitafidis G, Kanakakis I, et al. Contemporary antiplatelet treatment in acute coronary syndrome patients undergoing percutaneous coronary intervention: 1-year outcomes from the GReek AntiPlatElet (GRAPE) Registry. J Thromb Haemost. 2016;14:1146–54.

17. Park K-H, Jeong MH, Ahn Y, Ahn TH, Seung KB, Oh DJ, et al. Comparison of short-term clinical outcomes between ticagrelor versus clopidogrel in patients with acute myocardial infarction undergoing successful revascularization; from Korea Acute Myocardial Infarction Registry-National Institute of Health. Int J Cardiol. 2016;215:193–200.

18. D'Ascenzo F, Moretti C, Bianco M, Bernardi A, Taha S, Cerrato E, et al. Meta-analysis of the duration of dual antiplatelet therapy in patients treated with second-generation drug-eluting stents. Am J Cardiol. 2016;117:1714–23.

19. Thygesen K, Alpert JS, Jaffe AS, Simoons ML, Chaitman BR, White HD, et al. Third universal definition of myocardial infarction. J Am Coll Cardiol. 2012;60:1581–98.

20. Appleby MA, Angeja BG, Dauterman K, Gibson CM. Angiographic assessment of myocardial perfusion: TIMI myocardial perfusion (TMP) grading system. Heart. 2001;86:485–6.

21. Mehran R, Rao SV, Bhatt DL, Gibson CM, Caixeta A, Eikelboom J, et al. Standardized bleeding definitions for cardiovascular clinical trials: a consensus report from the Bleeding Academic Research Consortium. Circulation. 2011; 123:2736–47.

22. Steg G, James SK, Atar D, Badano LP, Blömstrom-Lundqvist C, Borger MA, et al. ESC guidelines for the management of acute myocardial infarction in patients presenting with ST-segment elevation. Eur Heart J. 2012;33:2569–619.

23. O'Gara PT, Kushner FG, Ascheim DD, Casey DE, Chung MK, de Lemos JA, et al. 2013 ACCF/AHA guideline for the management of ST-elevation myocardial infarction: executive summary. Circulation. 2013;127:529–55.

24. Cutlip DE, Windecker S, Mehran R, Boam A, Cohen DJ, van Es G-A, et al. Clinical end points in coronary stent trials: a case for standardized definitions. Circulation. 2007;115:2344–51.

25. Biondi-Zoccai G, Romagnoli E, Agostoni P, Capodanno D, Castagno D, D'Ascenzo F, et al. Are propensity scores really superior to standard multivariable analysis? Contemp Clin Trials. 2011;32:731–40.

26. Rassen JA, Glynn RJ, Brookhart MA, Schneeweiss S. Covariate selection in high-dimensional propensity score analyses of treatment effects in small samples. Am J Epidemiol. 2011;173:1404–13.

27. Hosmer DW, Lemeshow S. Applied logistic regression. New York: Wiley; 1989.

28. Hamm CW, Bassand J-P, Agewall S, Bax J, Boersma E, Bueno H, et al. ESC guidelines for the management of acute coronary syndromes in patients presenting without persistent ST-segment elevation: the Task Force for the management of acute coronary syndromes (ACS) in patients presenting without persistent ST-segment elevation of the European Society of Cardiology (ESC). Eur Heart J. 2011;32:2999–3054.

29. Hobl EL, Stimpfl T, Ebner J, Schoergenhofer C, Derhaschnig U, Sunder-Plassmann R, et al. Morphine decreases clopidogrel concentrations and effects: a randomized, double blind, placebo-controlled trial. J Am Coll Cardiol. 2014;63:630–5.

30. Alexopoulos D, Xanthopoulou I, Gkizas V, Kassimis G, Theodoropoulos KC, Makris G, et al. Randomized assessment of ticagrelor versus prasugrel antiplatelet effects in patients with ST-segment-elevation myocardial infarction. Circ Cardiovasc Interv. 2012;5:797–804.

31. Cattaneo M, Schultz R, Nylander S. Adenosine-mediated effects of ticagrelor. Evidence and potential clinical relevance. J Am Coll Cardiol. 2014;63:2503–9.

32. Alexopoulos D, Theodoropoulos KC, Stavrou EF, Xanthopoulou I, Kassimis G, Tsigkas G, et al. Prasugrel versus high dose clopidogrel to overcome early high on clopidogrel platelet reactivity in patients with ST elevation myocardial infarction. Cardiovasc Drugs Ther. 2012;26:393–400.

33. Mehta SR, Tanguay J-F, Eikelboom JW, Jolly SS, Joyner CD, Granger CB, et al. Double-dose versus standard-dose clopidogrel and high-dose versus low-dose aspirin in individuals undergoing percutaneous coronary intervention for acute coronary syndromes (CURRENT-OASIS 7): a randomised factorial trial. Lancet. 2010;376:1233–43.

34. Bellemain-Appaix A, Brieger D, Beygui F, Silvain J, Pena A, Cayla G, et al. New P2Y12 inhibitors versus clopidogrel in percutaneous coronary intervention: a meta-analysis. J Am Coll Cardiol. 2010;56:1542–51.

35. James SK, Roe MT, Cannon CP, Cornel JH, Horrow J, Husted S, et al. Ticagrelor versus clopidogrel in patients with acute coronary syndromes intended for non-invasive management: substudy from prospective randomised PLATelet inhibition and patient Outcomes (PLATO) trial. BMJ. 2011;342:d3527.

36. Kunadian V, James SK, Wojdyla DM, Zorkun C, Wu J, Storey RF, et al. Angiographic outcomes in the PLATO trial (Platelet Inhibition and Patient Outcomes). JACC Cardiovasc Interv. 2013;6:671–83.

26

Comparison of global myocardial strain assessed by cardiovascular magnetic resonance tagging and feature tracking to infarct size at predicting remodelling following STEMI

Abhishek M. Shetye[1,2], Sheraz A. Nazir[1], Naveed A. Razvi[1,3], Nathan Price[1,4], Jamal N. Khan[1], Florence Y. Lai[1], Iain B. Squire[1], Gerald P. McCann[1] and Jayanth R. Arnold[1*]

Abstract

Background: To determine if global strain parameters measured by cardiovascular magnetic resonance (CMR) acutely following ST-segment Elevation Myocardial Infarction (STEMI) predict adverse left ventricular (LV) remodelling independent of infarct size (IS).

Methods: Sixty-five patients with acute STEMI (mean age 60 ± 11 years) underwent CMR at 1–3 days post-reperfusion (baseline) and at 4 months. Global peak systolic circumferential strain (GCS), measured by tagging and Feature Tracking (FT), and global peak systolic longitudinal strain (GLS), measured by FT, were calculated at baseline, along with IS. On follow up scans, volumetric analysis was performed to determine the development of adverse remodelling – a composite score based on development of either end-diastolic volume index [EDVI] ≥20% or end-systolic volume index [ESVI] ≥15% at follow-up compared to baseline.

Results: The magnitude of GCS was higher when measured using FT ($-21.1 \pm 6.3\%$) than with tagging (-12.1 ± 4.3; $p < 0.001$ for difference). There was good correlation of strain with baseline LVEF (r 0.64–to 0.71) and IS (ρ -0.62 to–0.72). Baseline strain parameters were unable to predict development of adverse LV remodelling. Only baseline IS predicted adverse remodelling – Odds Ratio 1.05 (95% CI 1.01–1.10, $p = 0.03$), area under the ROC curve 0.70 (95% CI 0.52–0.87, $p = 0.04$).

Conclusion: Baseline global strain by CMR does not predict the development of adverse LV remodelling following STEMI.

Keywords: Cardiac magnetic resonance, Tagging, Feature tracking, Strain, Remodelling, ST-elevation myocardial infarction

* Correspondence: jra14@le.ac.uk
[1]Department of Cardiovascular Sciences, University of Leicester, Glenfield Hospital, Groby Road, Leicester LE3 9QF, UK
Full list of author information is available at the end of the article

Background

Adverse left ventricular (LV) remodelling is associated with poor outcome following ST-segment Elevation Myocardial Infarction (STEMI) [1–3]. Therefore, early recognition of at risk patients may enable targeted therapeutic intervention to attenuate adverse remodelling, and thereby reduce the progression to heart failure, and improve clinical outcome.

Myocardial strain describes the relative change in length of myocardial segments and provides an objective measure of LV function [4]. We have previously conducted a systematic review of seven studies that showed global longitudinal strain (GLS) as measured by speckle-tracking echocardiography predicts clinical outcome and LV remodelling following STEMI [5]. Infarct size (IS) has been shown to be a powerful predictor of adverse remodelling and prognosis following STEMI [6, 7]. However, IS cannot be quantified using routine echocardiography. Another disadvantage with echocardiography is that strain analysis may be hampered by variable image quality and the limited number of short axis views that are acquired [8], precluding the reliable assessment of global circumferential strain (GCS).

CMR is the gold standard non-invasive technique for the assessment of LV volumes and IS quantification [9, 10]. Myocardial tissue tagging has traditionally been regarded as the reference method for the quantification of peak systolic strain [11, 12]. Feature Tracking (FT) is a novel post-processing strain quantification technique that can be performed on routinely acquired steady-state free precession cine sequences. This avoids the difficulties of tagging, which requires additional image acquisitions with prolonged breath holding and time-consuming post-processing analysis [13, 14]. In a previous study of 24 patients following STEMI, FT was shown to be more robust and quicker to analyse, providing stronger correlation with IS and superior intra- and inter-observer variability when compared with tagging [14].

In one study of 74 patients following STEMI [15], GCS by FT predicted global functional recovery (left ventricular ejection fraction [LVEF] >50%) at follow-up but its utility in identifying patients who subsequently develop adverse remodelling was not demonstrated. Furthermore, there was no adjustment for IS, and strain as measured by FT was not compared with the established standard of tagging.

To date, there have been no reports assessing whether CMR-measured global strain is associated with adverse LV remodelling independent of IS. The primary aim of this study was to determine whether global strain parameters as assessed by CMR-tagging and FT could predict the development of adverse LV remodelling and whether they provide any incremental value to IS.

Methods

Study population

In a previously published study assessing the prevalence and extent of microvascular obstruction following STEMI, we recruited patients presenting to a single, regional cardiac centre in the UK with a first STEMI between January 2010 and December 2012 – the inclusion and exclusion criteria have been previously defined [16]. For the present study, the functional data derived from this earlier study were analysed. Baseline CMR was performed 1–3 days post reperfusion, with follow-up CMR, 4 months after admission. The study was conducted according to the Declaration of Helsinki, was approved by the local research ethics committee (Derbyshire Research Ethics Committee, **09/H0401/21**) and all patients provided written informed consent.

Imaging protocol

CMR was performed on a 1.5 T scanner (Siemens Avanto, Erlangen, Germany) using a 6-channel phased-array cardiac receiver coil – see Fig. 1 for study imaging protocol

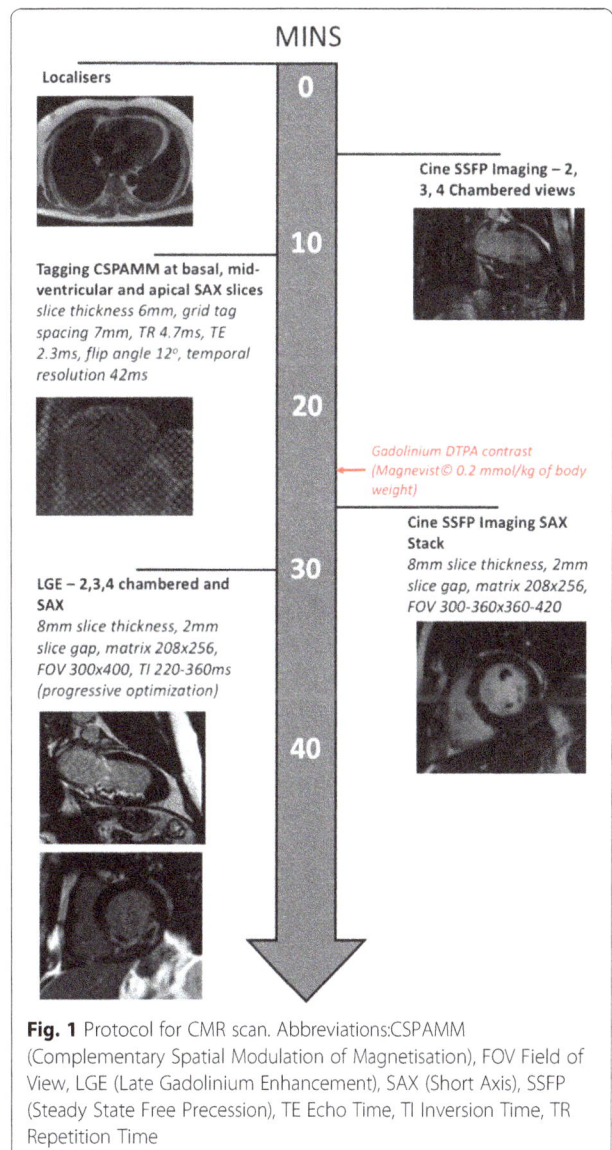

Fig. 1 Protocol for CMR scan. Abbreviations:CSPAMM (Complementary Spatial Modulation of Magnetisation), FOV Field of View, LGE (Late Gadolinium Enhancement), SAX (Short Axis), SSFP (Steady State Free Precession), TE Echo Time, TI Inversion Time, TR Repetition Time

for CMR scan (common at both baseline and follow-up). Cine and late gadolinium enhancement imaging were performed as previously described [16]. Three equidistant tagging short axis (SAX) cine images were acquired using complementary spatial modulation of magnetisation (CSPAMM) at base, mid-ventricle and apex.

Image analysis

All images were anonymised and, following completion of the study, were analysed offline by experienced operators blinded to all clinical information. Volumetric analysis and IS quantification were performed at the time of the original study whilst global strain assessment by tagging and FT was performed post-hoc after the original study had been completed.

Myocardial tagging

Strain was evaluated on SAX tagging images (NP) acquired at baseline using the SinMOD algorithm – *InTag* post-processing plugin (Creatis, Lyon, France) for *OsiriX* (Pixmeo, Switzerland) [13] – see Fig. 2. GCS was derived as an average of the values assessed at the three SAX slices as previously described [17]. Tagging images were not acquired in long axis views and consequently, only circumferential strain analysis was performed.

Feature tracking (ft)

Strain analysis on FT was performed using the *Diogenes Feature Tracking V6.3* (TomTec Imaging Systems, Munich, Germany) (AS) as previously described [14, 17, 18]. Briefly, endocardial contours were defined at end-diastole on SAX and long axis cine steady state free precession images and propagated – see Fig. 2. To determine GCS,

three equidistant SAX slices that best represented the base, mid-ventricle and apex were selected from the SAX stack similar to those used for tagging. To determine GLS, analysis was performed using the 2, 3 and 4-chamber long axis views.

Volumetric analysis & infarct size quantification

Volumetric, functional and IS assessment were performed using *QMass V7.1* (Medis, Leiden, Netherlands) (NAR and JNK). All volumes were indexed to Body Surface Area. IS was quantified semi-automatically using the full-width half-maximum technique as previously described [19]. Adverse LV remodelling was calculated as a composite score based on development of either a relative increase in end-systolic volume index of 15% or a relative increase in end-diastolic volume index of 20% at follow-up compared with baseline [1, 20]

Statistical analysis

Normality was assessed using the Shapiro-Wilk test, histograms and Q-Q plots. Normally distributed data are expressed as mean ± SD whilst non-normally distributed data are shown as median (interquartile range). Comparison of normally distributed data was performed using paired *t*-test, and non-normally distributed data, using Mann–Whitney *U*-test, and categorical data, using Chi-Squared test. Correlation between parameters was assessed using either Pearson's correlation coefficient (r) or Spearman's rank coefficient (ρ) where appropriate.

Logistic regression was performed to assess predictors of the LV remodelling parameters. Receiver operator characteristic curve analysis was performed for all significant predictors of adverse LV remodelling. All values

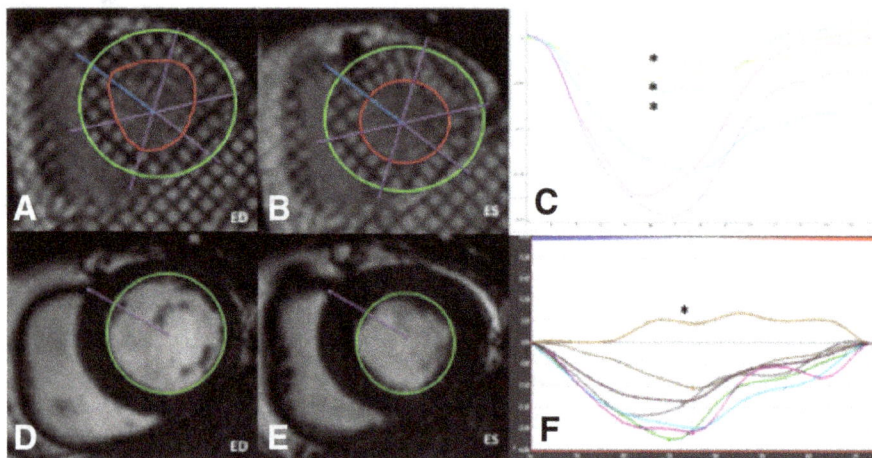

Fig. 2 Comparison of strain analysis by tagging and feature tracking (FT) at short axis (SAX). (**a**, **b**) Tagged complementary spatial modulation of magnetisation (CSPAMM) basal short axis slice shown with endocardial and epicardial contours at *end-diastole* (*ED*) *end-systole* (*ES*) in a patient following inferior MI. (**c**) The resultant peak systolic circumferential strain curve at each segment with severely hypokinetic segments denoted by an (*). (**d**, **e**) Feature Tracking (FT) on cine Steady State Free Precession (SSFP) SAX slice with endocardial borders defined is shown at *ED* (**d**) and *ES* (E). (**f**) Segmental peak systolic circumferential strain curve by FT with dyskinetic segment denoted by an asterisk (*)

with $p < 0.05$ were considered statistically significant. Statistical analysis was performed using *SPSS version 22.0* (Chicago, IL)

Results

Baseline characteristics

Table 1 summarised the baseline characteristics of the study population. Sixty-five patients underwent baseline and follow-up CMR scans. Patients were treated as follows: primary PCI ($n = 39$, 60%), thrombolysis ($n = 13$, 20%), rescue PCI ($n = 8$, 12%) and late-PCI ($n = 5$, 8%). Thrombolysis was performed with tissue plasminogen

Table 1 Key patient characteristics

Demographics			
Age, years	59.5 ± 11.0		
Male sex, n (%)	60 (92)		
Current/previous smoker, n (%)	28 (43.1)		
Hypercholesterolaemia, n (%)	15 (23.1)		
Hypertension, n (%)	19 (29.2)		
Admission HR, beats per minute	76 ± 12		
Admission Systolic BP, mmHg	124 ± 26		
Admission Diastolic BP, mmHg	75 ± 15		
Peak Creatine Kinase, iU/L	1064 (418–2588)		
Anterior STEMI, n (%)	30 (46)		
Discharge Medications			
Aspirin, n (%)	57 (88)		
Clopidogrel, n (%)	59 (91)		
Warfarin, n (%)	6 (9)		
Statin, n (%)	63 (97)		
Beta-blocker, n (%)	64 (99)		
ACEi/ARA, n (%)	63 (97)		
Loop/Thiazide Diuretic, n (%)	5 (8)		
Spironolactone/ Eplerenone, n (%)	7 (11)		
CMR Parameters	Baseline	Follow-up	p-value
LVEDVI, ml/m^{-2}	91.1 (84.5–102.2)	93.5 (85.0–106)	0.454
LVESVI, ml/m^{-2}	53.5 (47.6–65.9)	47.7 (39.8–61.6)	0.001
LVEF, %	41.0 ± 8.40	47.2 ± 8.46	<0.001
IS, % (of LV mass)	22.3 (14.5–35.5)	17.0 (12.3–22.8)	<0.001

Abbreviations: *ACEi* (Angiotensin Converting Enzyme Inhibitor), *ARB* (Angiotensin-II Receptor Blocker), *BP* (Blood Pressure), *CAD* (Coronary Artery Disease), *HR* (Heart Rate), *IS* (Infarct Size), *LV* (Left Ventricular), *LVEDVI* (Left Ventricular End Diastolic Volume), *LVEF* (Left Ventricular Ejection Fraction), *LVESVI* (Left Ventricular End Systolic Volume), *N/A* (Not Applicable), *STEMI* (ST-segment Elevation Myocardial Infarction)

activator analogues where facilities for primary PCI were not available within a two-hour period of symptom-onset. Rescue PCI was performed in patients in whom ST-segment resolution of >50% post-thrombolysis was not achieved. Late PCI describes primary PCI >12 h after symptom onset in the presence of ECG and/or clinical evidence of continuing ischaemia.

Cmr findings

Key patient characteristics are shown in Table 1. Compared with baseline, there was a decrease in LV end-systolic volume index at follow up (47.7 ml.m^{-2} versus 53.5 ml.m^{-2}, mean difference –5.6 ml.m^{-2}, $p < 0.001$) and an increase in LVEF (47.2 ± 8.5 versus 41.0 ± 8.4%, mean difference 6.2%, $p < 0.001$). Eleven (16.9%) patients had developed adverse LV remodelling – nine (13.8%) patients had an increase in LV end-systolic volume index ≥15%, and six (9.2%) patients had an increase in LV end-diastolic volume index ≥20%.

Strain at baseline

Strain analysis was possible in all ($n = 65$) patients with FT and in 64 patients with tagging (one patient had non-analysable images). GCS was significantly higher with FT than with tagging (–21.1 ± 6.3% versus –12.1 ± 4.3%, $p < 0.001$). GLS by FT was –13.2 ± 5.5%.

Correlation of strain with baseline lvef & is

There was good correlation of GCS, measured by both FT and tagging, with baseline IS ($\rho = -0.72$ for tagging and $\rho = -0.61$ for FT) and LVEF ($r = 0.70$ for tagging and $r = 0.71$ for FT). GLS (FT) also had similar correlation with baseline IS and LVEF (Table 2).

Prediction of adverse lv remodelling

None of the baseline strain parameters was able to predict the development of adverse LV remodelling (Table 3). Only baseline IS predicted the development of adverse LV remodelling with statistical significance, albeit modestly – Odds Ratio 1.05 (1.01–1.10, $p = 0.03$, i.e. the odds of a patient having developed adverse LV remodelling increased

Table 2 Correlation of baseline strain parameters with LVEF and IS

	Infarct size (IS)	Ejection Fraction (LVEF)
Tagging (n = 64)		
GCS	–0.72**	0.70**
Feature Tracking		
GCS	–0.61**	0.71**
GLS	–0.62**	0.64**

Abbreviations: *EF* (Ejection Fraction), *GCS* (Global Circumferential Strain), *GLS* (Global Longitudinal Strain), *IS* (Infarct Size)
Note: Spearman's Rank coefficient (ρ) for IS, Pearson's correlation coefficient (r) for EF
**$p < 0.01$

Table 3 Global Strain and IS to predict development of LV remodelling

Baseline Variable	Prediction of Adverse Remodelling – OR (95% CI, p-value)
GCS (FT), %	0.92 (0.83–1.03, p = 0.16)
GLS (FT), %	0.90 (0.79–1.03, p = 0.14)
GCS (Tagging), %	0.88 (0.74–1.05, p = 0.15)
IS, %	1.05 (1.01–1.10, p = 0.03)*

Abbreviations: CI (Confidence Interval), FT (Feature Tracking), GCS (Global Circumferential Strain), GLS (Global Longitudinal Strain), IS (Infarct Size) OR (Odds Ratio)
*p < 0.05

by 0.05% for every unit increase in baseline IS). In predicting adverse remodelling, the area-under-the curve with receiver operator characteristic curve analysis for baseline IS was moderate – 0.70 (0.52–0.87, p = 0.04) (Fig. 3).

Discussion

This is the first study to evaluate the role of CMR-based strain assessment (using both tagging and FT) in predicting adverse LV remodelling following STEMI. Our data showed that although global strain parameters appear to have a good correlation with baseline IS, none of them can significantly predict the development of remodelling. The only significant predictor of adverse LV remodelling appears to be baseline IS and this is consistent with previous results [7].

The only other study to evaluate the role of CMR-based global strain at predicting endpoints post-STEMI evaluated FT in isolation (without tagging) and showed

that GCS was associated with the development of LVEF > 50% at follow-up [15]. However, this study identified 'low risk' subjects with global functional LV recovery and rather than those with adverse LV remodelling.

Previous studies have shown that strain, as evaluated by both tagging and FT, appears to be decreased in the myocardial segments in the infarcted region compared with non-infarcted segments [21, 22]. This may explain the good correlation between baseline strain parameters and IS. However, unlike IS, which is purely a measure of myocardial scar burden, global strain is influenced by both infarct- and non-infarct-related myocardial segments. Consequently, there may have been hyperkinetic wall motion in the non-infarct related segments leading to a 'preserved' overall global strain value in some patients. This may explain the superiority of IS in predicting adverse LV remodelling given that, unlike global strain, it is purely a measure of the extent of myocardial damage post-infarction. Furthermore, segmental strain analysis by both tagging and FT has been shown to have high intra- and inter-observer variability and therefore may not be a reliable measure of LV function in a clinical setting [14].

Our results suggest that CMR-based global strain may not have a significant role to play in the setting of acute STEMI as has previously been suggested [15]. Larger studies will be required to determine whether acutely measured strain by CMR is predictive of clinical endpoints (such as mortality and/or development of Major Adverse Cardiac Events, MACE) and provides incremental prognostic data compared with IS assessment alone.

Limitations

This study had a relatively small sample size with a small proportion of patients developing remodelling. This may partly represent the beneficial effects of secondary prevention measures (angiotensin-converting enzyme inhibitors, beta-blockers and statins) which were prescribed in the majority of patients and known to prevent remodelling post-STEMI [23]. Additionally, other markers of poor post-STEMI outcomes, such as age and infarct location, could not be accounted for in the regression model without risk of 'over-fitting' [24, 25]. Our patients were predominantly male so further studies are required in cohorts with larger numbers of female patients [26]. Technical limitations of CMR-based strain assessment include sub-optimal tracking of endocardial motion on some post-contrast SSFP images due to reduced contrast-to-noise ratio between the blood pool and myocardium (FT) and image degradation due to poor breath-holding and ectopy (tagging) [14]. Tagging sequences were not acquired in long axis views and hence the value of GLS after STEMI could not be assessed.

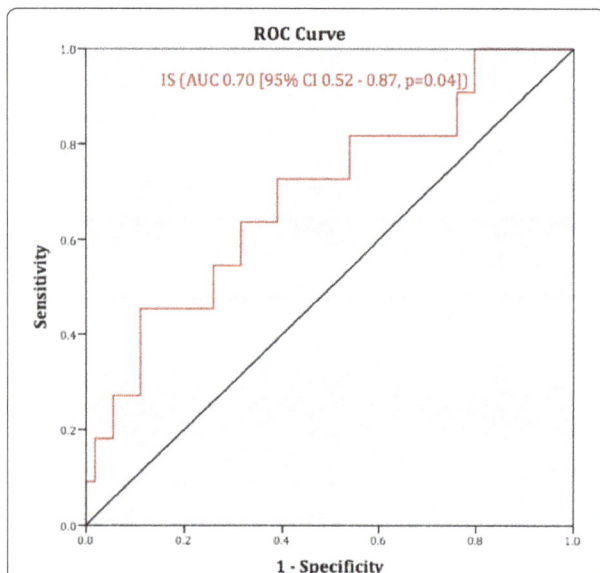

Fig. 3 Receiver Operator Characteristic *Curve* for baseline Infarct Size to predict LV End-Systolic Volume Index ≥15% at follow-up versus baseline. Abbreviations: AUC (Area Under the *Curve*); CI (95% Confidence Interval); IS (Infarct Size)

Conclusions

CMR measured global strain was correlated with baseline IS following STEMI but had no significant value in predicting adverse LV remodelling. Further work is needed to determine if this holds true for the prediction of clinical endpoints post-STEMI.

Abbreviations

CMR: Cardiac magnetic resonance imaging; FT: Feature tracking; GCS: Global circumferential strain; GLS: Global longitudinal strain; IS: Infarct size; LV: Left ventricular; LVEF: Left ventricular ejection fraction; PCI: Percutaneous coronary intervention; SAX: Short axis; STEMI: ST-segment elevation myocardial Infarction.

Acknowledgements

Not applicable.

Funding

British Heart Foundation (BHF), National Institute for Health Research (NIHR), and the University of Leicester, United Kingdom. This work is part of a student (AS) Bachelor of Science project funded by the University of Leicester and the NIHR (GPM is supported by a NIHR Postdoctoral Research Fellowship). All patients were recruited as part of a previous project grant funded by the BHF (Title: *Plasma matrix metalloproteinase and tissue inhibitor of metalloproteinase after acute myocardial infarction in man: a cardiac magnetic resonance study of left ventricular remodelling* – Grant number: *PG /08/082/ 2572*) and the NIHR Leicester Cardiovascular Biomedical Research Unit.

Authors' contributions

GPM, SAN, JRA and IS designed the concept of the study; NAR recruited the patients; NAR and GPM supervised patient scans; NP performed tagging analysis on all patients; NAR and JNK performed volumetric analysis and infarct size quantification on all scans; AS performed Feature Tracking analysis on all patients, statistical analysis and wrote the manuscript; FYL performed statistical analysis on the data; JRA helped in writing the manuscript along with any key revisions needed; All the authors reviewed the manuscript, provided key revisions as necessary and approved the final version of the manuscript.

Competing interests

The authors declare that they have no competing interests.

Author details

[1]Department of Cardiovascular Sciences, University of Leicester, Glenfield Hospital, Groby Road, Leicester LE3 9QF, UK. [2]Oxford University Hospitals NHS Trust, Oxford OX3 9DU, UK. [3]Ipswich Hospital NHS trust, Ipswich IP4 5PD, UK. [4]Leeds Institute of Cardiovascular and Metabolic Medicine (LICAMM), University of Leeds, Leeds LS2 9JT, UK.

References

1. Cohn JN, Ferrari R, Sharpe N. Cardiac remodeling–concepts and clinical implications: a consensus paper from an international forum on cardiac remodeling. Behalf of an International Forum on Cardiac Remodeling. J Am Coll Cardiol. 2000;35(3):569–82.
2. Bolognese L, Neskovic AN, Parodi G, Cerisano G, Buonamici P, Santoro GM, Antoniucci D. Left ventricular remodeling after primary coronary angioplasty: patterns of left ventricular dilation and long-term prognostic implications. Circulation. 2002;106(18):2351–7.
3. Konstam MA, Kramer DG, Patel AR, Maron MS, Udelson JE. Left ventricular remodeling in heart failure: current concepts in clinical significance and assessment. J Am Coll Cardiol Img. 2011;4(1):98–108.
4. Zwanenburg JJM. Mapping Asynchrony of Circumferential Shortening in the Human Heart with High Temporal Resolution MRI Tagging. Amsterdam: Vrije University; 2005.
5. Shetye A, Nazir SA, Squire IB, McCann GP. Global myocardial strain assessment by different imaging modalities to predict outcomes after ST-elevation myocardial infarction: A systematic review. World J Cardiol. 2015; 7(12):948–60.
6. Ezekowitz JA, Armstrong PW, Granger CB, Theroux P, Stebbins A, Kim RJ, Patel MR. Predicting chronic left ventricular dysfunction 90 days after ST-segment elevation myocardial infarction: An Assessment of Pexelizumab in Acute Myocardial Infarction (APEX-AMI) Substudy. Am Heart J. 2010;160(2):272–8.
7. Chareonthaitawee P, Christian TF, Hirose K, Gibbons RJ, Rumberger JA. Relation of initial infarct size to extent of left ventricular remodeling in the year after acute myocardial infarction. J Am Coll Cardiol. 1995;25(3):567–73.
8. Feigenbaum H, Mastouri R, Sawada S. A practical approach to using strain echocardiography to evaluate the left ventricle. Circ J. 2012;76(7):1550–5.
9. Flachskampf FA, Schmid M, Rost C, Achenbach S, DeMaria AN, Daniel WG. Cardiac imaging after myocardial infarction. Eur Heart J. 2011;32(3):272–83.
10. Pattynama PM, De Roos A, Van der Wall EE, Van Voorthuisen AE. Evaluation of cardiac function with magnetic resonance imaging. Am Heart J. 1994; 128(3):595–607.
11. Khan JN, Wilmot EG, Leggate M, Singh A, Yates T, Nimmo M, Khunti K, Horsfield MA, Biglands J, Clarysse P, et al. Subclinical diastolic dysfunction in young adults with Type 2 diabetes mellitus: a multiparametric contrast-enhanced cardiovascular magnetic resonance pilot study assessing potential mechanisms. Eur Heart J Cardiovasc Imaging. 2014;15(11):1263–9.
12. Clark NR, Reichek N, Bergey P, Hoffman EA, Brownson D, Palmon L, Axel L. Circumferential myocardial shortening in the normal human left ventricle. Assessment by magnetic resonance imaging using spatial modulation of magnetization. Circulation. 1991;84(1):67–74.
13. Clarysse P, Basset C, Khouas L, Croisille P, Friboulet D, Odet C, Magnin IE. Two-dimensional spatial and temporal displacement and deformation field fitting from cardiac magnetic resonance tagging. Med Image Anal. 2000; 4(3):253–68.
14. Khan JN, Singh A, Nazir SA, Kanagala P, Gershlick AH, McCann GP: Comparison of cardiovascular magnetic resonance feature tracking and tagging for the assessment of left ventricular systolic strain in acute myocardial infarction. Eur J Radiol. 2015;84(5):840–8.
15. Buss SJ, Krautz B, Hofmann N, Sander Y, Rust L, Giusca S, Galuschky C, Seitz S, Giannitsis E, Pleger S, et al. Prediction of functional recovery by cardiac magnetic resonance feature tracking imaging in first time ST-elevation myocardial infarction. Comparison to infarct size and transmurality by late gadolinium enhancement. Int J Cardiol. 2015;183C:162–70.
16. Khan JN, Razvi N, Nazir SA, Singh A, Masca NG, Gershlick AH, Squire I, McCann GP. Prevalence and extent of infarct and microvascular obstruction following different reperfusion therapies in ST-elevation myocardial infarction. J Cardiovasc Magn Reson. 2014;16:38.
17. Singh A, Steadman CD, Khan JN, Horsfield MA, Bekele S, Nazir SA, Kanagala P, Masca NG, Clarysse P, McCann GP: Intertechnique agreement and interstudy reproducibility of strain and diastolic strain rate at 1.5 and 3 tesla: A comparison of feature-tracking and tagging in patients with aortic stenosis. J Magn Reson Imaging. 2015;41(4):1129–37.
18. Hor KN, Baumann R, Pedrizzetti G, Tonti G, Gottliebson WM, Taylor M, Benson W, Mazur W: Magnetic resonance derived myocardial strain assessment using feature tracking. J Vis Exp. 2011;12(48). doi:10.3791/2356.
19. Khan JN, Nazir SA, Horsfield MA, Singh A, Kanagala P, Greenwood JP, Gershlick AH, McCann GP. Comparison of semi-automated methods to quantify infarct size and area at risk by cardiovascular magnetic resonance imaging at 1.5T and 3.0T field strengths. BMC Res Notes. 2015;8(1):52.
20. Cong T, Sun Y, Shang Z, Wang K, Su D, Zhong L, Zhang S, Yang Y: Prognostic Value of Speckle Tracking Echocardiography in Patients with ST-Elevation Myocardial Infarction Treated with Late Percutaneous Intervention. Echocardiography. 2015;32(9):1384–91.
21. Marcus JT, Gotte MJ, Van Rossum AC, Kuijer JP, Heethaar RM, Axel L, Visser CA. Myocardial function in infarcted and remote regions early after infarction in man: assessment by magnetic resonance tagging and strain analysis. Magn Reson Med. 1997;38(5):803–10.
22. Maret E, Todt T, Brudin L, Nylander E, Swahn E, Ohlsson JL, Engvall JE. Functional measurements based on feature tracking of cine magnetic

resonance images identify left ventricular segments with myocardial scar. Cardiovasc Ultrasound. 2009;7:53.

23. Task Force on the management of STseamiotESoC, Steg PG, James SK, Atar D, Badano LP, Blomstrom-Lundqvist C, Borger MA, Di Mario C, Dickstein K, Ducrocq G, et al. ESC Guidelines for the management of acute myocardial infarction in patients presenting with ST-segment elevation. Eur Heart J. 2012;33(20):2569–619.

24. Babyak MA. What you see may not be what you get: a brief, nontechnical introduction to overfitting in regression-type models. Psychosom Med. 2004;66(3):411–21.

25. Pocock SJ, Wang D, Pfeffer MA, Yusuf S, McMurray JJ, Swedberg KB, Ostergren J, Michelson EL, Pieper KS, Granger CB. Predictors of mortality and morbidity in patients with chronic heart failure. Eur Heart J. 2006; 27(1):65–75.

26. Andre F, Steen H, Matheis P, Westkott M, Breuninger K, Sander Y, Kammerer R, Galuschky C, Giannitsis E, Korosoglou G, et al. Age- and gender-related normal left ventricular deformation assessed by cardiovascular magnetic resonance feature tracking. J Cardiovasc Magn Reson. 2015;17(1):25.

Permissions

The contributors of this book come from diverse backgrounds, making this book a truly international effort. This book will bring forth new frontiers with its revolutionizing research information and detailed analysis of the nascent developments around the world.

We would like to thank all the contributing authors for lending their expertise to make the book truly unique. They have played a crucial role in the development of this book. Without their invaluable contributions this book wouldn't have been possible. They have made vital efforts to compile up to date information on the varied aspects of this subject to make this book a valuable addition to the collection of many professionals and students.

This book was conceptualized with the vision of imparting up-to-date information and advanced data in this field. To ensure the same, a matchless editorial board was set up. Every individual on the board went through rigorous rounds of assessment to prove their worth. After which they invested a large part of their time researching and compiling the most relevant data for our readers.

The editorial board has been involved in producing this book since its inception. They have spent rigorous hours researching and exploring the diverse topics which have resulted in the successful publishing of this book. They have passed on their knowledge of decades through this book. To expedite this challenging task, the publisher supported the team at every step. A small team of assistant editors was also appointed to further simplify the editing procedure and attain best results for the readers.

Apart from the editorial board, the designing team has also invested a significant amount of their time in understanding the subject and creating the most relevant covers. They scrutinized every image to scout for the most suitable representation of the subject and create an appropriate cover for the book.

The publishing team has been an ardent support to the editorial, designing and production team. Their endless efforts to recruit the best for this project, has resulted in the accomplishment of this book. They are a veteran in the field of academics and their pool of knowledge is as vast as their experience in printing. Their expertise and guidance has proved useful at every step. Their uncompromising quality standards have made this book an exceptional effort. Their encouragement from time to time has been an inspiration for everyone.

The publisher and the editorial board hope that this book will prove to be a valuable piece of knowledge for researchers, students, practitioners and scholars across the globe.

List of Contributors

Yu-Tsung Cheng, Tsun-Jui Li u, Hui-Chin Lai, Wen-Lieng Lee, Hung-Yun Ho, Chieh-Shou Su and Kuo-Yang Wang
Cardiovascular Center and Department of Anesthesiology, Taichung Veterans General Hospital, Taichung, Taiwan

Tsun-Jui Liu, Hui-Chin Lai, Wen-Lieng Lee, Chieh-Shou Su and Kuo-Yang Wang
Departments of Medicine and Surgery, Yang-Ming University School of Medicine, Taipei, Taiwan

Chia-Ning Liu
Taipei First Girls High School, Taipei, Taiwan

Kuo-Yang Wang
Chung-Shan Medical University School of Medicine, Taichung, Taiwan

Tongtong Yu, Yuanyuan Dong, Jiahe Zhu, Chunyang Tian, Zhijun Sun and Zhaoqing Sun
Department of Cardiology, Shengjing Hospital of China Medical University, Shenyang, Liaoning, People's Republic of China

Jeremy Adams and Harindra C. Wijeysundera
Division of Cardiology, Schulich Heart Centre, Sunnybrook Health Sciences Centre, 2075 Bayview Avenue, Suite A202, Toronto, ON M4N3M5, Canada

eremy Adams, Brian Wong and Harindra C. Wijeysundera
Department of Medicine, Sunnybrook Health Sciences Centre, University of Toronto, Toronto, ON, Canada

Brian Wong
Centre for Quality Improvement and Patient Safety, University of Toronto, Toronto, ON, Canada

Harindra C. Wijeysundera
Institute of Health Policy, Management and Evaluation, University of Toronto, Toronto, ON, Canada
Institute for Clinical Evaluative Sciences (ICES), Toronto, ON, Canada
Li Ka Shing Knowledge Institute of St. Michael Hospital, University of Toronto, Toronto, ON, Canada

Zhang-Wei Chen, Zi-Qing Yu, Hong-Bo Yang, Ju-Ying Qian, Xian-Hong Shu and Jun-Bo Ge
Department of Cardiology, Shanghai Institute of Cardiovascular Diseases, Zhongshan Hospital, Fudan University, 180 Fenglin Road, Shanghai 200032, PR China

Ying-Hua Chen
Department of Endocrinology Medicine, East Hospital, Tongji University School of Medicine, Shanghai 200120, China

Yoshito Kadoya
Department of Internal Medicine, Kyotambacho Hospital, Kyotambacho, Kyoto, Japan

Tsuneaki Kenzaka
Division of Community Medicine and Career Development, Kobe University Graduate School of Medicine, Kobe, Japan

Ruwanthi Bandara, Ruwan Munasinghe, Nandana Dinamithra, Amila Subasinghe, Jayantha Herath, Mahesh Ratnayake and Buddhini Imbulpitiya
Professorial Medical Unit, Teaching Hospital Peradeniya, Peradeniya, Sri Lanka

Arjuna Medagama and Ameena Sulaiman
Department of Medicine, Faculty of Medicine, University of Peradeniya, Peradeniya, Sri Lanka

Yotsawee Chotechuang
Clinical Epidemiology Program, Faculty of Medicine, Chiang Mai University, Chiang Mai 50200, Thailand

Yotsawee Chotechuang
Cardiology Division, Internal Medicine Department, Lampang Hospital, Lampang 52000, Thailand

Arintaya Phrommintikul, Srun Kuanprasert, Noparat Thanachikun, Thanawat Benjanuwatra and Apichard Sukonthasarn
Cardiology Division, Department of Internal Medicine, Faculty of Medicine, Chiang Mai University, Chiang Mai 50200, Thailand

Roungtiva Muenpa
Pharmaceutical Care Unit, Pharmacy Department, Lampang Hospital, Lampang 52000, Thailand

Jayanton Patumanond
Center of Excellence in Applied Epidemiology, Faculty of Medicine, Thammasat University, Bangkok 12121, Thailand

Tuanchai Chaichuen
Cardiac catheterization laboratory Unit, Maharaj Nakorn Chiang Mai Hospital, Chiang Mai, Thailand

Hong Zhang, Yong-chun Cui, Yi Tian, Wei-min Yuan, Jian-zhong Yang, Peng Peng, Kai Li, Xiao-peng Liu, Dong Zhang, Ai-li Wu and Yue Tang
Animal Experiment Center & Beijing Key Laboratory of Pre-clinical Research and Evaluation for Cardiovascular Implant Materials, Beijing 100037, People's Republic of China

Zhou Zhou
Center of Clinical Laboratory, State Key Laboratory of Cardiovascular Disease, Fu Wai Hospital, National Center for Cardiovascular Diseases, Chinese Academy of Medical Sciences and Peking Union Medical College, Beijing 100037, China

Hans-Josef Feistritzer, Sebastian Johannes Reinstadler, Gert Klug, Martin Reindl, Sebastian Wöhrer, Christoph Brenner, Johannes Mair and Bernhard Metzler
University Clinic of Internal Medicine III, Cardiology and Angiology, Medical University of Innsbruck, Anichstraße 35, A-6020 Innsbruck, Austria

Agnes Mayr
Department of Radiology, Medical University of Innsbruck, Anichstraße 35, A-6020 Innsbruck, Austria

Chunlai Shao, Jing Zhu, Jianchang Chen and Weiting Xu
Department of Cardiology, The Second Affiliated Hospital of Soochow University, Sanxiang Street 1055, Suzhou, China

Wang Yunyun, Li Tong, Liu Yingwu, Liu Bojiang, Wang Yu, Hu Xiaomin, Li Xin and Peng Wenjin
Cardiac Center, Third Central Hospital of Tian Jin, Tian Jin 300170, China

JinFang Li
Essen Medical Associates, P.C.2015 Grand concourse, Bronx, NY 10453, USA

Peng-cheng He, Yuan-hui Liu, Xue-biao Wei and Shu-guang Lin
Department of Cardiology, Guangdong Cardiovascular Institute, Guangdong Provincial Key Laboratory of Coronary Heart Disease Prevention, Guangdong General Hospital, Guangdong Academy of Medical Sciences, Guangzhou 510080, Guangdong, China

Chong-yang Duan
State Key Laboratory of Organ Failure Research, National Clinical Research Center for Kidney Disease, Guangzhou, China

Chong-yang Duan
Department of Biostatistics, School of Public Health, Southern Medical University, Guangzhou 510515, China

Yuan Gao, Lina Ren, Dandan Fan and Guoxian Qi
Department of Cardiology, First Affiliated Hospital of China Medical University, Shenyang, Liaoning 110001, China

Daming Jiang
Department of Cardiology, Dandong Center Hospital, Dandong, Liaoning 118000, China

Bo Zhang
Department of Cardiology, First Affiliated Hospital, Dalian Medical University, Dalian, Liaoning 116011, China

Yujiao Sun
Department of Geriatric Cardiology, First Affiliated Hospital of China Medical University, Shenyang, Liaoning 110001, China

Ibrahim Akin and Uzair Ansari
Universitäts medizin Mannheim, Mannheim, Germany

Henrik Schneider
Universitätsklinikum Rostock und Hanseklinikum Wismar, Rostock, Germany

Christoph A. Nienaber
Universitätsklinikum Rostock, Rostock, Germany

Werner Jung and Mike Lübke
Schwarzwald-Baar Klinikum Villingen-Schwenningen, Villingen-Schwenningen, Germany

Andreas Rillig
Asklepios Klinikum St. Georg Hamburg, Hamburg, Germany

Nina Wunderlich
Universitätsklinikum Rostock und Kardiovaskuläres Zentrum Darmstadt, Darmstadt, Germany

Ralf Birkemeyer
Universitätsklinikum Rostock und Herzklinik Ulm, Ulm, Germany

Ibrahim Akin
Medical Faculty Mannheim, University Heidelberg, Theodor-Kutzer Ufer 1-3, 68167 Mannheim, Germany

Regina El Dib
Department of Anaesthesiology, Botucatu Medical School, Unesp – Univ Estadual Paulista, São Paulo, Brazil

Regina El Dib
McMaster Institute of Urology, McMaster University, Hamilton, Ontario, Canada

Frederick Alan Spencer
Division of Cardiology, Department of Medicine, McMaster University, St. Joseph's Healthcare - 50 Charlton Avenue East, Hamilton, Ontario, Canada

Erica Aranha Suzumura
Research Institute - Hospital do Coração (HCor), São Paulo, Brazil

Huda Gomaa
Department of Pharmacy, Tanta Chest Hospital, Tanta, Egypt

Joey Kwong
Division of Cardiology and Heart Education And Research Training (HEART) Centre, Department of Medicine and Therapeutics, Prince of Wales Hospital and Institute of Vascular Medicine, The Chinese University of Hong Kong, Shatin, Hong Kong

Gordon Henry Guyatt
Department of Clinical Epidemiology and Biostatistics, McMaster University, Hamilton, Ontario, Canada
Department of Medicine, McMaster University, Hamilton, Ontario, Canada

Per Olav Vandvik
Department of Medicine, Innlandet Hospital Trust-Division Gjøvik, Oppland, Norway
Institute for Health and Society, Faculty of Medicine, University of Oslo, Oslo, Norway

Mohammad Azizul Karim, Abdullah Al Shafi Majumder and Khandaker Qamrul Islam
National Institute of Cardiovascular Diseases (NICVD), Dhaka, Bangladesh

Muhammad Badrul Alam
Rangpur Medical College, Rangpur, Bangladesh

Makhan Lal Paul
Central Medical College, Comilla, Bangladesh

Mohammad Shafiqul Islam
Trishal Health Complex, Mymensingh, Bangladesh

Kamrun N. Chowdhury
Department of Epidemiology, National Centre for Control of Rheumatic Fever and Heart Disease, Dhaka, Bangladesh

Sheikh Mohammed Shariful Islam
International Center for Diarrhoeal Disease Research, Bangladesh, Center for Control of Chronic Diseases, Dhaka, Bangladesh
Center for International Health, University of Munich, Munich, Germany
Cardiovascular Division, The George Institute for Global Health, Sydney, Australia

Aiqun Ma
Shaanxi Key Laboratory of Molecular Cardiology (Xi'an Jiaotong University), Xi'an, China

Aiqun Ma
Key Laboratory of Environment and Genes Related to Diseases (Xi'an Jiaotong University), Ministry of Education, Xi'an, China

J. Schmucker, S. Seide, H. Wienbergen, E. Fiehn, J. Stehmeier, R. Hambrecht and A. Fach
The Bremer Institut für Herz- und Kreislaufforschung (BIHKF) am Klinikum Links der Weser, Bremen, Germany

K. Günther, W. Ahrens and H. Pohlabeln
The Leibniz-Institut für Präventionsforschung und Epidemiologie Bremen – BIPS, Bremen, Germany

Olga L. Barbarash, Irina S. Bykova, Vasiliy V. Kashtalap, Mikhail V. Zykov, Oksana N. Hryachkova, Victoria V. Kalaeva, Kristina S. Shafranskaya, Victoria N. Karetnikova and Anton G. Kutikhin
Research Institute for Complex Issues of Cardiovascular Diseases, Sosnovy Boulevard 6, 650002 Kemerovo, Russian Federation

Olga L. Barbarash, Vasiliy V. Kashtalap and Victoria N. Karetnikova
Kemerovo State Medical University, Voroshilova Street 22a, 650029 Kemerovo, Russian Federation

Yonggu Lee, Eunjin Kim and Jeong-Hun Shin
Division of Cardiology, Department of Internal Medicine, Hanyang University Guri Hospital, 153, Gyeongchun-ro, Guri-si, Gyeonggi-do 11923, South Korea

Bae Keun Kim
Department of Cardiology, Sungae Hospital, Seoul, Republic of Korea

Josip Vincelj
Clinical Hospital Dubrava, Zagreb, Republic of Croatia

Xhevdet Krasniqi, Blerim Berisha, Masar Gashi, Dardan Koçinaj and Fisnik Jashari
University Clinical Center of Kosova, Mother Theresa n.n, 10000 Prishtina, Republic of Kosovo

Núria Ribas, Cosme García-García, Oona Meroño, Lluís Recasens, Víctor Bazán, Neus Salvatella, Julio Martí-Almor and Jordi Bruguera
Cardiology Department, Hospital del Mar, Passeig Marítim, 25-29, 08003 Barcelona, Spain

Núria Ribas, Oona Meroño, Lluís Recasens, Neus Salvatella, Julio Martí-Almor and Jordi Bruguera
Heart Diseases Biomedical Research Group, IMIM (Hospital del Mar Medical Research Institute), Barcelona, Spain

Núria Ribas
Medicine Department, Program in Internal Medicine, Universitat Autònoma de Barcelona, Barcelona, Spain

Cosme García-García
Hospital Universitari Germans Trias i Pujol, Badalona, Spain

Silvia Pérez-Fernández and Roberto Elosua
IMIM (Hospital del Mar Medical Research Institute). Cardiovascular Epidemiology and Genetics Group (EGEC), REGICOR Study Group, Barcelona, Spain
CIBER de Enfermedades Cardiovasculares (CIBERCV), Barcelona, Spain

Ching-Yu Julius Chen and Po-Yuan Chang
Cardiovascular Center and Division of Cardiology, Department of Internal Medicine, National Taiwan University Hospital, 7 Chung-Shan South Road, 100 Taipei, Taiwan

Ching-Yu Julius Chen
Division of Cardiology, Department of Internal Medicine, National Taiwan University College of Medicine, No.1, Ren-Ai Road Section 1, 100 Taipei, Taiwan

Tzu-Ching Yang and Shao-Chun Lu
Department of Biochemistry and Molecular Biology, National Taiwan University College of Medicine, No.1, Ren-Ai Road Section 1, 100 Taipei, Taiwan

Christopher Chang
Taipei American School, 800 Chung Shan North Road Section 6, Taipei 11152, Taiwan

C . García-García, N. Ribas, L. L. Recasens, O. Meroño, A. Fernández, A. Pérez, F. Miranda, H. Tizón-Marcoss, J. Martí-Almor and J. Bruguera
Cardiology Department, Hospital del Mar, Parc de Salut Mar-IMIM, Barcelona, Spain

C . García-García
Cardiology Department, Hospital Universitari Germans Trias i Pujol, Carretera Canyet s/n, 08916 Badalona, Spain

C . García-García and I. Subirana
CIBER de Enfermedades Cardiovasculares (CIBERCV), Barcelona, Spain

N. Ribas and R. Elosua
Ph Program in Internal Medicine, Universitat Autònoma de Barcelona, Barcelona, Spain

N. Ribas, L. L. Recasens, O. Meroño, H. Tizón-Marcos, J. Martí-Almor and J. Bruguera
Heart Diseases Biomedical Research Group, IMIM (Hospital del Mar Medical Research Institute), Barcelona, Spain

I. Subirana
IMIM (Hospital del Mar Medical Research Institute), Cardiovascular Epidemiology and Genetics Group (EGEC), REGICOR Study Group, Barcelona, Spain

Hélder Pereira and Daniel Caldeira
Serviço de Cardiologia, Hospital Garcia de Orta EPE, Avenida Prof. Torrado da Silva, 2801-951 Almada, Portugal
Centro Cardiovascular da Universidade de Lisboa (CCUL), CAML, Faculdade de Medicina, Universidade de Lisboa, Avenida Professor Egas Moniz, Lisboa 1649-028, Portugal

Daniel Caldeira
Unidade de Farmacologia Clínica, Instituto de Medicina Molecular; Laboratório de Farmacologia Clínica e Terapêutica, Faculdade de Medicina, Universidade de Lisboa, Avenida Professor Egas Moniz, Lisboa 1649-028, Portugal

Rui Campante Teles
Hospital de Santa Cruz, Centro Hospitalar de Lisboa Ocidental, EPE, Lisboa, Portugal
Registo Nacional de Cardiologia de Intervenção, APIC-CNCDC, Lisboa, Portugal

Pedro Farto e Abreu
Hospital Professor Doutor Fernando da Fonseca EPE, Amadora, Portugal

Ricardo Santos
Hospital de São Bernardo, Centro Hospitalar de Setúbal EPE, Setúbal, Portugal

António Drummond
Hospital do Funchal, Madeira, Portugal

Renato Fernandes
Hospital do Espírito Santo, Évora, Portugal

Rui Cruz Ferreira
Hospital de Santa Marta, Centro Hospitalar Lisboa Central EPE, Lisboa, Portugal

Sousa Ramos
Hospital CUF Infante Santo, Lisboa, Portugal

Matteo Vercellino and Gioel Gabrio Secco
Interventional Cardiology, Santi Antonio, Biagio e Cesare Arrigo Hospital, Alessandria, AL, Italy

Federico Ariel Sànchez
Coronary Care Unit, Sanremo Hospital, Sanremo, IM, Italy

Valentina Boasi
Interventional Cardiology, Sanremo Hospital, Sanremo, IM, Italy

Dino Perri and Stefano Cattunar
Sanremo Hospital, Sanremo, IM, Italy

Chiara Tacchi
Emergency Room, Sanremo Hospital, Sanremo, IM, Italy

Gianfranco Pistis
Cardiology Unit, Santi Antonio, Biagio e Cesare Arrigo Hospital, Alessandria, AL, Italy

Giovanni Mascelli
Cardiology Unit, Sanremo Hospital, Sanremo, IM, Italy

Abhishek M. Shetye, Sheraz A. Nazir, Naveed A. Razvi, Nathan Price, Jamal N. Khan, Florence Y. Lai, Iain B. Squire, Gerald P. McCann and Jayanth R. Arnold
Department of Cardiovascular Sciences, University of Leicester, Glenfield Hospital, Groby Road, Leicester LE3 9QF, UK

Abhishek M. Shetye
Oxford University Hospitals NHS Trust, Oxford OX3 9DU, UK

Naveed A. Razvi
Ipswich Hospital NHS trust, Ipswich IP4 5PD, UK

Nathan Price
Leeds Institute of Cardiovascular and Metabolic Medicine (LICAMM), University of Leeds, Leeds LS2 9JT, UK

Index